#845

CLINICAL SIMULATIONS

SELECTED PROBLEMS IN PATIENT MANAGEMENT

SECOND EDITION

CLINICAL SIMULATIONS

SELECTED PROBLEMS IN PATIENT MANAGEMENT

SECOND EDITION

AN ACCESS® BOOK

PREPARED BY

THE COLLEGE COMMITTEE ON STUDENT APPRAISAL

University of Illinois College of Medicine
Chicago, Illinois

EDITED BY

CHRISTINE H. McGUIRE, M.A.

Professor of Medical Education, Associate Director and Chief, Research and Evaluation Section, Center for Educational Development

LAWRENCE M. SOLOMON, M.D., F.R.C.P.

Professor and Head, Department of Dermatology, Abraham Lincoln School of Medicine; Adjunct Professor of Medical Education, Center for Educational Development

PHILLIP M. FORMAN, M.D.

Associate Professor of Pediatrics and Neurology, Abraham Lincoln School of Medicine; Associate Professor of Medical Education and Director, Center for Educational Development

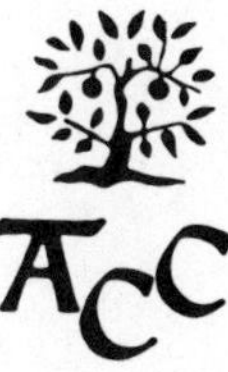

APPLETON-CENTURY-CROFTS/NEW YORK

Copyright © 1976 by APPLETON-CENTURY-CROFTS
A Publishing Division of Prentice-Hall, Inc.

All rights reserved. This book, or any parts thereof, may not be used or reproduced in any manner without written permission. For information address Appleton-Century-Crofts, 292 Madison Avenue, New York, New York 10017

78 79 80 / 10 9 8 7 6 5 4 3 2

The ACCESS® latent image process utilized in this publication is produced under license from New Century Education Corporation.

This process is covered by one or more of the following: United States Pat. Nos. 3,363,336; 3,363,337; 3,363,338; 3,438,927; 3,516,177; 3,650,046; Patented in Canada, 1969, 1971, 1972; Patented in France, Nos. 1,503,270; 7,013,287; Patented in Germany, No. 1,497,722; Patented in Great Britain, No. 1,171,149; Patented in Japan, No. 634,455; Other U.S. and foreign patents pending.

Printed in the United States of America
0-8385-1161-9

CONTRIBUTORS

CHARLES F. ABILDGAARD, M.D., Professor of Pediatrics, University of California School of Medicine at Davis, Davis, California

ALEXANDER S. ANDERSON, M.D., Associate Professor of Medicine, John A. Burns School of Medicine, University of Hawaii at Manoa, Honolulu, Hawaii

ROBERT J. BAKER, M.D., Professor of Surgery; Chief, General Surgery; Abraham Lincoln School of Medicine, University of Illinois College of Medicine, Chicago, Illinois

HARRY BROWN, M.D.
Toronto, Canada

GERARD M. CERCHIO, M.D., Associate Dean and Associate Professor of Medicine, Abraham Lincoln School of Medicine, University of Illinois College of Medicine, Chicago, Illinois

ROBERT E. CONDON, M.D., M.S., F.A.C.S., Professor of Surgery, Medical College of Wisconsin; Chief, Surgical Service, Wood Veterans Administration Hospital, Milwaukee, Wisconsin

J. B. DRORI, M.D., F.A.C.P., Assistant Clinical Professor of Neurology, University of California Medical Center, San Francisco, California

PHILLIP M. FORMAN, M.D., Associate Professor of Pediatrics and Neurology, Abraham Lincoln School of Medicine; Associate Professor of Medical Education and Director, Center for Educational Development, University of Illinois College of Medicine, Chicago, Illinois

LEWIS A. HAMILTON, JR., M.D., F.A.C.O.G., Senior Surgeon, Pregnancy Research Branch, National Institute of Child Health and Human Development, National Institutes of Health, Bethesda, Maryland

GEORGE R. HONIG, M.D., Professor of Pediatrics, Director of Hematology, Children's Memorial Hospital, Chicago, Illinois

CHARLES A. HORN, Physician Assistant, Chicago, Illinois

MARILYN A. HRUBY, M.D., Department of Hematology, Children's Memorial Hospital, Chicago, Illinois

EDSEL K. HUDSON, M.D., Associate Professor of Medicine and Medical Director, Ambulatory Care Services, Rush-Presbyterian-St. Lukes Hospital, Chicago, Illinois

EUGENE W. ISAACS, M.D., Pediatrician, Highland Park, Illinois

HAROLD L. KLAWANS, M.D., Director, Division of Neurology, Michael Reese Hospital and Medical Center; Professor, Department of Medicine (Neurology), University of Chicago, Pritzer School of Medicine, Chicago, Illinois

SIDNEY LEVITSKY, M.D., Professor of Surgery, Chief, Division of Cardiothoracic Surgery, Abraham Lincoln School of Medicine, University of Illinois College of Medicine, Chicago, Illinois

ARTHUR LOEWY, M.D., Professor of Otolaryngology, Abraham Lincoln School of Medicine, University of Illinois College of Medicine, Chicago, Illinois

DAVID M. LONG, M.D., Ph.D., Cardiovascular and Thoracic Surgeon, La Mesa, California

WILLIAM H. McCARTHY, M.D., Department of Surgery, University of Sydney, Sydney Hospital, Sydney, New South Wales, Australia

JO MILLER, M.D., F.R.C.S. (C), F.A.C.S., Orthopedic Surgeon-in-Chief, The Montreal General Hospital; Associate Professor of Surgery, McGill University, Montreal, Canada

ROBERT A. MILLER, M.D., Professor of Pediatrics, Abraham Lincoln School of Medicine, University of Illinois College of Medicine; Chairman, Pediatrics, Cook County Children's Hospital, Chicago, Illinois

ROY M. PITKIN, M.D., Professor of Obstetrics and Gynecology, University of Iowa College of Medicine, Iowa City, Iowa

EDWARD SAVAGE, M.D., Professor and Chief, Division of Gynecology, Martin Luther King, Jr. General Hospital, Los Angeles, California

LAWRENCE M. SOLOMON, M.D., F.R.C.P., Professor and Head, Department of Dermatology, Abraham Lincoln School of Medicine; Adjunct Professor of Medical Education, Center for Educational Development, University of Illinois College of Medicine, Chicago, Illinois

NICHOLAS TOROK, M.D., Professor of Otolaryngology, Abraham Lincoln School of Medicine, University of Illinois College of Medicine, Chicago, Illinois

LAWRENCE TREMONTI, M.D., Assistant Dean; Assistant Professor of Medicine, Abraham Lincoln School of Medicine, University of Illinois College of Medicine, Chicago, Illinois

ANGELO TOIGO, M.D.*

DHARMAPURI VIDYASAGAR, M.D., Associate Professor of Pediatrics, Abraham Lincoln School of Medicine; Director of the Newborn Nursery, University of Illinois College of Medicine, Chicago, Illinois

RICHARD S. WEBB, JR., M.D., F.A.C.S., Clinical Associate Professor of Surgery, University of Illinois College of Medicine, Chicago, Illinois; Attending Physician, Rockford Memorial Hospital, Rockford, Illinois

***Deceased**

PREFACE

We are extremely pleased that our first effort in publishing these problem-solving exercises has received such warm welcome and beckoned the birth of this second edition.

This edition has been considerably altered from the first although the patients' problems remain the same. In the past five years many changes have occurred in the approach to a number of the issues raised in these problems, and we have attempted to bring the recommended management of each patient into concert with current concepts. As a result, five of the twenty problems have been completely rewritten, another five have been altered in a major fashion and the remaining ten problems have undergone considerable revision. Twenty additional reviewers have commented on the content of the problems.

We have added a section of standard laboratory values so that the normal may be referred to. In this regard we have used a variety of techniques, units, and equivalent measures because they exist in practice as one travels from hospital to hospital or uses different laboratories.

The commentary to each problem has been enlarged and some appropriate bibliographic material added.

Finally, although the management of certain disease states such as shock and diabetes in pregnancy have undergone specialty transformation, and certain diagnostic procedures and patient managements have become more complicated, we would like the student to consider himself as the physician on whom the patient is relying for help. In solving the problem a learning process takes place which fills in the gap for the next such patient encountered. In other words, if you would not normally manage a given problem by yourself, do so under these circumstances; there is no harm to it and you may enjoy the experience.

A reviewer in commenting on another volume of simulations said: "There is no way to skim it. You can't even read it; you have to think it." That is the essence of what this edition is all about. Think your way through and have fun.

Christine H. McGuire
Lawrence M. Solomon
Phillip M. Forman

Chicago, 1976

PREFACE TO FIRST EDITION

Over the decade 1961 to 1970 more than 100 members of the clinical faculty of the University of Illinois College of Medicine and more than a dozen experts in educational evaluation of the Center for Educational Development cooperated in designing, constructing, and editing the library of simulated problems in patient management on which this publication is based.

To single out those authors, reviewers, and committee members who participated most directly and most recently in the preparation of the simulations contained in this book serves only to suggest the numerous others whose many and varied contributions to the development and evaluation of such materials have made this volume possible. Among these latter, far too numerous to cite individually, the editors want especially to express appreciation to the following: the late Dr. Frederick Lewy and his successor as Director of Medical Education of the American Heart Association, Dr. Richard E. Hurley, whose concern for the efficiency and effectiveness of programs of continuing education led them to underwrite with both time and money the initial development of the first set of branched simulations for the assessment of educational programs and the diagnosis of educational needs; both current and former members of the American Board of Orthopedic Surgery who, in a joint study with the Center for Educational Development (supported by the Bureau of Health Professions Education and Manpower Training of the United States Public Health Service), undertook the basic research essential to the validation of simulation technique as a method of professional self-assessment; Dr. William J. Grove who, in his role as the first chairman of the newly created Appraisal Committee, provided the creative leadership essential in shaping the policies that have guided the Committee's development and who, subsequently, in his capacity as Dean of the College of Medicine, has given unstintingly in the support of the work of that Committee as it has evolved; Dr. George E. Miller who, as Director of the Center for Educational Development, not only built and trained a technical staff to work with faculty, but also provided the energetic stimulus and imaginative guidance essential in making such cooperative undertakings productive, and without whose invaluable assistance and advice this book could not have been produced; Mrs. Tommie Royce who provided editorial assistance in the early stages of the preparation of the manuscript; Miss Helen Pauckstys who furnished some of the illustrative materials for the book; Miss Theresa Cochran and Miss Franki Legette whose energy, skill, and patience in deciphering the authors' intentions made the first draft legible and who, together with Miss Linda Wilson, Miss Jill Soula, and Mrs. Kay Hanson, worked tirelessly to ready the final manuscript for the printer.

Finally, the enthusiastic reception and constructive criticism by the many thousand students, house staff, and clinicians who have responded to these problems have served to encourage their improvement and refinement. We look forward to such assistance from our readers, to be incorporated in the next volume of problems. Meanwhile, the authors and editors hope that you will find the study of the problems that constitute the present volume as challenging and stimulating as has been our task of writing and editing them.

C.H.M.
L.M.S.

CONTENTS

THE PROBLEMS

APPENDICES

FOREWORD

Early in Dr. Granville Bennett's tenure as Dean of the University of Illinois College of Medicine (1954-67) a series of meetings was conducted at which departments outlined their curricula and their methods for evaluating results of their teaching efforts. It soon became evident that all departments were having similar problems with respect to student and faculty morale. Although many opinions were voiced as to the reasons for the less than optimal "esprit," criticism of the examination system was heard most often. Yet no one was clear about how to improve—help was needed.

In 1958 the faculty endorsed the recommendation that an Office of Research in Medical Education be established within the College to study their problems through research into the educational process. Through the efforts of Dean Bennett and Lester J. Evans, M.D., support for the office was obtained from the Commonwealth Fund, and George E. Miller, M.D., was appointed Director. Meanwhile, the standing Faculty Committee on Examinations had been administering a "comprehensive examination system" that had been established more than twenty years earlier. The system consisted of two examinations, one administered at the end of the sophomore year and the other at the end of the senior year. The examinations were composed of a series of essay questions provided by the departments, which usually centered around several selected topics. As might be expected, the scoring of these examinations was difficult even though an elaborate system of multiple scorers had been developed.

The Committee on Examinations, seeking to improve the system of appraisal and promotion, turned to the newly-established Office of Research in Medical Education. The Committee on Examinations and other faculty committees undertook a series of studies concerning the "climate for learning." These studies showed that the prevailing system of student examination, grading, and promotion failed to record accurately student achievement with respect to many of the most important goals of medical education. The system, in fact, appeared to increase the tendencies toward fragmentation of learning, focus student attention on trivial detail, and stimulate unhealthy competition among students for grades and among departments for the students' time and attention.

After extensive discussion and often heated debate the faculty concurred that the setting of standards for certification was an institutional rather than a departmental function. Invoking this principle, the Committee on Examinations recommended that a college-wide system of comprehensive examinations of a new type be established on an experimental basis. It further recommended that the Committee on Examinations be reorganized as the Faculty Committee on Student Appraisal with the assigned task of constructing, administering, and reporting all instruments used for the purpose of official student assessment. The results of these examinations were to be forwarded to the Faculty Committee on Promotions, to students, and to departmental faculties.

The newly created committee spent most of its time during its first year of existence reviewing official documents and carrying on extensive discussions with departmental representatives in an effort to develop a comprehensive set of institutional goals and standards in terms of which student progress could be assessed. The resulting behavioral objectives were then classified into the familiar cognitive, manipulative, and affective domains. Comprehensive written examinations were to be used to measure the cognitive goals. Practical laboratory and clinical examinations were to be used to measure certain psychomotor skills. The affective domain was to be assessed by systematic accumulation of anecdotal records.

One of the important objectives requiring assessment was the development of clinical judgment. Patient management problems were the result of the effort to develop more reliable and valid methods of assessing this objective. Patient management problems are simulated exercises to test the complex skill of gathering data and making judgments. The simulations began in a rather crude written form but are now available in a highly sophisticated computerized form. Over the years the patient management problems have been modified in response to suggestions of both students and faculty and their use has been extended from that of appraisal for certification to self-assessment for learning purposes and to the diagnosis of educational needs.

Finally, virtually all who have used the simulated clinical encounters, no matter in what form, have suggested that they would be superb self-instructional materials. It is in response to this suggestion that the present volume has been prepared.

WILLIAM J. GROVE, M.D.
Vice-Chancellor for Academic Affairs
University of Illinois at the Medical Center

INTRODUCTION

THE NATURE AND PURPOSE OF CLINICAL SIMULATIONS

A simulated clinical problem, like the simulators used by NASA in training astronauts or by large corporations in training business executives, is designed to imitate life—its challenges and emergencies—while at the same time providing protection from the hazards of even a momentary lapse in judgment that inexperience or inattention may cause. Thus it offers the student or physician an opportunity to test his judgment and skill in dealing with the complexities of reality, to get realistic feedback on the consequences of each decision he makes, and to learn from his successes and failures, without subjecting himself or his patients to any risk. Unlike clinical practice where the consequences of a diagnostic or therapeutic intervention are usually delayed and often difficult to interpret, feedback in a simulated clinical problem is prompt and specific; hence the physician need not wait a lifetime—either his own or his patient's—to gain the benefits of a lifetime of experience in sharpening his clinical acumen. Further, a simulated problem affords the luxury of "wiping the slate clean" and of trying new tactics whenever the first approach to a clinical situation fails to achieve the desired effects; in so doing it supplies a means of improving management skills through extraclinical practice. Finally, as presented here each simulation is accompanied by an explanatory comment and recommended plan of management which allows the reader to compare his own views with those of the authors. This feature of the simulations thus provides access to the thinking of authoritative consultants with whom the reader can, in effect, "discuss" his decisions regarding every step in the management of each of the patients in his simulated practice.

The twenty men, women, and children who compose that practice, ie, who appear as patients in this book, have been selected to illustrate important issues that merit careful consideration in the work-up and management of patients with such commonly encountered complaints as headache, fever, abdominal pain, injury, and the like. Some of the problems posed by these patients stress interpretive skills, others management skills; some focus on diagnosis, others on therapy; in some the critical issues are whether and when to intervene surgically, in others, when to delay and when to act promptly. While the optimal resolution of each case involves, as it does in life, certain unique aspects, the fundamental methods are those any physician uses in his day-to-day office and hospital practice.

Description of a Clinical Simulation

Each problem is introduced with a brief statement of a complaint such as the physician might elicit from the patient himself, from a friend or relative who accompanied him, or from a colleague who had referred him. Here, as elsewhere throughout the volume, information about the patient's condition is couched in realistic terms appropriate to its source: it is *not* presented in classic textbook or conference style. For example, information derived from a patient's description of his symptoms, history, and present illness is supplied in layman's language suitable to that patient's age, education, and occupation; information derived from diagnostic procedures is typically supplied in the language of the clinical record.

Following the statement of the problem is a list of specific interventions or of general strategies. From these the initial approach can be selected, eg, further history, physical examination, laboratory evaluation, or immediate therapy. As each decision is made, information regarding the results of that decision is provided, along with instructions pointing to the next section appropriate to the problem. In each new section possible interventions that may yield further information about the patient are listed. The reader can select as many or as few as seem appropriate in light of the specific circumstances at that stage of the problem. Once again, the results of each intervention are presented in realistic verbal or visual form. It then becomes necessary to decide what further steps would seem to be indicated on the basis of these new data. In this manner the problem is carried through many more stages, in each of which the reader must make further choices based on the *specific* responses of the patient which were evoked by *his own* earlier decisions.

As noted above, the stages in the work-up and the responses to each intervention are designed to simulate an actual clinical situation and are reported in a form resembling that encountered in the office or hospital setting. For example, an order for a specific test reveals a laboratory report; an order for an x-ray, audiogram, electrocardiogram, and the like may direct the reader to a photographic reproduction of the x-ray or tracing; a color plate may be provided in response to an order for a smear, culture, or biopsy; the patient's reaction is reported in response to medication. Unless a consultation is requested, no interpretation of these data is offered and none is explicitly demanded of the reader; as in a conventional clinical setting, data are ordinarily provided in response to any request and these data are available for consideration in making subsequent decisions about the management of a patient.

The complications which must be managed will depend (as they do in the office or clinic) on the unique combination of specific procedures elected at earlier stages. These decisions may lead to an instruction to skip one or more sections of a problem entirely because the reader's approach has been effective in avoiding potential complications. If, however, this approach entails harmful interventions at any stage or fails to encompass measures essential to the recovery of the patient, feedback is given regarding the complication that has developed and opportunity is provided to take appropriate measures to rectify the patient's condition. If these remedial measures are inadequate, the problem may be terminated and the reader advised that the patient has suffered a relapse and has been sent to another hospital, or has been referred to a consultant, or has died. Alternatively, if the corrective measures are adequate the reader is directed to a new section of the problem representing the next stage in the work-up and management of that patient.

The Approach to a Clinical Simulation

Each simulation is composed of many sections which correspond to various stages in the diagnostic work-up and treatment of the patient described. At each stage alternate sections are often included to provide for the differing approaches that students or physicians may wish to follow. However, the fact that a section is available does not necessarily imply that it would be included in the optimal management of the patient described and in most problems many more sections are provided than any one individual will find it necessary to use.

At the conclusion of each problem, the reader is directed to the appropriate Appendix, which contains an explanatory comment and the consultants' advice regarding the management of the patient. Some problems deal with an emergency situation for which only a minimal initial diagnostic work-up is recommended. Other problems involve conditions that require thorough evaluation prior to any decision about therapy; in these, diagnostic shortcuts may lead to inadequate or inappropriate treatment decisions. In still other problems, where the diagnosis is quite obvious, it may be necessary to avoid indulging in an over-elaborate work-up and to make a decision regarding the point at which adequate confirmation of a working diagnosis has been achieved. Some problems concern the long-term management of chronic disease where it is necessary to monitor the consequences of therapy, reevaluate the patient, and modify the therapeutic regime. In others, once the diagnosis has been made, there may be little or nothing that can be done to reverse the course of the illness; in such situations it will be necessary to resist the temptation of intervening uselessly. In short, the recommended approaches to these patients are flexible and varied to suit the situation, as they are in any practice setting.

In considering the Appendix, it is important for the reader to recognize that some differences in opinion among clinicians are inevitable simply as a consequence of diversity in philosophies of management and rationales for therapy; others may occur due to variation of newer diagnostic and therapeutic procedures, while still others may result from genuine discrepancies in competence in dealing with rapidly developing, highly specialized areas. In each case, however, the explanatory comment is designed to reveal the consultants' reasons for the approach they recommend, an approach which the reader is free to accept or reject.

Responding to a Clinical Simulation

The balance of this book consists of twenty simulated clinical problems. Each problem is composed of several sections corresponding to various stages in the diagnostic work-up and treatment of the patient described. In each section a list of possible procedures is presented in the left hand column; from this list you are to select *all* the interventions you regard as significant in the care of *this patient* at the specific stage of the problem represented by that section. Indicate your choices by *gently* rubbing the special marker (supplied with this volume) over the blank area to the right of the number corresponding to each item of your choice. In a few seconds printed material will appear in that area; this material will provide you with additional information describing the results of your decision, will refer you to one of the photographs in the back of the book, or will direct you to the next appropriate section of the problem. In order to obtain all the information available in response to each decision be sure to rub the marker over the *entire area* for any choice you make. Be careful not to reveal information in adjacent areas; it would be inappropriate to the choice you have made and thus might mislead you. (Note: Each response is enclosed in a pair of brackets, [ ], which will appear as you rub the marker over the appropriate area. When these symbols appear you will know that you have obtained all the information relevant to your choice.)

The various sections of each problem are arranged in random order and it is therefore necessary for you to *skip back and forth precisely as directed by the instructions you receive in each section*. Occasionally you will be directed to skip entirely one or more sections of a problem either because your approach would be effective in avoiding potential complications with which these sections are concerned or because it has obviated entirely the necessity of dealing with certain aspects of the problem. *Be sure to follow these instructions exactly;* failure to do so will cause you to obtain feedback that may be inappropriate to your decisions.

The problems are constructed to simulate a clinical situation as closely as possible; they are not designed to test whether you can arrive at a diagnosis with a minimum amount of information. Alternatively, the fact that an option is offered or that a section is printed does not necessarily imply that it would be included in the optimal management of the patient described. If you choose to take a history or to perform a physical examination you should bear in mind that you are expected to select only those items you regard as pertinent. Similarly, in your recommendations regarding laboratory evaluation and therapeutic management, you should select only those items you regard as indicated under the circumstances described in the problem. In summary, you should make every intervention you regard as indicated and you should avoid making any intervention that you regard as noncontributory or inappropriate. You should approach the simulated patient in precisely the same way as you would approach a similar patient whom you might see in your office or hospital practice.

In listing possible lines of inquiry the editors have attempted to use a standard nomenclature; abbreviations are limited to those points at which a clear context is provided. In reporting the results of each laboratory test a standard set of units and of normal values is employed throughout. These values can be checked by reference to Appendix U.

Finally, it should be noted that in any office or clinic setting many problems are resolved through consultation and discussion with colleagues. Consequently, in some problems you are offered the opportunity to request one or more consultations. However, the "report" provided *in the text* of a response to such a request should not necessarily be interpreted as representing the authors' and editors' views of the specialty, since on occasion it has been necessary to depart somewhat from reality in order to maintain the problem format and to give you maximum opportunity to manage the simulated problem yourself. However, at the conclusion of each problem you are referred to the appropriate Appendix which consists of a brief comment explaining the more important points in the consultants' thinking about the problem, together with a detailed map outlining the sequence of steps they recommend in the management of the patient described. At each stage in this recommended approach those interventions considered *especially* critical and those regarded as *particularly* wasteful or harmful are listed. These lists are not intended as a comprehensive guide to the care of the patient; rather they are offered as further clarification and specification of the consultants' views.

And now you are ready to work; the authors and editors hope you will find it a challenging and rewarding experience.

How To Use ACCESS®

The response areas in this book are printed with an invisible ink process called ACCESS.® When you rub in these areas with your ACCESS® marker, the printed answer will appear.

The selections in this book are listed in the left hand column and numbered, with the same number appearing directly next to it in the right hand column. By rubbing the space next to the number in the right hand column your response will appear. Each answer will begin with a bracket and end with a bracket.

Rub here for your response.

24	Blood urea nitrogen	24	[16 mg/100 ml.]
25	Serum uric acid	25	[4 mg/100 ml.]

Rub here for your response.

26	Urine coproporphyrin	26	[10 μg/24 hours.]
27	Blood lead level	27	[0.010 mg/100 ml.]

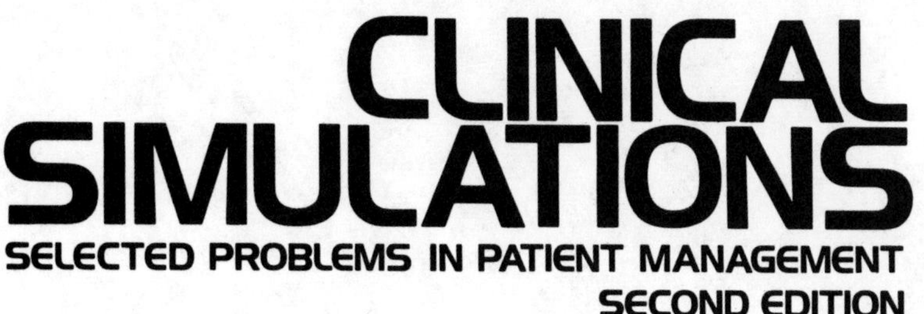

CLINICAL SIMULATIONS

SELECTED PROBLEMS IN PATIENT MANAGEMENT

SECOND EDITION

PROBLEM I

THE PALE, LETHARGIC CHILD

The patient is a two-year-old black child, brought to the Emergency Room by his mother because of increasing irritability and poor appetite for several weeks. She says that he had been well and until recently was eating table foods with the family. In addition to the above complaint, his mother says that he has been less active in the past month, but she had not been aware of any pallor until the physician in the Emergency Room brought it to her attention. He has had no fever or other evidence of recent infection. Four older siblings are in good health.

Physical examination reveals an irritable black child who appears well nourished. Rectal temperature – 99F, Pulse – 110 per minute, Respirations – 25 per minute, Blood pressure 95/60 mm Hg. Except for pallor of the palms, sole, and mucous membranes, a spleen felt 2 cm below the left costal margin, and a blowing systolic murmur along the left sternal border, the examination is within normal limits.

Initial laboratory results from the Emergency Room were recorded as: hemoglobin – 3.0 g/100 ml; hematocrit – 13%; white blood cell count – 12,000/mm^3; differential: Bands – 4%, segmented neutrophils – 36%, eosinophils – 3%, monocytes – 2%, and lymphocytes – 55%.

The patient is admitted to the hospital for further evaluation.

NOW CONTINUE WITH SECTION 1-A

SECTION 1-A

YOU WOULD NOW REQUEST (SELECT AS MANY AS YOU CONSIDER INDICATED):

1	More detailed family history	1	[Mother, age – 38 years, well; father – age 45 years, has hypertension; sister – age 4, and three brothers – ages 7, 9, and 10 years, all entirely well; no history of anemia in family but paternal grandmother once had "yellow jaundice."]
2	More detailed dietary history	2	[The mother reported that the boy ate well until the recent decrease in appetite. He has been fed cow's milk since 2 months of age and now drinks 1 to 2 quarts per day. His diet also includes meat, potatoes, cereal, and other vegetables; he has had no supplemental vitamins. Last summer he was observed eating dirt in the back yard on two occasions.]
3	More detailed past history	3	[Birth weight 8 lb 8 oz; normal pregnancy and delivery; development normal; has had all the usual immunizations except smallpox vaccination and measles vaccine.]
4	Chest film	4	[Clear chest, minimal cardiomegaly.]
5	Tuberculin skin test	5	[3 mm induration at 48 hours.]
6	Urinalysis	6	[Clear, yellow; specific gravity 1.018; protein – negative; sugar – negative; acetone – trace; sediment – rare red blood cell.]

7	Serum protein electrophoresis	**7**	[Total protein 6.9 g/100 ml; Albumin – 65%; Alpha$_1$ globulin – 5%, Alpha$_2$ – 9%, Beta – 9%, Gamma – 12%.]
8	Hemoglobin electrophoresis	**8**	[Hemoglobin AS.]
9	Blood smear for morphology	**9**	[SEE FIGURE 8, PAGE 411.]
10	Platelet count	**10**	[45,000/mm^3.]
11	Sickle cell preparation	**11**	[SEE FIGURE 12, PAGE 411.]
12	Bone marrow aspiration	**12**	[SEE FIGURE 16, PAGE 412.]
13	Serum iron and iron binding capacity	**13**	[Serum iron 23 μg/100 ml; iron binding capacity 350 μg/100 ml.]
14	Serum B_{12}	**14**	[230 pgm/ml.]
15	Serum folic acid	**15**	[15 ng/ml.]
16	Osmotic fragility of red cells	**16**	[Hemolysis starts at 0.45% saline; complete at 0.30% saline.]
17	Prothrombin time	**17**	[12 seconds (control – 14 seconds).]
18	Partial thromboplastin time	**18**	[40 seconds.]
19	Bleeding time	**19**	[14 minutes (Ivy technique).]
20	Reticulocyte count	**20**	[3%.]
21	Serum bilirubin	**21**	[Direct 0.2 mg/100 ml, indirect 0.7 mg/100 ml.]
22	Red cell survival study with radioactive chromium (patient's cells)	**22**	[^{51}Cr T 1/2 – 28 days.]

23	Bone marrow biopsy (surgical)	23	[Done, specimen sent to pathology lab; you await interpretation.]
24	Blood urea nitrogen	24	[15 mg/100 ml.]
25	Serum uric acid	25	[3 mg/100 ml.]
26	Urine coproporphyrin (24 hours)	26	[100 µg/24 hours.]
27	Blood lead level	27	[0.001 mg/100 ml.]
28	Coombs test	28	[Negative.]
29	Lupus erythematosus cell preparation	29	[Negative.]
30	Erythrocyte glucose-6-phosphate dehydrogenase screening test	30	[Negative.]
31	Stool guaiac	31	[2+ positive.]

UNLESS OTHERWISE DIRECTED IN THE RESPONSE COLUMN CONTINUE WITH SECTION 1-B

SECTION 1-B

YOUR PROGNOSIS FOR THIS PATIENT IS AS FOLLOWS (CHOOSE ONLY ONE):

32	Excellent with proper medical therapy	32	[Mother so advised.]
33	Excellent with proper surgical therapy	33	[Mother so advised.]
34	Should respond to proper management of acute episode, but is unlikely to have normal longevity	34	[Mother so advised.]

35	May respond to medical management but is most likely to die of disease within months to a few years	**35**	[Mother so advised.]
36	Unlikely to survive present episode	**36**	[Mother so advised.]

UNLESS OTHERWISE DIRECTED IN THE RESPONSE COLUMN CONTINUE WITH SECTION 1-C

SECTION 1-C

37	Record your diagnostic impressions below ____________ ____________ ____________ ____________ ____________	**37**	[The complete diagnosis as recorded on the patient's chart was (i) iron deficiency anemia; (ii) sickle cell trait. SEE APPENDIX E FOR ADDITIONAL COMMENT AND RECOMMENDED MANAGEMENT. END OF PROBLEM 1.]

NOW DEVELOP RESPONSE 37 FOR ADDITIONAL INFORMATION AND INSTRUCTIONS

PROBLEM 2

THE PALE, LETHARGIC CHILD

The patient is a four-year-old black child, brought to the Emergency Room because of marked weakness and lethargy developing over a two-day period. Prior to this illness he has never received medical attention, nor has he been seriously ill. Since the child's mother did not accompany him to the hospital, a more detailed history is not immediately available.

Physical examination reveals a thin child with marked pallor who appears acutely ill. Rectal temperature — 100F, Pulse — 130 per minute, Respirations — 40 per minute, Blood pressure — 70/30 mm Hg. In addition to the obvious pallor, he is found to have a liver edge palpable 1 cm below the right costal margin and the spleen is felt to extend below the umbilicus (10 cm below the left costal margin). The apex impulse is felt in the 5th intercostal space at the anterior axillary line and a harsh systolic murmur is heard over the precordium, maximal at the apex.

Blood count in the Emergency Room was recorded as: hemoglobin — 3.0 g/100 ml; hematocrit — 10%; white blood cell count — 14,000/mm^3; differential: Bands — 5%, segmented neutrophils — 60%, eosinophils — 1%, lymphocytes — 34%.

The patient is admitted to the hospital for further evaluation.

NOW CONTINUE WITH SECTION 2-A

SECTION 2-A

YOU WOULD NOW REQUEST (SELECT AS MANY AS YOU CONSIDER INDICATED):

1	More detailed family history	1	[Mother — age 23 years, living and well; father — age 24 years, also well; one brother — age 2 years, apparently well; no family history of anemia.]

2	More detailed dietary history	2	[Patient has always been a "poor eater" but has been offered a fairly well balanced diet; no history of pica.]
3	More detailed past history	3	[He was the product of a normal pregnancy; birth weight 6 lbs. Although there are no other siblings for comparison, his mother believes that he has always been thin and less active than other children his age. No other specific symptoms were elicited.]
4	Chest film	4	[Lung fields clear; moderate enlargement of the heart is present.]
5	Tuberculin skin test	5	[No induration at 48 hours.]
6	Urinalysis	6	[Small amount of amber urine obtained; specific gravity – 1.009; protein 1+; sugar – negative; acetone – trace; sediment – occasional red blood cells, few granular casts.]
7	Serum protein electrophoresis	7	[Total protein – 6.3 g/100 ml; Albumin – 65%; Alpha$_1$ globulin – 5%; Alpha$_2$ – 9%; Beta – 9%; Gamma – 12%.]
8	Hemoglobin electrophoresis	8	[SS hemoglobin.]
9	Blood smear for morphology	9	[SEE FIGURE 9, PAGE 411.]
10	Platelet count	10	[23,000/mm^3.]
11	Sickle cell preparation	11	[SEE FIGURE 12, PAGE 411.]
12	Bone marrow aspiration	12	[SEE FIGURE 17, PAGE 412.]

13	Serum iron and iron binding capacity	13
14	Serum B_{12}	14
15	Serum folic acid	15
16	Osmotic fragility of red cells	16
17	Prothrombin time	17
18	Partial thromboplastin time	18
19	Bleeding time	19
20	Reticulocyte count	20
21	Serum bilirubin	21
22	Red cell survival study with radioactive chromium (patient's cells)	22
23	Bone marrow biopsy (surgical)	23
24	Blood urea nitrogen	24
25	Serum uric acid	25
26	Urine coproporphyrin (24 hours)	26
27	Blood lead level	27
28	Coombs test	28
29	Lupus erythematosus cell preparation	29

30	Erythrocyte glucose-6-phosphate dehydrogenase screening test		
31	Stool guaiac		

UNLESS OTHERWISE DIRECTED IN THE RESPONSE COLUMN CONTINUE WITH SECTION 2-B

SECTION 2-B

YOUR PROGNOSIS FOR THIS PATIENT IS AS FOLLOWS (CHOOSE ONLY ONE):

32	Excellent with proper medical therapy	**32**	
33	Excellent with proper surgical therapy	**33**	
34	Should respond to proper management of acute episode, but is unlikely to have normal longevity	**34**	
35	May respond to medical management, but is most likely to die of disease within months to a few years	**35**	
36	Unlikely to survive present episode	**36**	

UNLESS OTHERWISE DIRECTED IN THE RESPONSE COLUMN CONTINUE WITH SECTION 2-C

SECTION 2-C

37 Record your diagnostic impressions below ______________

____

____

____

____

37 [The complete diagnosis as recorded on the patient's chart was (i) sickle cell anemia (ii) red cell sequestration. SEE APPENDIX B FOR ADDITIONAL COMMENT AND RECOMMENDED MANAGEMENT. END OF PROBLEM 2.]

NOW DEVELOP RESPONSE 37 FOR ADDITIONAL INFORMATION AND INSTRUCTIONS

PROBLEM 3

THE PALE, LETHARGIC CHILD

The patient is a six-year-old black child, brought to the Emergency Room because he has gradually developed pallor and easy fatigue during the last two months. He had previously been in good health. He has had no fever and his appetite is fair but unchanged. Despite the above symptoms he has been attending school and has remained active. He has no other complaints.

Physical examination reveals a well-developed black child in no acute distress. Oral temperature – 98F, Pulse – 100 per minute, Respirations – 20 per minute, Blood pressure – 100/60 mm Hg. Moderate pallor is present. Except for a spleen tip which on deep inspiration descends 2 cm below the left costal margin, the remainder of the examination is within normal limits.

The initial blood count in the Emergency Room was recorded as: hemoglobin – 4.2g/100 ml; hematocrit – 12%; white blood cell count – 6,000/mm^3; differential: Bands – 1%, segmented neutrophils – 24%, lymphocytes – 75%.

The patient is admitted to the hospital for further evaluation.

NOW CONTINUE WITH SECTION 3-A

SECTION 3-A

YOU WOULD NOW REQUEST (SELECT AS MANY AS YOU CONSIDER INDICATED):

1	More detailed family history	1	[Mother – age 30 years has diabetes; father killed in auto accident; brother – age 8, and sister – age 5 years, both well.]

2	More detailed dietary history	2
3	More detailed past history	3
4	Chest film	4
5	Tuberculin skin test	5
6	Urinalysis	6
7	Serum protein electrophoresis	7
8	Hemoglobin electrophoresis	8
9	Blood smear for morphology	9
10	Platelet count	10
11	Sickle cell preparation	11
12	Bone marrow aspiration	12
13	Serum iron and iron binding capacity	13
14	Serum B_{12}	14
15	Serum folic acid	15

16 Osmotic fragility of red cells

17 Prothrombin time

18 Partial thromboplastin time

19 Bleeding time

20 Reticulocyte count

21 Serum bilirubin

22 Red cell survival study with radioactive chromium (patient's cells)

23 Bone marrow biopsy (surgical)

24 Blood urea nitrogen

25 Serum uric acid

26 Urine coproporphyrin (24 hours)

27 Blood lead level

28 Coombs test

29 Lupus erythematosus cell preparation

30 Erythrocyte glucose-6-phosphate dehydrogenase screening test

31 Stool guaiac

UNLESS OTHERWISE DIRECTED IN THE RESPONSE COLUMN CONTINUE WITH SECTION 3-B

SECTION 3-B

YOUR PROGNOSIS FOR THIS PATIENT IS AS FOLLOWS (CHOOSE ONLY ONE):

32	Excellent with proper medical therapy	**32**	[Mother so advised.]
33	Excellent with proper surgical therapy	**33**	[Mother so advised.]
34	Should respond to proper management of acute episode, but is unlikely to have normal longevity	**34**	[Mother so advised.]
35	May respond to medical management but is most likely to die of disease within months to a few years	**35**	[Mother so advised.]
36	Unlikely to survive present episode	**36**	[Mother so advised.]

UNLESS OTHERWISE DIRECTED IN THE RESPONSE COLUMN CONTINUE WITH SECTION 3-C

SECTION 3-C

37	Record your diagnostic impressions below ____________ ____________________ ____________________ ____________________ ____________________	**37**	[The complete diagnosis as recorded on the patient's chart was acute leukemia. SEE APPENDIX C FOR ADDITIONAL COMMENT AND RECOMMENDED MANAGEMENT. END OF PROBLEM 3.]

NOW DEVELOP RESPONSE 37 FOR ADDITIONAL INFORMATION AND INSTRUCTIONS

PROBLEM 4

THE PALE, LETHARGIC CHILD

The patient is an eight-year-old black child, brought to the Emergency Room because of fatigue and pallor which has developed over a one-week period. He also complains of occasional abdominal pain, but denies nausea or vomiting. Prior to this episode the boy had been in apparent good health, but occasionally was thought to be pale compared to his sister, especially following infections (colds, sore throats). Three weeks prior to admission he had tonsillitis and received an antibiotic for one week. The symptoms and fever associated with this latter episode improved within 3 to 4 days after starting the drug.

Physical examination reveals a well developed moderately pale black child in no acute distress. Oral temperature – 99.6F, Pulse – 98 per minute, Respirations – 26 per minute, Blood pressure – 108/68 mm Hg. The spleen is palpable 3 cm below the left costal margin; the liver is not felt. Slight diffuse abdominal tenderness without rebound is present. The remainder of the examination is entirely within normal limits.

The initial blood count was recorded in the Emergency Room as follows: hemoglobin – 3.0 g/100 ml; hematocrit – 10%; white blood cell count – 13,000/mm^3; differential: Bands – 2%, segmented neutrophils – 58%, lymphocytes – 40%.

The patient is admitted to the hospital for further evaluation.

NOW CONTINUE WITH SECTION 4-A

SECTION 4-A

YOU WOULD NOW REQUEST (SELECT AS MANY AS YOU CONSIDER INDICATED):

1	More detailed family history	1
2	More detailed dietary history	2
3	More detailed past history	3
4	Chest film	4
5	Tuberculin skin test	5
6	Urinalysis	6
7	Serum protein electrophoresis	7
8	Hemoglobin electrophoresis	8
9	Blood smear for morphology	9
10	Platelet count	10

11	Sickle cell preparation	11
12	Bone marrow aspiration	12
13	Serum iron and iron binding capacity	13
14	Serum B_{12}	14
15	Serum folic acid	15
16	Osmotic fragility of red cells	16
17	Prothrombin time	17
18	Partial thromboplastin time	18
19	Bleeding time	19
20	Reticulocyte count	20
21	Serum bilirubin	21
22	Red cell survival study with radioactive chromium (patient's cells)	22
23	Bone marrow biopsy (surgical)	23
24	Blood urea nitrogen	24
25	Serum uric acid	25
26	Urine coproporphyrin (24 hours)	26
27	Blood lead level	27
28	Coombs test	28

29	Lupus erythematosus cell preparation	**29**	[Negative.]
30	Erythrocyte glucose-6-phosphate dehydrogenase screening test	**30**	[Negative.]
31	Stool guaiac	**31**	[Negative.]

UNLESS OTHERWISE DIRECTED IN THE RESPONSE COLUMN CONTINUE WITH SECTION 4-B

SECTION 4-B

YOUR PROGNOSIS FOR THIS PATIENT IS AS FOLLOWS (CHOOSE ONLY ONE):

32	Excellent with proper medical therapy	**32**	[Mother so advised.]
33	Excellent with proper surgical therapy	**33**	[Mother so advised.]
34	Should respond to proper management of acute episode, but is unlikely to have normal longevity	**34**	[Mother so advised.]
35	May respond to medical management but is most likely to die of disease within months to a few years	**35**	[Mother so advised.]
36	Unlikely to survive present episode	**36**	[Mother so advised.]

UNLESS OTHERWISE DIRECTED IN THE RESPONSE COLUMN CONTINUE WITH SECTION 4-C

SECTION 4-C

37 Record your diagnostic impressions below ______________

____

____

____

____

37 [The complete diagnosis as recorded on the patient's chart was hereditary spherocytosis, aplastic phase. SEE APPENDIX D FOR ADDITIONAL COMMENT AND RECOMMENDED MANAGEMENT. END OF PROBLEM 4.]

NOW DEVELOP RESPONSE 37 FOR ADDITIONAL INFORMATION AND INSTRUCTIONS

PROBLEM 5

AN ACUTE ABDOMEN

Thirty minutes after a light luncheon, and during a board of directors' meeting, a 50-year-old woman executive develops severe abdominal pain. The chairman of the board calls you and asks that you see her as soon as possible. At your request he agrees to arrange for her immediate transfer to a nearby hospital.

When you arrive there thirty minutes later you find the patient lying on a cart in the Emergency Room. She appears to be in severe pain and begs you for relief.

NOW CONTINUE WITH SECTION 5-A

SECTION 5-A

YOU WOULD NOW (CHOOSE ONLY ONE):

1	Obtain further history	**1**	[TURN TO SECTION 5-F, PAGE 31.]
2	Perform a physical examination	**2**	[TURN TO SECTION 5-H, PAGE 39.]
3	Hospitalize patient for immediate surgery	**3**	[TURN TO SECTION 5-C, PAGE 21.]
4	Hospitalize patient for urgent surgery after preoperative preparation	**4**	[TURN TO SECTION 5-I, PAGE 42.]
5	Hospitalize patient for conservative management without further evaluation	**5**	[TURN TO SECTION 5-E, PAGE 25.]

6 Hospitalize patient for further evaluation 6

SECTION 5-B

YOU WOULD NOW (CHOOSE ONLY ONE):

7 Obtain further history 7

8 Perform a physical examination 8

9 Institute medical management 9

10 Arrange for immediate surgery 10

11 Arrange for surgery after pre-operative preparation 11

SECTION 5-C

IF YOU HAVE BEEN DIRECTED TO THIS SECTION, CONSIDER THE PROCEDURES LISTED BELOW, AND INDICATE THOSE YOU WISH TO HAVE PERFORMED ON YOUR PATIENT AT THIS TIME (SELECT AS MANY AS YOU CONSIDER INDICATED):

12 Appendectomy 12

13 Drainage of appendiceal abscess 13

14 Cholecystectomy 14

15	Cholecystostomy	**15**	[Mushroom catheter is placed into slightly thickened gallbladder and brought out through stab wound in right upper quadrant.]
16	Exploration of common bile duct	**16**	[Common bile duct is normal in diameter and contains no calculi; a T-tube is inserted.]
17	Transverse colostomy	**17**	[Loop of transverse colon is brought out over a glass rod.]
18	Sigmoid colostomy	**18**	[Loop of sigmoid colon is brought out over a glass rod.]
19	Cecostomy	**19**	[Long tube placed in cecum, fixed with purse string sutures; brought out through stab wound in right lower quadrant.]
20	Closure of perforated viscus	**20**	[Anterior perforation of duodenum is closed with silk sutures over small piece of attached omentum.]
21	Biopsy of perforated viscus	**21**	[Frozen section is reported showing inflammatory tissue.]
22	Drainage of peritoneal cavity	**22**	[Two soft rubber drains are placed in peritoneal cavity and brought out through a stab wound.]
23	Drainage of subphrenic abscess	**23**	[No abscess is found.]
24	Inguinal or femoral herniorrhaphy	**24**	[No hernia is found.]

The operative procedure is tolerated fairly well. Two hours after the patient is returned to the recovery room, the nurse reports that the blood pressure has dropped to 60 systolic and 40 diastolic. The pulse rate is 96 per minute. The rectal temperature is 102.4F. The patient is awake and does not appear disoriented. Breath sounds are normal with a few basilar rales. Abdominal examination is not remarkable.

YOU WOULD NOW (SELECT AS MANY AS YOU CONSIDER INDICATED:

25	Order portable chest x-ray	**25**	[SEE FIGURE 40, PAGE 417.]
26	Order portable flat film of abdomen	**26**	[SEE FIGURE [illegible]8, PAGE 419.]
27	Order blood volume study	**27**	[One hour later blood volume is reported as 3800 cc; the blood pressure and pulse rate remain unchanged.]
28	Start intravenous therapy with 20 mg of metaraminol in 500 cc 5% dextrose in water	**28**	[Transient elevation of blood pressure to [illegible]/50 mm Hg occurs but, despite increasing the rate of drip, after 30 minutes the blood pressure falls to 50/30 mm Hg.]
29	Administer atropine sulfate 0.6 mg intramuscularly	**29**	[There is no improvement after 30 minutes.]
30	Return patient to operating room and reexplore operative wound	**30**	[Patient dies on the operating table in profound shock; nothing is found to explain the etiology of the shock. IGNORE INSTRUCTIONS AT END OF THIS SECTION AND TURN NOW TO SECTION [illegible], PAGE 49.]
31	Transfuse immediately with 500 cc of matched whole blood	**31**	[Blood pressure rises to 90/70 mm Hg but after 30 minutes falls quickly to 50/30 mm Hg; pulse rate remains about 96 per minute.]
32	Infuse 500 cc of dextran immediately	**32**	[Blood pressure rises to 90/70 mm Hg but after 30 minutes falls quickly to 50/30 mm Hg.]

33 Administer 15 mg morphine sulfate intramuscularly 33

34 Administer 100 mg meperidine intramuscularly 34

35 Administer 200 mg methylprednisolone intravenously at the rate of 100 mg/8 hours. 35

36 Administer 50 mg cortisone acetate intramuscularly 36

UNLESS OTHERWISE DIRECTED IN THE RESPONSE COLUMN CONTINUE WITH SECTION 5-D

SECTION 5-D

IN VIEW OF YOUR DIAGNOSIS YOU WOULD ADVISE THE PATIENT THAT (SELECT AS MANY AS YOU CONSIDER INDICATED):

37 She will develop recurrence of her symptoms and require surgery sometime in the future. 37

38 She will develop recurrence of her symptoms but will very likely respond to medical management. 38

39 Recurrence is unlikely and further surgery will not be necessary. 39

40 She will need another operation within the next six months. 40

41 Recurrence is unlikely if she remains on a fat free diet. 41

42 Recurrence is unlikely if she remains on a bland diet. 42

43 Her condition is incurable. 43

44 She must change her occupation and move to a different area of the country. 44

45 Record your diagnoses below: 45

____

____

____

____

____

NOW DEVELOP RESPONSE 45 FOR ADDITIONAL INFORMATION AND INSTRUCTIONS

SECTION 5-E

YOU WOULD NOW ORDER (SELECT AS MANY AS YOU CONSIDER INDICATED):

46 Nasogastric suction 46

47	Tap water enema	**47**	[Done with considerable discomfort for patient; moderate return of brown stool.]
48	Foley retention catheter	**48**	[Inserted; 50 cc clear urine removed.]
49	Collection of urine specimen four times a day for glucose determination	**49**	[Done; urine positive for glucose 2+.]
50	Urine culture and antibiotic sensitivities	**50**	[Urine sent to lab.]
51	Gastric lavage with saline solution	**51**	[Terminated quickly because of agonizing, generalized pain.]
52	Nothing by mouth	**52**	[Order posted on bed.]
53	Clear liquids only	**53**	[Done, but patient unable to retain fluid.]
54	Soft bland diet	**54**	[Food refused by patient.]
55	Record intake and output	**55**	[Recorded.]
56	Oxygen per nasal catheter at 12 liters per minute flow	**56**	[Catheter blows off oxygen tubing.]
57	Oxygen per nasal catheter at 6 liters per minute flow	**57**	[Done.]
58	Oxygen tent with high humidity	**58**	[Done.]
59	Intragastric cold milk drip	**59**	[Terminated quickly because of marked increase in pain.]
60	Morphine sulfate 5 mg intramuscularly every four hours as needed	**60**	[Done; nurse notifies you two hours later that patient still has severe pain.]

61	Morphine sulfate 15 mg intramuscularly every four hours as needed	61	
62	Meperidine 25 mg intramuscularly every four hours as needed	62	
63	Meperidine 100 mg intramuscularly every four hours as needed	63	
64	Procaine penicillin G in therapeutic dose intramuscularly every 12 hours	64	
65	Ampicillin trihydrate in therapeutic dose intravenously every six hours	65	
66	Streptomycin in therapeutic dose intramuscularly every 12 hours.	66	
67	Streptomycin in therapeutic dose orally every 12 hours	67	
68	Tetracycline in therapeutic dose orally every six hours	68	
69	Tetracycline in therapeutic dose intramuscularly every six hours	69	
70	Tetracycline in therapeutic dose intravenously every six hours	70	
71	Clindamycin and gentamycin in therapeutic doses intravenously every six hours	71	

	Order		Response
72	Atropine sulfate 5 mg intramuscularly every six hours	72	[Given; five minutes after first dose, pulse rate is 180 per minute, pupils become markedly dilated; marked restlessness and convulsion ensue, followed by coma and death. IGNORE INSTRUCTIONS AT END OF THIS SECTION AND TURN NOW TO SECTION 8-L, PAGE 49.]
73	Altropine sulfate 0.4 mg intramuscularly every six hours	73	[Given.]
74	Tincture of belladonna 10-12 drops in water three times a day before meals and at night	74	[First dose given and promptly vomited.]
75	Propantheline 15 mg orally three times a day and at bedtime	75	[First dose given and promptly vomited.]
76	Propantheline 5 mg orally three times a day and at night	76	[First dose given and promptly vomited.]
77	Propantheline 15 mg intramuscularly every six hours	77	[Given.]
78	Propantheline 5 mg intramuscularly every six hours	78	[Given.]
79	Phenobarbital 30 mg orally four times a day	79	[First dose given and promptly vomited.]
80	Phenobarbital 30 mg intramuscularly four times a day	80	[Given.]
81	Phenobarbital 100 mg intramuscularly at night for sleep as needed	81	[Given; patient sleeps restlessly.]
82	Chlorpromazine 25 mg intramuscularly every six hours	82	[Given.]

83	Chlorpromazine 50 mg intramuscularly every six hours	**83**
84	Lanatoside C 1.6 mg intravenously in divided doses	**84**
85	Digoxin 0.4 mg intravenously or intramuscularly	**85**
86	Aluminum hydroxide gel suspension 10 cc before each meal and between meals	**86**
87	Magnesium trisilicate suspension (Gelusil) 10 cc before each meal and between meals	**87**
88	Chlorpropamide 250 mg daily (Diabinese)	**88**
89	Tolbutamide 0.5 g twice a day (Orinase)	**89**
90	Regular insulin subcutaneously every six hours	**90**
91	Hydrocortisone 500 mg intravenously	**91**
92	Hydrocortisone 25 mg intravenously	**92**
93	Cortisone acetate 25 mg intramuscularly every six hours	**93**
94	Cortisone acetate 50 mg intramuscularly every six hours	**94**
95	1000 cc of 5% dextrose in water	**95**
96	1000 cc of 5% dextrose in 0.25% saline solution	**96**

97	1000 cc of 5% dextrose in isotonic saline	97	[Started.]
98	500 cc of 1/6 molar sodium lactate solution	98	[Started.]
99	Add 20 mEq potassium chloride to intravenous fluid	99	[Done.]
100	Add 40 mEq potassium chloride to intravenous fluid	100	[Done.]
101	Add 80 mEq potassium chloride to intravenous fluid	101	[Done.]
102	Add regular insulin 20 units to each liter of fluid	102	[Done.]
103	Add regular insulin 100 units to each liter of fluid	103	[Done.]
104	Add 20 mg of metaraminol to intravenous fluid	104	[Done.]
105	Add 10 mg metaraminol to intravenous fluid	105	[Done.]
106	Add 10 mg neosynephrine to intravenous fluid	106	[Done.]
107	Type and crossmatch 1000 cc blood	107	[Done.]
108	500 cc of dextran	108	[Started.]
109	500 cc whole blood	109	[Started.]
110	250 cc serum albumin	110	[Started.]
111	3000 cc Ringer's lactate solution	111	[Started.]

112	3000 cc Ringer's lactate solution with 50 cc 7.5% sodium bicarbonate in each liter	**112**	[Started.]

UNLESS OTHERWISE DIRECTED IN THE RESPONSE COLUMN TURN TO SECTION 5-K WHEN YOU HAVE COMPLETED THIS SECTION

SECTION 5-F

IN OBTAINING THE HISTORY YOU WOULD BE PARTICULARLY INTERESTED TO INQUIRE ABOUT (SELECT AS MANY AS YOU CONSIDER ESPECIALLY PERTINENT; YOU CAN RETURN TO THIS SECTION AT ANY TIME TO OBTAIN ANY ADDITIONAL HISTORICAL INFORMATION YOU MAY REQUIRE):

113	Duration of present illness	**113**	[Became ill just about an hour ago.]
114	Headache	**114**	[Occasional headache, relieved by aspirin.]
115	Visual disturbances	**115**	[None.]
116	Hearing disturbances	**116**	[None.]
117	Epistaxis	**117**	[None.]
118	Chest pain	**118**	[Occasional burning substernal pain, relieved by drinking glass of milk.]
119	Dyspnea and orthopnea	**119**	[Becomes "short of breath" after climbing two flights of stairs.]
120	Wheezing respiration	**120**	[None.]
121	Paroxysmal nocturnal dyspnea	**121**	[None.]
122	Cough	**122**	[Coughs on arising in the morning, producing moderate amount of green sputum.]
123	Dizziness and vertigo	**123**	[None.]

124	Blood pressure	**124**	[Blood pressure was "150 over 90" one year ago.]
125	Ankle swelling	**125**	[Some ankle swelling at the end of the day; disappears by morning.]
126	Hemoptysis	**126**	[None.]
127	Hematemesis	**127**	[None.]
128	Dysphagia	**128**	[Occasionally experiences sensation of food sticking in her throat.]
129	Appetite	**129**	[Appetite has been good.]
130	Nausea and vomiting	**130**	[Occasional nausea with no relationship to her meals; she vomited once after onset of her pain.]
131	Nature of vomitus	**131**	[Partially digested food she had eaten at lunch.]
132	Bowel habits	**132**	[Has one bowel movement every other day.]
133	Nature of stools	**133**	[Stools are frequently hard, "normal" in color.]
134	Type of pain	**134**	[Pain has been severe and constant since its onset; it is not relieved by position and is aggravated by moving around.]
135	Onset of pain	**135**	[Sudden; she remembers exactly what she was doing when it occurred; she volunteers that she had just lighted a cigarette.]

136	Location of pain	136	[It began in upper abdomen, but a few minutes later she developed pain in the right side of her abdomen.]
137	Diet	137	[Four years ago she was given a diet which she has not followed exactly most of the time.]
138	Weight and height	138	[Usual weight is 150 pounds; presently weighs about 140 pounds; height 5' 4".]
139	Jaundice	139	[None.]
140	Urinary symptoms	140	[None.]
141	Color of urine	141	[Light yellow and clear.]
142	Back pain	142	[Has some low back pain at the end of the day.]
143	Joint pains	143	[She has had pain in her wrists and fingers for about two years but this was relieved by some medicine.]
144	Skin diseases	144	[None.]
145	Bleeding tendency	145	[Has an occasional nose bleed.]
146	Trauma	146	[Broke right arm as a child.]
147	Previous hospitalizations	147	[Hospitalized five years earlier with vague upper abdominal pain, but "nothing was found."]
148	Other illness	148	[Told she had diabetes four years ago.]

149	Previous surgery	**149**	[Breast biopsy at age 35; physician told her it was "nothing to worry about."]
150	Allergy history	**150**	[Sensitive to penicillin and sulfa drugs.]
151	Drug history	**151**	[Until six months ago she had been taking some pills prescribed for her "arthritis"; she had taken these pills for about one year; she has also been taking two other white tablets a day for the past four years.]
152	Venereal disease	**152**	[Denied.]
153	Menstrual history	**153**	[Her periods have been irregular in frequency, duration and amount for two years.]
154	Smoking habits	**154**	[She smokes about 30 cigarettes a day.]
155	Alcoholic intake	**155**	[She usually has one or two cocktails before supper; today she had one martini before the luncheon.]
156	Neurologic history	**156**	[No neurologic symptoms.]

YOU WOULD NOW (CHOOSE ONLY ONE):

157	Perform physical examination	**157**	[TURN TO SECTION 5-H, PAGE 39.]
158	Arrange for immediate surgery	**158**	[TURN TO SECTION 5-C, PAGE 21.]
159	Arrange for urgent surgery after preoperative preparation	**159**	[TURN TO SECTION 5-I, PAGE 42.]

160	Institute medical management without further evaluation	**160**	[TURN TO SECTION 5-E, PAGE 25.]
161	Arrange for inpatient evaluation	**161**	[CONTINUE WITH SECTION 5-[illegible]]

SECTION 5-G

YOU WOULD NOW ORDER THE FOLLOWING DETERMINATIONS (SELECT AS MANY AS YOU CONSIDER INDICATED):

162	Hematocrit	**162**	[illegible]
163	Hemoglobin	**163**	[13.5 g/100 ml.]
164	White blood cell count	**164**	[illegible]
165	Differential white blood cell count	**165**	[Neutrophils — 70%; lymphocytes — 20%; monocytes — 5%; eosinophils — 3%; basophils — 2%; adequate platelets.]
166	Urinalysis	**166**	[Specific gravity 1.022; 2+ glucose, negative protein, negative acetone; microscopic examination reveals a few epithelial cells.]
167	Urine culture	**167**	[No growth.]
168	Stool guaiac test	**168**	[Negative.]
169	Stool benzidene test	**169**	[Negative.]
170	Erythrocyte sedimentation rate	**170**	[20 mm per hour (corrected).]
171	Serum electrolyte determinations	**171**	[Na — 140 mEq/L; K — 4.4 mEq/L; Cl — 100 mEq/L; CO_2 — 26 mEq/L.]
172	Blood urea nitrogen	**172**	[12 mg/100 ml.]

173	Serum protein electrophoresis	173	[Total protein — 7.4 g/100 ml, Albumin — 60%; Alpha$_1$ globulin — 7%, Alpha$_2$ — 10%, Beta — 10%, Gamma — 13%.]
174	Serum cholesterol	174	[480 mg/100 ml.]
175	Serum creatinine	175	[1.0 mg/100 ml.]
176	Bromsulphalein retention	176	[4% retention after 45 minutes.]
177	Serum bilirubin	177	[1.0 mg/100 ml.]
178	Thymol turbidity (serum)	178	[3 units.]
179	Cephalin flocculation (serum)	179	[Negative.]
180	Serum glutamic oxalacetic transaminase	180	[50 IU/L.]
181	Prothrombin time	181	[15.4 seconds (control — 14.5 seconds).]
182	Partial thromboplastin time	182	[38 seconds.]
183	Serum alkaline phosphatase	183	[170 IU/L.]
184	Serum acid phosphatase	184	[1.4 units (King-Armstrong).]
185	Serum amylase	185	[380 units/100 ml (Somogyi).]
186	Urinary amylase	186	[1360 mg glucose/24 hours (Somogyi).]
187	Blood sugar (random sample)	187	[185 mg/100 ml.]
188	Serum calcium and phosphorus	188	[Calcium — 5.0 mEq/L; phosphorus — 1.0 mEq/L.]
189	STS	189	[Nonreactive.]

190	Call patient's pharmacist and physician for further information about patient	**190**	[Patient has been taking prednisone 5 mg per day until two months ago; four years ago phenformin, one tablet twice a day, was prescribed.]

Radiographic Studies

191	Chest x-ray	**191**	[SEE FIGURE 39, PAGE 417.]
192	Flat film of abdomen	**192**	[SEE FIGURE 47, PAGE 419.]
193	Upright film of abdomen	**193**	[Patient unable to stand up.]
194	Lateral decubitus x-ray of abdomen	**194**	[SEE FIGURE 49, PAGE 420.]
195	Barium enema	**195**	[Done; no evidence of obstruction.]
196	Upper gastrointestinal series	**196**	[Patient promptly vomits and complains of increase in her pain.]
197	Intravenous pyelogram	**197**	[Interpreted as normal.]
198	Cholecystogram	**198**	[Patient vomits the tablets.]
199	Intravenous cholangiogram	**199**	[Gallbladder and common duct visualized.]

Other Studies

200	Proctoscopy	**200**	[Patient unable to tolerate position for proctoscopy.]
201	Electrocardiogram	**201**	[Patient sedated. SEE FIGURE 1, PAGE 404.]

202	Circulation times	**202**	[Eight seconds, arm to lung time with ether; 13 seconds arm to tongue with dehydrocholic acid (Decholin).]
203	Central venous pressure	**203**	[120 mm of saline with manometer at level of right atrium.]
204	Pulmonary artery wedge pressure	**204**	[5 mm Hg.]
205	Lumbar puncture	**205**	[Patient is unable to tolerate the position; procedure terminated without success.]
206	Tuberculin skin test	**206**	[Done.]

YOU WOULD NOW (CHOOSE ONLY ONE):

207	Observe the patient for a few hours	**207**	[TURN TO SECTION 5-J, PAGE 46.]
208	Institute medical management	**208**	[TURN TO SECTION 5-E, PAGE 25.]
209	Arrange for immediate surgery	**209**	[TURN TO SECTION 5-C, PAGE 21.]
210	Arrange for urgent surgery after preoperative preparation	**210**	[TURN TO SECTION 5-I, PAGE 42.]
211	Discharge patient for observation at home; you tell her that you will see her at home later in the evening	**211**	[When you arrive that evening you find that patient's family took her to another hospital for care. TURN TO SECTION 5-L, PAGE 49.]

SECTION 5-H

IN PERFORMING THE PHYSICAL EXAMINATION YOU WOULD BE PARTICULARLY INTERESTED TO CHECK (SELECT AS MANY AS YOU CONSIDER ESPECIALLY PERTINENT; YOU CAN RETURN TO THIS SECTION AT ANY TIME TO OBTAIN ANY ADDITIONAL INFORMATION YOU MAY REQUIRE ABOUT THE INITIAL PHYSICAL FINDINGS):

212	Extraocular movements	**212**	[Normal.]
213	Pupils	**213**	[React to light and accomodation.]
214	Funduscopic examination	**214**	[Normal.]
215	Ears	**215**	[Normal.]
216	Scalp	**216**	[Normal.]
217	Nose	**217**	[Deviated septum; normal mucosa.]
218	Mouth and pharynx	**218**	[False dentures; no mucosal lesions; lips appear lightly cyanotic.]
219	Neck	**219**	[Thyroid nonpalpable; no cervical adenopathy; trachea in midline; no [illegible] distension.]
220	Heart	**220**	[Size normal to percussion; S-1 and S-2 normal; no murmurs heard.]
221	Lungs	**221**	Few basilar rales heard; these clear with coughing.]
222	Breasts	**222**	[Bilateral diffuse nodularity; nontender; no dominant masses; [illegible] healed scar in upper inner quadrant of [illegible] breast.]
223	Peripheral pulses	**223**	[All present and symmetrically equal. No bruits.]

224	Blood pressure (right arm)	**224**	[100/65 mm Hg.]
225	Pulse rate	**225**	[110 per minute; regular.]
226	Respiratory rate	**226**	[32 per minute.]
227	Temperature	**227**	[100.4F rectally.]
228	Valsalva maneuver	**228**	[Patient is unable to perform this maneuver because of severe pain.]
229	Abdomen	**229**	[Flat; difficult to palpate because of exquisite tenderness throughout all quadrants, marked muscle spasm, particularly in epigastrium and right side of abdomen.]
230	Liver	**230**	[Unable to palpate because of exquisite tenderness.]
231	Spleen	**231**	[Unable to palpate because of exquisite tenderness.]
232	Bowel sounds	**232**	[After listening for five minutes, only rare bowel sounds are heard.]
233	Inguinal areas	**233**	[No evidence of hernia.]
234	External genitalia	**234**	[Normal.]
235	Upper extremities, range of motion	**235**	[Normal.]
236	Upper extremities, motor strength	**236**	[Normal.]
237	Lower extremities, range of motion	**237**	[Normal.]
238	Lower extremities, motor strength	**238**	[Normal.]

239	Spine	**239**	[Examined with considerable difficulty because patient is unable to cooperate due to pain.]
240	Range of motion of back	**240**	[Patient is unable to stand because of severe pain; complains bitterly when asked to roll over on her side.]
241	Straight leg raising	**241**	[Above 45° elevation patient complains of severe abdominal pain.]
242	Skin	**242**	[Spotty pigmentation and macular atrophy noted along lower tibial area of both legs; varices bilaterally.]
243	Sensation	**243**	[Patient is unable to concentrate well; sensation is grossly normal.]
244	Romberg test	**244**	[Patient unable to stand because of severe abdominal pain.]
245	Finger to nose test	**245**	[Normal.]
246	Heel to knee test	**246**	[Normal.]
247	Rectal examination	**247**	[Small external hemorrhoids; no intrinsic masses; marked tenderness in both adnexal regions; firm smooth mass anteriorly.]
248	Pelvic examination	**248**	[Normal cervix with small os; patient complains of severe pain when bimanual examination is attempted; impossible to determine size of uterus or palpate adnexa.]

YOU WOULD NOW (CHOOSE ONLY ONE):

249	Obtain further history	**249**	[TURN TO SECTION 5-F, PAGE 31.]

250	Observe patient for a few hours	250	[TURN TO SECTION 5-J, PAGE 46.]
251	Arrange for further inpatient evaluation and treatment	251	[TURN TO SECTION 5-G, PAGE 35.]
252	Arrange for urgent surgery after preoperative preparation	252	[CONTINUE WITH SECTION 5-I.]
253	Arrange for immediate surgery	253	[TURN TO SECTION 5-C, PAGE 21.]
254	Institute medical management without further evaluation	254	[TURN TO SECTION 5-E, PAGE 26.]
255	Administer narcotic and discharge to care of family; see patient on house call later in the evening	255	[When you arrive that evening, you find that the patient's family took her to another hospital for care. TURN TO SECTION 5-L, PAGE 49.]

SECTION 5-I

IN PREPARING YOUR PATIENT FOR SURGERY YOU WOULD NOW ORDER (SELECT AS MANY AS YOU CONSIDER INDICATED):

256	Nasogastric suction	256	[Levine tube inserted and intermittent suction started.]
257	Tap water enema	257	[Done with considerable discomfort to the patient; moderate return of brown feces.]
258	"Fleet" enema or oil retention enema	258	[Done with considerable discomfort to the patient; moderate return of brown feces.]
259	Foley retention catheter	259	[Inserted; 50 cc clear urine removed.]

260	Measure urinary output every two hours	260	[Done.]
261	Gastric lavage	261	[Terminated because of agonizing pain.]
262	Nothing by mouth	262	[Order posted on bed.]
263	Record intake and output	263	[Started.]
264	Oxygen per nasal catheter at 12 liters per minute flow	264	[Nasal catheter blows off oxygen tubing.]
265	Oxygen per nasal catheter at 6 liters per minute flow	265	[Nasal catheter inserted and oxygen started.]
266	Oxygen tent with high humidity	266	[Done.]
267	Morphine sulfate 5 mg intramuscularly	267	[Given with little relief from pain.]
268	Morphine sulfate 15 mg intramuscularly	268	[Given with considerable relief from pain.]
269	Meperidine 50 mg intramuscularly	269	[Given with little relief from pain.]
270	Meperidine 100 mg intramuscularly	270	[Given with considerable relief from pain.]
271	Procaine penicillin G intramuscularly in therapeutic dose	271	[Patient develops severe acute urticarial reaction which responds to adrenalin administered subcutaneously.]
272	Ampicillin trihydrate intravenously in therapeutic dose	272	[Patient develops severe acute urticarial reaction which responds to adrenalin administered subcutaneously.]
273	Streptomycin 0.5 g intramuscularly	273	[Given.]

274	Streptomycin 1.0 g intramuscularly	274	[Given.]
275	Tetracycline orally in usual therapeutic dose	275	[Given, but capsules are promptly vomited.]
276	Tetracycline intramuscularly in therapeutic dose	276	[Given.]
277	Tetracycline intravenously in therapeutic dose	277	[Given.]
278	Clindamycin and gentamycin intravenously in therapeutic doses	278	[Given.]
279	Atropine sulfate 5 mg intramuscularly	279	[Patient collapses five minutes later, has a convulsion and dies. IGNORE INSTRUCTIONS AT END OF THIS SECTION AND TURN NOW TO SECTION 5-L, PAGE 49.]
280	Atropine sulfate 0.6 mg intramuscularly	280	[Given.]
281	Atropine sulfate 0.1 mg intramuscularly	281	[Given.]
282	Scopolamine 5 mg intramuscularly	282	[Patient collapses ten minutes later, has a convulsion and dies. IGNORE INSTRUCTIONS AT END OF THIS SECTION AND TURN NOW TO SECTION 5-L, PAGE 49.]
283	Scopolamine 0.4 mg intramuscularly	283	[Given.]
284	Scopolamine 0.1 mg intramuscularly	284	[Given.]

285	Aluminum hydroxide gel suspension 10 cc	**285**	[Given and promptly vomited.]
286	Magnesium trisilicate suspension (Gelusil), 10 cc	**286**	[Given and promptly vomited.]
287	Chlorpropamide 250 mg stat (Diabinese)	**287**	[Given and promptly vomited.]
288	Tolbutamide 0.5 g stat (Orinase)	**288**	[Given and promptly vomited.]
289	Regular insulin 25 mg subcutaneously	**289**	[Given.]
290	Methylprednisolone 500 mg intravenously	**290**	[Given.]
291	Methylprednisolone 25 mg intravenously	**291**	[Given.]
292	Cortisone acetate 25 mg intramuscularly	**292**	[Given.]
293	Cortisone acetate 50 mg intramuscularly	**293**	[Given.]
294	Lanatoside C 1.6 mg intravenously in divided doses	**294**	[Given.]
295	Digoxin 0.4 mg intravenously	**295**	[Given.]
296	Phytonadione 10 mg intravenously (Mephyton)	**296**	[Given.]
297	1000 cc 5% dextrose in water	**297**	[Started.]
298	1000 cc 5% dextrose in 0.25% saline solution	**298**	[Started.]
299	500 cc 1/6 molar sodium lactate solution	**299**	[Started.]
300	1000 cc lactated Ringer's solution	**300**	[Started.]

301	500 cc 3% saline solution	**301**	[Started.]
302	Add 20 mEq potassium chloride to intravenous fluid	**302**	[Done.]
303	Add 40 mEq potassium chloride to intravenous fluid	**303**	[Done.]
304	Add 80 mEq potassium chloride to intravenous fluid	**304**	[Done.]
305	Add aqueous solution of multi-vitamins to intravenous fluid	**305**	[Done.]
306	Add 20 mg metaraminol to intravenous fluid	**306**	[Done.]
307	Add 8.0 cc of levarterenol bitartrate solution to intravenous fluid	**307**	[Done.]
308	500 cc of dextran	**308**	[Given.]
309	250 cc plasma	**309**	[Given.]
310	500 cc whole blood (type 0, Rh negative)	**310**	[Given.]
311	Type and cross-match 1000 cc blood	**311**	[Done.]

UNLESS OTHERWISE DIRECTED IN THE RESPONSE COLUMN TURN TO SECTION 5-C WHEN YOU HAVE COMPLETED THIS SECTION

SECTION 5-J

Two hours later the patient appears to be much worse. The pulse rate is 120 per minute. Blood pressure is 90 systolic and 60 diastolic. The severe pain has not abated. All other findings are unchanged.

YOU WOULD NOW (CHOOSE ONLY ONE):

312	Obtain further laboratory determinations	**312**	[TURN TO SECTION 5-G, PAGE 35.]
313	Institute medical management	**313**	[TURN TO SECTION 5-E, PAGE 25.]
314	Arrange for surgery with pre-operative preparation	**314**	[TURN TO SECTION 5-I, PAGE 42.]
315	Arrange for immediate surgery	**315**	[TURN TO SECTION 5-C, PAGE 21.]
316	Discharge patient	**316**	[You are notified by another physician that the patient is admitted to another hospital at the insistence of her family. TURN TO SECTION 5-L, PAGE 49.]
317	Continue observation in the emergency room	**317**	[Patient's condition continues to deteriorate with profound hypotension and a pulse rate of 180 per minute. Three hours later she expires. TURN TO SECTION 5-L, PAGE 49.]

SECTION 5-K

Two hours later you are called back because the patient's condition has become much worse. The blood pressure is now 80/50 mm Hg; the pulse rate is 120 per minute; and the respiratory rate is 30 per minute. Respirations are shallow and the patient is perspiring profusely. Urinary output in the past two hours has totaled 50 cc.

YOU WOULD NOW (SELECT AS MANY AS YOU CONSIDER INDICATED):

318	Transfuse with 1000 cc whole blood as rapidly as possible	**318**	[Given; blood pressure responds for one hour, rising to 100/60 mm Hg but pulse rate remains the same. Patient dies two hours later. IGNORE INSTRUCTIONS AT END OF THIS SECTION AND TURN NOW TO SECTION 5-L, PAGE 49.]
319	Start levarterenol bitartrate drip with two ampules (4.0 cc each) diluted in 1000 cc 5% dextrose in water	**319**	[Drip started with blood pressure rising to 110/80 mm Hg for two hours; pulse rate remains the same; after two hours, patient dies suddenly. IGNORE INSTRUCTIONS AT END OF THIS SECTION AND TURN NOW TO SECTION 5-L, PAGE 49.]
320	Start metaraminol drip with 20 mg diluted in 1000 cc 5% dextrose in water	**320**	[Drip started with blood pressure rising to 110/80 mm Hg for two hours; pulse rate remains the same; after two hours, patient dies suddenly. IGNORE INSTRUCTIONS AT END OF THIS SECTION AND TURN NOW TO SECTION 5-L, PAGE 49.]
321	Administer mannitol, 100 cc of 12.5% solution intravenously	**321**	[Given; condition of patient remains unchanged.]
322	Obtain chest x-ray stat	**322**	[As patient is put in a sitting position for taking the film, blood pressure becomes unobtainable and patient dies. IGNORE INSTRUCTIONS AT END OF THIS SECTION AND TURN NOW TO SECTION 5-L, PAGE 49.]
323	Obtain flat film of abdomen stat	**323**	[SEE FIGURE 48, PAGE 419.]

324	Continue present regimen without change	**324**	[Patient expires one hour later. IGNORE INSTRUCTIONS AT END OF THIS SECTION AND TURN NOW TO SECTION 5-L.]
325	Administer methylprednisolone 500 mg intravenously and continue pharmacologic regimen	**325**	[Blood pressure responds dramatically rising to 120/80 mm Hg, pulse rate drops to 100; patient continues to do well for four hours, but condition suddenly deteriorates rapidly and patient dies. IGNORE INSTRUCTIONS AT END OF THIS SECTION AND TURN NOW TO SECTION 5-L.]
326	Administer methylprednisolone 500 mg intravenously and arrange for immediate surgery	**326**	[TURN TO SECTION 5-C, PAGE 21.]
327	Arrange for prompt surgery	**327**	[TURN TO SECTION 5-C, PAGE 21.]

UNLESS OTHERWISE DIRECTED IN THE RESPONSE COLUMN TURN TO SECTION 5-C WHEN YOU HAVE COMPLETED THIS SECTION

SECTION 5-L

328	Record your diagnoses below: ____________________ ____________________ ____________________ ____________________ ____________________ ____________________ ____________________	**328**	[The diagnosis as recorded on the chart for this patient was (i) duodenal ulcer with perforation (ii) diabetes mellitus (iii) probable rheumatoid arthritis for which the patient was taking corticosteroids (iv) sensitivity to penicillin and also possibly sulfonamides. SEE APPENDIX A FOR ADDITIONAL COMMENT AND RECOMMENDED MANAGEMENT. END OF PROBLEM 5.]

NOW DEVELOP RESPONSE 328 FOR ADDITIONAL INFORMATION AND INSTRUCTIONS

PROBLEM 6

A "NERVOUS" PATIENT WITH A SORE THROAT

You have been asked to see a 37-year-old woman with fever and severe sore throat of three days' duration. She has also had excessive sweating and extreme tiredness for the last two months, as well as unusual numbness and tingling of the fingers. An accompanying letter from the surgeon, who had not seen the patient since he discharged her two years ago, states that her temperature in his office today was 100.4F and her pulse rate was 144 per minute. He detected a nontender swelling in her neck and prescribed an antibiotic.

NOW CONTINUE WITH SECTION 6-A

SECTION 6-A

YOU WOULD NOW (CHOOSE ONLY ONE):

1	Perform physical examination	**1**	[CONTINUE WITH SECTION 6-B.]
2	Obtain a throat culture stat	**2**	[TURN TO SECTION 6-G, PAGE 61.]
3	Obtain history	**3**	[TURN TO SECTION 6-D, PAGE 56.]
4	Initiate appropriate therapy	**4**	[TURN TO SECTION 6-E, PAGE 59.]

SECTION 6-B

IN PERFORMING THE PHYSICAL EXAMINATION YOU WOULD BE PARTICULARLY INTERESTED TO CHECK (SELECT AS MANY AS YOU CONSIDER ESPECIALLY PERTINENT; YOU CAN RETURN TO THIS SECTION AT ANY TIME TO OBTAIN ANY ADDITIONAL INFORMATION YOU MAY REQUIRE ABOUT THE INITIAL PHYSICAL FINDINGS):

5	Blood pressure	**5**	[138/82 mm Hg. Contraction of the flexor muscles of the arm and hand occurred as the pressure was taken.]
6	Temperature	**6**	[100.8F oral.]
7	Respiratory rate	**7**	[20 per minute.]
8	Pulse rate	**8**	[144 per minute, regular.]
9	General observation	**9**	[Patient restless and crying during examination.]
10	Skin	**10**	[Warmth increased, fine texture, increased perspiration.]
11	Eye lids	**11**	[Slight retraction.]
12	Extraocular muscle movement	**12**	[Decreased ocular convergence.]
13	Pupils	**13**	[Equal; react equally to light.]
14	Funduscopic examination	**14**	[The ocular discs are normal; the vessels are full with no sign of arteriosclerosis.]
15	Conjunctiva	**15**	[Chemosis bilaterally.]
16	Scalp	**16**	[Scalp normal; hair, fine texture; there is a diffuse loss of hair seen on close inspection.]
17	External auditory canals	**17**	[The skin is normal.]

18	Tympanic membranes	**18**	[Both drums are clear; there is a normal light reflex present bilaterally [illegible]]
19	Nose	**19**	[The nasal mucosa is normal; there is no obstruction or septal deviation.]
20	Teeth	**20**	[illegible]
21	Tongue	**21**	[Normal in size, color and papillation; [illegible] tremor of the tongue.]
22	Pharynx	**22**	[Diffuse erythema; [illegible]]
23	Inspection of the neck	**23**	[SEE FIGURE [illegible], PAGE 424.]
24	Palpation of the neck	**24**	[Asymmetric thyroid gland, nontender, with right lobe diffusely enlarged about three times normal; isthmus slightly enlarged and left lobe not well palpated.]
25	Auscultation of the neck	**25**	[Bruit heard over right paratracheal mass.]
26	Percussion of the neck	**26**	[No abnormal resonance elicited.]
27	Inspection of the chest	**27**	[Expansion full and symmetrical; increased cardiac pulsation seen.]
28	Palpation of the chest	**28**	[Increased force of cardiac pulsation; no increased fremitus or thrills.]
29	Percussion of the chest	**29**	[Left border cardiac dullness in 4th intercostal space inside midclavicular line; lung fields resonant throughout.]

30 Auscultation of the chest 30

31 Inspection of the abdomen 31

32 Palpation of the abdomen 32

33 Percussion of the abdomen 33

34 Auscultation of the abdomen 34

35 Inspection of the extremities 35

36 Palpation of the extremities 36

37 Auscultation of the extremities 37

38 External genitalia 38

39 Pelvic examination 39

40 Rectal examination 40

41 Cranial nerve examination 41

42 Muscle strength 42

43 Deep tendon reflexes 43

44 Vibratory sensation 44

45 Trousseau sign 45

46	Plantar responses	**46**	[Down-going bilaterally.]

YOU WOULD NOW (CHOOSE ONLY ONE):

47	Request a consultation	**47**	[Patient agrees [illegible] TURN TO SECTION 6-H, PAGE 62.]
48	Obtain history	**48**	[TURN TO SECTION 6-D, PAGE [illegible].]
49	Initiate laboratory evaluation	**49**	[CONTINUE WITH SECTION 6-C.]
50	Initiate definitive therapy	**50**	[TURN TO SECTION 6-E, PAGE 59.]

SECTION 6-C

YOU WOULD NOW ORDER THE FOLLOWING DETERMINATIONS (SELECT AS MANY AS YOU CONSIDER INDICATED):

51	Blood culture	**51**	[Minimal turbidity in broth in 48 hours. No growth on innoculated blood agar pour plate.]
52	Gastric analysis	**52**	[Acid output – 3.4 mEq/hour; Diagnex Blue – 1 mg excreted/2 hours, Volume – 70 ml; pH – 1.2.]
53	Basal metabolic rate	**53**	[+31%, +30%, +33%, (three determinations).]
54	Surgical biopsy of neck lesion	**54**	[Done; much bleeding ensues, patient rapidly deteriorates. DO NOT MAKE ANY MORE CHOICES IN THIS SECTION; TURN NOW TO SECTION 6-H.

55	Serum calcium and phosphorus	**55**	[Ca = 3.8 mEq/L, P = 2.2 mEq/L.]
56	Fasting blood sugar	**56**	[110 mg/100 ml.]
57	Pharyngeal culture	**57**	[Coagulase-negative staphylococcus aureus.]
58	Serum thyroxine, (Pattee-Murphy) concentration	**58**	[15 μg/100 ml.]
59	Circulation time (arm to tongue)	**59**	[8 seconds.]
60	Stool culture	**60**	[Nonmotile gram-negative fermenter of lactose and glucose.]
61	Qualitative urine calcium	**61**	[Negative.]
62	Serum cholesterol (total)	**62**	[150 mg/100 ml.]
63	Serum creatinine	**63**	[0.8 mg/100 ml.]
64	White blood cell count and differential	**64**	[WBC – 5000/mm^3; differential; segmented neutrophils – 57%, lymphocytes – 40%, monocytes – 3%.]
65	Radioactive iodine (I^{131}) uptake	**65**	[56% in 24 hours.]
66	Cerebrospinal fluid examination	**66**	[No cells, protein 50 mg/100 cc.]
67	Urine culture	**67**	[Aerobacter aerogenes less than 1000 colonies/cc.]
68	Stool guaiac test	**68**	[Negative.]
69	Tri-iodothyronine uptake (resin)	**69**	[50%.]
70	Thyroid scan	**70**	[Enlarged right lobe with homogenous uptake; very little uptake on left side.]
71	Tri-iodothyronine daily for one week followed by ^{131}I uptake	**71**	[Radioactive iodine uptake 53% in 24 hours.]

YOU WOULD NOW (CHOOSE ONLY ONE):

72	Obtain history	**72**
73	Perform physical examination	**73**
74	Initiate definitive therapy	**74**
75	Request a consultation	**75**

SECTION 6-D

YOU WOULD BE PARTICULARLY INTERESTED TO INQUIRE ABOUT (SELECT AS MANY AS YOU CONSIDER ESPECIALLY PERTINENT; YOU CAN RETURN TO THIS SECTION AT ANY TIME TO OBTAIN ANY ADDITIONAL HISTORICAL INFORMATION YOU MAY REQUIRE):

76	Nature of the sore throat	**76**
77	Reaction to physical activity	**77**
78	Location of pain	**78**
79	Childhood illnesses	**79**
80	Previous surgical procedures	**80**

81	Pathologist's report on specimen from previous surgical intervention	81
82	Allergies	82
83	Family history of illness	83
84	Marital status	84
85	Occupation	85
86	Smoking habits	86
87	Medications	87
88	Alcohol intake	88
89	Palpitation	89
90	Chest pain	90
91	Dyspnea	91
92	Orthopnea	92
93	Paroxysmal nocturnal dyspnea	93
94	Cough	94

95	Insomnia	**95**	[Yes, for past two weeks and during illness two years ago.]
96	Ankle swelling	**96**	[None.]
97	Abdominal pain	**97**	[None.]
98	Bowel habits	**98**	[Four to six bowel movements daily for three weeks.]
99	Food intolerances	**99**	[None.]
100	Vomiting	**100**	[None.]
101	Nausea	**101**	[None.]
102	Jaundice	**102**	[None.]
103	Dysphagia	**103**	[None.]
104	Nature of stools	**104**	[Soft but formed.]
105	Headache	**105**	[None.]
106	Visual disturbance	**106**	[Watering and burning of eyes for past three or four weeks.]
107	Color of urine	**107**	[Yellow and clear.]
108	Joint pain	**108**	[None.]
109	Emotional disturbances	**109**	[Crying, irritable, and nervous.]
110	Weight change	**110**	[Five-pound loss in two weeks.]
111	Appetite	**111**	[Good -- increased food intake.]
112	Pregnancies	**112**	[One, uneventful, 15 years ago.]
113	Menstrual history	**113**	[Last menstrual period four months ago -- scant.]
114	Venereal disease	**114**	[None.]

115 Urinary symptoms **115**

116 Muscle weakness **116**

YOU WOULD NOW (CHOOSE ONLY ONE):

117 Initiate laboratory evaluation **117**

118 Perform physical examination **118**

119 Request a consultation **119**

120 Initiate definitive therapy **120**

SECTION 6-E

ON THE BASIS OF THE INFORMATION NOW AVAILABLE YOU SUSPECT THAT THIS PATIENT HAS (CHOOSE ONE OR MORE):

121 An inflammatory disease **121**

122 A metabolic and endocrine disorder **122**

123 A disease due to a microbiologic agent **123**

124	A neoplastic disorder	124	[REVIEW AVAILABLE DATA THEN TURN TO SECTION 6-H, PAGE 62.]
125	A psychiatric disorder	125	[REVIEW AVAILABLE DATA THEN TURN TO SECTION 6-H, PAGE 62.]
126	A congenital disease	126	[REVIEW AVAILABLE DATA THEN TURN TO SECTION 6-H, PAGE 62.]
127	A disease of unknown etiology	127	[IF THIS HAS BEEN YOUR ONLY CHOICE IN THIS SECTION, PLEASE MAKE ANOTHER CHOICE.]

Record your specific diagnosis here: ______________________________

UNLESS OTHERWISE DIRECTED IN THE RESPONSE COLUMN CONTINUE WITH SECTION 6-F

SECTION 6-F

YOU WOULD THEREFORE RECOMMEND (SELECT AS MANY AS YOU CONSIDER INDICATED):

128	Phenoxymethyl penicillin	128	[Patient develops temperature 104F (oral) and generalized urticara.]
129	Propylthiouracil	129	[Patient improves.]
130	Calcium gluconate orally	130	[Trousseau's sign disappears.]
131	Digitalis lanata	131	[No response to the usual therapeutic dose.]
132	Patient be reassured and asked to return in three months	132	[Patient consults another physician. TURN NOW TO SECTION 6-H, PAGE 62.]

133	Surgical intervention	**133**	[Patient dies of severe exacerbation of disease. TURN NOW TO SECTION 6-H, PAGE 62.]
134	Prednisone 30 mg per day	**134**	[Sore throat subsides rapidly but all other symptoms persist.]
135	Vitamin D	**135**	[Trousseau's sign disappears.]
136	Opium tincture	**136**	[Diarrhea abates temporarily; other symptoms persist.]
137	Methimazole	**137**	[Patient improves.]

UNLESS OTHERWISE DIRECTED IN THE RESPONSE COLUMN TURN TO SECTION 6-H WHEN YOU HAVE COMPLETED THIS SECTION

SECTION 6-G

138	Develop response 138 opposite for report of culture from throat	**138**	[Coagulese negative staphylococcus aureus.]

WITH THIS INFORMATION YOU WOULD NOW (CHOOSE ONLY ONE):

139	Initiate definitive therapy	**139**	[TURN TO SECTION 6-E, PAGE 59.]
140	Obtain history	**140**	[TURN TO SECTION 6-D, PAGE 56.]
141	Perform physical examination	**141**	[TURN TO SECTION 6-B, PAGE 51.]
142	Request a consultation	**142**	[Patient agrees to visit another physician. CONTINUE WITH SECTION 6-H.]
143	Initiate laboratory investigation	**143**	[TURN TO SECTION 6-C, PAGE 54.]

SECTION 6-H

144 Record your diagnostic impressions below:

____

____

____

____

____

144 [The diagnosis as recorded on the chart for this patient was (i) recurrent postoperative thyrotoxicosis; (ii) hypoparathyroidism, secondary to surgery; (iii) acute pharyngitis. SEE APPENDIX 1 FOR ADDITIONAL COMMENTS AND RECOMMENDED MANAGEMENT. END OF PROBLEM 6.]

NOW DEVELOP RESPONSE 144 FOR ADDITIONAL INFORMATION AND INSTRUCTIONS

PROBLEM 7

LOW BACK PAIN

You are a family practitioner in a group practice with other family practitioners.

A patient was admitted to the hospital yesterday evening. You have never seen this patient before; he was referred to you because of a problem of low back pain, by a former colleague who recently retired.

The hospital chart now includes the routine admission papers and a history and physical done by the intern which is very short and sketchy, followed by the diagnosis "low back pain, possible disc, patient in no acute distress."

There is also a letter from the referring physician which reads as follows:

> Dear Doctor:
> This is to introduce Mr. J. Smith, age 49 years, who has a history of two years of recurrent low back pain, which recently is worse and prevents him from doing his work. My diagnosis is herniated disc.
>
> Sincerely,
> Dr. Hippocrates

The patient is in bed in Room 421.

NOW CONTINUE WITH SECTION 7-A

SECTION 7-A

YOU WOULD NOW (CHOOSE ONLY ONE):

1	Visit the patient and take a history	**1**	[TURN TO SECTION 7-F, PAGE 77.]

2	Visit the patient and perform a physical examination	**2**	[TURN TO SECTION 7-C, PAGE 69.]
3	Order laboratory tests, special investigations and x-ray studies	**3**	[TURN TO SECTION 7-J, PAGE 8[illegible].]
4	Seek consultation	**4**	[CONTINUE WITH SECTION 7-B.]
5	Initiate definitive treatment	**5**	[TURN TO SECTION 7-D, PAGE 76.]

SECTION 7-B

YOU WOULD NOW REQUEST THE FOLLOWING CONSULTATIONS (SELECT AS MANY AS YOU CONSIDER INDICATED):

6	Allergist	**6**	[It is my opinion that this patient does not have a major allergic problem. His postnasal drip and mild rhinitis may be on an allergic basis, but do not concern the patient. His other problems seem more pressing.]
7	Cardiologist	**7**	[This patient has a history of angina which is well controlled by medication. His electrocardiogram suggests moderate ischemia. He is not disabled by his symptoms and within reasonable limits, he should continue his work. His age and symptoms together with elevated cholesterol levels suggest generalized arterial disease.]

8 Dermatologist

8 [This patient has no dermatologic complaints other than mild seborrhea. His low back pain does not have the distribution of herpes zoster. Thank you for the consultation.]

9 Endocrinologist

9 [This patient has no apparent hormone imbalance on the basis of the history, physical examination, or those investigations which have been done.]

10 Neurosurgeon

10 [This is an unclear [illegible] problem and may represent an atypical disc syndrome. I would be happy to accept the patient on transfer with the thought that surgical management might be indicated after further investigation. IF YOU WISH TO TRANSFER THE PATIENT, DEVELOP RESPONSE 11 BELOW FOR INSTRUCTIONS. IF YOU DO NOT WISH TO TRANSFER THE PATIENT, SKIP RESPONSE 11 AND SIMPLY CONTINUE WITH THIS SECTION.]

11 [This patient has been transferred to the neurosurgical service and is lost to follow-up. DO NOT MAKE ANY MORE CHOICES IN THIS SECTION. INSTEAD TURN NOW TO SECTION 7-G, PAGE 93.]

12 Ophthalmologist

12 [This patient has no acute eye problem; funduscopic examination suggests [illegible]sclerosis; no treatment is recommended.]

13 Orthopedic Surgeon

13 [This patient may represent one of the unusual situations where one [illegible] protruding [illegible] without nerve [illegible] It is interesting to [illegible] completely pain- [illegible] but gives [illegible] con- [illegible] recommend [illegible] it should be [illegible] surgery may [illegible] be required. IF YOU WISH TO TRANSFER THE PATIENT, DEVELOP RESPONSE 14 BELOW FOR INSTRUCTIONS; IF YOU DO NOT WISH TO TRANSFER THE PATIENT SKIP RESPONSE 14 AND SIMPLY CONTINUE WITH THIS SECTION.]

14 [This patient has been transferred to the orthopedic service and is lost to follow-up. DO NOT MAKE ANY MORE CHOICES IN THIS SECTION; INSTEAD TURN NOW TO SECTION 7-G, PAGE 8[illegible].]

15 Otolaryngologist

15 [The patient has no serious problem. He has a mild rhinitis with posterior nasal drip, but no other gross abnormalities. His larynx is normal.]

16	Psychiatrist	16	[This patient's symptoms may well be of psychiatric origin; he has marked conflicts in many areas. If [illegible] find no organic explanation for the complaints, [illegible] transfer to psychiatric care. IF YOU WISH TO TRANSFER THE PATIENT, DEVELOP RESPONSE 17 BELOW FOR INSTRUCTIONS; IF YOU DO NOT WISH TO TRANSFER THE PATIENT [illegible] RESPONSE 17 AND [illegible] CONTINUE WITH THIS SECTION.]
		17	[This patient has been transferred to the psychiatric service and is lost to followup. DO NOT MAKE ANY MORE CHOICES IN THIS SECTION. INSTEAD TURN NOW TO SECTION 7-G.]
18	Surgeon (general)	18	[This patient's symptoms are probably not originating in an abdominal viscus. I cannot explain them without further data. This may be a spine disorder.]
19	Urologist	19	[This patient's complaints are probably not originating in the genitourinary system.]

20	Vascular surgeon	20	[This patient's complaints are related to obstruction of the internal iliac artery and are in the nature of intermittent claudication. I recommend transfer to my service for definitive treatment. IF YOU WISH TO TRANSFER THE PATIENT, DEVELOP RESPONSE 21 BELOW FOR INSTRUCTIONS; IF YOU DO NOT WISH TO TRANSFER THE PATIENT SKIP RESPONSE 21 AND SIMPLY CONTINUE WITH THIS SECTION.]
		21	[The patient has been transferred to the care of the vascular surgeon. You hear as a follow-up that the diagnosis has been confirmed and definitive treatment is being initiated. DO NOT MAKE ANY MORE CHOICES IN THIS SECTION; INSTEAD TURN NOW TO APPENDIX N FOR ADDITIONAL COMMENT AND RECOMMENDED MANAGEMENT. END OF PROBLEM 7.]

YOU WOULD NOW (CHOOSE ONLY ONE EACH TIME YOU ARE DIRECTED TO THIS SECTION):

22	Take a history if you have not done so previously	22	[TURN TO SECTION 7-F, PAGE 77.]
23	Perform a physical examination if you have not previously done so	23	[CONTINUE WITH SECTION 7-C.]
24	Order laboratory tests, special investigations and x-ray studies if you have not yet done so	24	[TURN TO SECTION 7-J, PAGE 86.]
25	Initiate definitive treatment	25	[TURN TO SECTION 7-D, PAGE 76.]

SECTION 7-C

IN PERFORMING THE PHYSICAL EXAMINATION YOU WOULD BE PARTICULARLY INTERESTED TO CHECK (SELECT AS MANY AS YOU CONSIDER ESPECIALLY PERTINENT; YOU CAN RETURN TO THIS SECTION AT ANY TIME TO OBTAIN ANY ADDITIONAL INFORMATION YOU MAY REQUIRE ABOUT INITIAL PHYSICAL FINDINGS):

General Examination

26	Nutrition	**26**	[Good.]
27	Weight	**27**	[190 pounds.]
28	Height	**28**	[5 feet, 10 inches.]
29	Physical type	**29**	[Mesomorphic.]
30	Complexion	**30**	[Fair.]
31	Race	**31**	[Caucasian.]
32	National background	**32**	[Nordic.]
33	Posture	**33**	[Erect with protruding abdomen.]
34	Gait	**34**	[Normal and effortless without limp or apparent pain.]
35	Movements while being examined	**35**	[Effortless and apparently painless.]
36	Intelligence and cooperativeness	**36**	[Good.]
37	Obvious deformities	**37**	[None.]

Head, Scalp, and Neck

38	Hair	**38**	[Blond with male pattern baldness.]

39	Scalp	**39**	[Normal; mild scaling.]
40	Skull shape	**40**	[No temporal or frontal bossing; symmetrical.]
41	Auscultation of skull	**41**	[Silent.]
42	Facial expression	**42**	[Symmetrical and normal.]
43	Neck palpation	**43**	[Trachea midline; thyroid not enlarged or nodular; no abnormality of lymph nodes.]

Ear, Nose, and Throat (For eye movements and funduscopic examination, see neurologic examination.)

44	External ears	**44**	[Normal.]
45	Mastoid area	**45**	[No scars or tenderness.]
46	Otoscopic visualization	**46**	[Canals clean and normal; tympanic membranes normal except for old scar on left side.]
47	Pupils and corneas	**47**	[Equal and round; no corneal opacity apparent.]
48	Nasal visualization	**48**	[Mucosa mildly inflammed with no evidence of polyps.]
49	Teeth	**49**	[All wisdom teeth missing — remainder in good repair.]
50	Tongue	**50**	[Slightly coated; no tremor or evidence of fasciculations; tonsils atrophic; posterior pharangeal wall shows evidence of postnasal discharge; palate symmetrical.]
51	Laryngeal visualization (mirror)	**51**	[Normal and symmetrical laryngeal function and appearance.]

Upper Limbs and Shoulder Girdle

52	General appearance	**52**	[No deformities.]
53	Color of hands	**53**	[Pink — no suggestion of cyanosis.]
54	Skin texture	**54**	[Hands heavily calloused.]
55	Nail beds	**55**	[Normal appearance with prompt capillary return.]
56	Radial pulses	**56**	[Firm, regular, and symmetrical.]
57	Radial pulses with the arms held in various positions	**57**	[Constant and symmetrical.]

Chest and Cardiovascular System

58	Blood pressure	**58**	[135/85 mm Hg (both arms).]
59	Pulse	**59**	[82 per minute.]
60	Respiration	**60**	[12 per minute.]
61	Observation of chest	**61**	[Symmetrical in shape and movements; no abnormal vascular pattern.]
62	Palpation of chest	**62**	[Symmetrical chest expansion; no thrills; apical impulse in midclavicular line.]
63	Percussion of chest	**63**	[Resonant throughout with full diaphragmatic excursion; heart is not enlarged.]
64	Auscultation of chest	**64**	[Breath sounds clear with no evidence of rales or consolidation and good aeration throughout.]

Abdomen

65 Inspection

65 [Protruding and moving freely and symmetrically with respirations; scar of appendectomy, right lower quandrant.]

66 Palpation

66 [Soft, no guarding, tenderness or masses; liver and spleen not palpable.]

67 Auscultation

67 [Bowel sounds present; not high pitched; no rushes heard.]

68 Inguinal region and genitalia

68 [No evidence of hernia; scrotum normal; testes descended; right varicocele.]

69 Rectal examination

69 [Sphincter normal; examination completed easily; no evidence of tumor, ulceration, or other abnormality; prostate not enlarged or nodular.]

70 Sigmoidoscopic examination

70 [Scope inserted to 20 cm; no abnormalities seen.]

Lower Limbs

71 General

71 [No deformities.]

72 Color

72 [Pink.]

73 Nutrition

73 [Good throughout; color and texture of skin and hair distribution are that of a normal male.]

74 Veins

74 [Single varicosity of right calf.]

75 Pedal pulses

75 [Present bilaterally, although slightly reduced on the left.]

76	Popliteal pulses	**76**	[Present bilaterally, although slightly reduced on the left.]
77	Femoral pulses	**77**	[Present bilaterally, but considerably less prominent on the left than on the right.]
78	Auscultation of femoral triangles	**78**	[Right normal; left has a prominent systolic bruit.]

Orthopedic Examination

79	Neck movements	**79**	[Full and free of pain.]
80	Upper limbs	**80**	[Full range of movement; no swelling or deformity of joints; full hand function.]
81	General	**81**	[Normal spine contour; no obvious gibbus.]
82	Movement	**82**	[Full range of back movements without pain or muscle spasm.]
83	Palpation	**83**	[No tenderness in back or sciatic regions; no sacroiliac tenderness or deformity.]
84	Straight leg raising	**84**	[To 90° bilaterally without pain.]
85	Trendelenburg test	**85**	[Negative.]
86	Range of movement	**86**	[Both hips have full range of movement without pain.]
87	Leg lengths	**87**	[Equal; both true and apparent.]
88	Thigh circumference	**88**	[Equal.]

89	Knees	89	[Knees are symmetrical and show no evidence of instability, internal derangement, or inflammatory disease.]
90	Ankles and feet	90	[Flat feet [illegible]]

Neurologic Examination

91	Cranial nerve I	91	[Not tested.]
92	Cranial nerve II	92	[Visual acuity roughly determined by reading newspaper easily.]
93	Cranial nerves III, IV, VI	93	[All eye movements are symmetrical; no double vision.]
94	Cranial nerve V	94	[Normal sensation over forehead, face, and mandibular skin.]
95	Cranial nerve VII	95	[Normal muscle tone and movement of all facial muscles.]
96	Cranial nerve VIII	96	[Apparently normal auditory acuity and symmetrical bone conduction.]
97	Cranial nerve IX	97	[Uvula in midline.]
98	Cranial nerve XI	98	[Symmetrical strength of shoulder shrug.]
99	Cranial nerve XII	99	[Tongue in midline.]
100	Upper limbs	100	[Sensation, power, and reflexes present and normal in both upper limbs.]
101	Sensation	101	[Symmetrical and normal.]

102	Motor system	**102**	[Power and tone of gluteal, quadriceps, and calf muscles are equal and symmetrical.]
103	Reflexes	**103**	[Achilles, patellar, and superficial reflexes present and symmetrical.]
104	Plantar response	**104**	[Down going.]
105	Fasciculations	**105**	[Absent.]
106	Myotonia	**106**	[Absent.]
107	Joint position sense	**107**	[Normal.]
108	Vibration, heat, and cold sensitivity	**108**	[Normal.]
109	Nystagmus	109	[None.]
110	Romberg test	**110**	[Negative.]
111	Eye grounds (ophthalmoscopic examination)	**111**	[Visualization of the eye grounds reveals some broadening of the blood column, the light reflex is widened, and there is a "copper wire" appearance to the vessels. There is evident some arteriovenous compression with deviation of the vein towards 90° at the crossings. The optic discs are normal.]
112	Pupils	**112**	[Pupils equal and round; respond equally to light and accommodation.]

YOU WOULD NOW (CHOOSE ONLY ONE):

113	Take a history if you have not yet done so	**113**	[TURN TO SECTION 7-F, PAGE 77.]

114 Order laboratory tests, special investigations, or x-ray studies if you have not already done so — **114** [TURN TO SECTION 7-J, PAGE [illegible].]

115 Seek consultation if you have not already done so — **115** [TURN TO SECTION [illegible], PAGE [illegible]

116 Initiate definitive treatment — **116** [CONTINUE WITH SECTION [illegible]

SECTION 7-D

YOU WOULD NOW RECOMMEND (CHOOSE ONLY ONE):

117 Nonsurgical management with the patient still in hospital — **117** [TURN TO SECTION 7-K, PAGE 93.]

118 An orthopedic surgical procedure — **118** [TURN TO SECTION 7-H, PAGE 83.]

119 Patient be discharged for home management — **119** [TURN TO SECTION 7-I, PAGE 85.]

SECTION 7-E

YOU WOULD NOW RECOMMEND (CHOOSE ONLY ONE):

120 An uninterrupted period of complete bed rest with pelvic traction to last seven to ten days — **120** [The patient is completely symptomfree during this period. On discharge however, he has a recurrence of symptoms. TURN TO SECTION 7-G, PAGE 83.]

121 Ten days of intensive physical therapy to include any combination of diathermy, massage, exercises, and intermittent traction 121

122 Manipulations of the spine carried out by yourself or the hospital physiatrist 122

SECTION 7-F

IN TAKING THE HISTORY YOU WOULD BE PARTICULARLY INTERESTED TO INQUIRE ABOUT (SELECT AS MANY AS YOU CONSIDER ESPECIALLY PERTINENT; YOU CAN RETURN TO THIS SECTION AT ANY TIME TO OBTAIN ANY ADDITIONAL HISTORICAL INFORMATION YOU MAY REQUIRE):

123 Chief complaint and history of present illness 123

124 Duration of present illness 124

125 Previous similar history 125

126	What increases the symptoms	**126** [illegible]
127	What decreases the symptoms	**127** [illegible] the pain eases if I sit down for a while, or lie down, or if I stop what I am doing and rest for a few minutes. It does not always go away completely. I often have cramps in my thigh and the left side of my back.]
128	Is your bed comfortable	**128** [It has an orthopedic mattress. I was quite uncomfortable in my old bed, which was saggy and I feel that I rest and sleep better in my present bed. I never have had much pain in bed.]
129	Exact location of pain	**129** [Here, (points to left sacroiliac region) and spreads here (left buttock and upper posterior thigh).]
130	Exacerbation of pain with coughing or sneezing	**130** [I don't know; I don't think so.]
131	Changes in appearance of legs or feet	**131** [No; I have a corn which bothers me sometimes.]
132	Numbness	**132** [I get a feeling in my thigh of coldness or crawling in the skin, but it is not really numb.]

133	Prior treatment for this condition	**133**

Past Health and Family History

134	Previous surgery	**134**
135	Serious illnesses and prior hospitalizations	**135**
		136

137	Mother's and father's health	137	[illegible]
138	Brothers and sisters	138	[illegible]

General Systemic Inquiry

139	Changes in weight in the past five years	139	[Only a pound or two in either direction.]
140	Any change in the level of activity and energy in the past few years	140	[Only as related to my [illegible] pain.]
141	Changes in personal habits and work capacity	141	[Really [illegible] I smoke a little more.]

Ear, Nose, and Throat

142	Any change in hearing	142	[None.]
143	Ear infections in the past	143	[Never.]
144	Chronic cough	144	[Smokers cough, worse when I smoke too much.]
145	Head colds and nasal discharge	145	[I get stuff in the back of my throat, don't you call that post-nasal drip?]

146	Sores or ulcers in mouth or tongue	**146**	[I get "cankers" now and then that last a few days; my gums don't bleed.]

Respiratory and Cardiovascular Systems

147	Any change in breathing in recent years	**147**	[Not really; of course, I'm not as energetic as I was 10 years ago.]
148	Any coughing up of blood	**148**	[No.]
149	Shortness of breath	**149**	[No; but this back pain certainly limits me. The chest pain that I told you about before used to be a problem, but is now less of a problem. (Details were given in history of past health.)]
150	Number of pillows for sleeping	**150**	[Two; I seem to sleep better in the last couple of years with two pillows rather than one.]
151	Leg pain	**151**	[Only the pain I was telling you about before in my back and left leg.]
152	Awareness of heart beat or racing	**152**	[Once in a great while.]
153	Leg pain at night	**153**	[No! I feel pretty good at night.]

Gastrointestinal System

154	Digestion	**154**	[Fine; I eat everything I like and have no stomach trouble.]
155	Changes in bowel habits or in size, shape and color of stool	**155**	[There has been no change.]
156	Blood in stools or in vomitus	**156**	[None.]

Genitourinary System

157	Ease of urination	**157**	[No problem.]
158	Difficulty in starting the stream	**158**	[None.]
159	Burning	**159**	[None.]
160	Frequency of urination at night	**160**	[I never have to get up except when I have been drinking a lot the evening before.]
161	Sores or discharge on genitals	**161**	[None.]

Neurologic System

162	Dizziness, headaches, visual disturbances, or changes in gait	**162**	[None.]

YOU WOULD NOW (CHOOSE ONLY ONE):

163	Perform a physical examination if you have not already done so	**163**	[TURN TO SECTION 7-C, PAGE 69.]
164	Order laboratory tests, special investigations and x-rays if you have not yet done so	**164**	[TURN TO SECTION 7-J, PAGE 86.]
165	Seek consultation	**165**	[TURN TO SECTION 7-B, PAGE 64.]
166	Initiate definitive treatment	**166**	[TURN TO SECTION 7-D, PAGE 76.]

SECTION 7-G

167 Record your diagnostic impressions below:

____

____

____

____

____

____

____

____

167 [Subsequent work-up revealed that the patient's complaints were related to obstruction of the internal iliac artery and were in the nature of intermittent claudication. The patient was transferred to the vascular surgeon. The diagnosis was confirmed and definitive treatment was initiated. SEE APPENDIX N FOR ADDITIONAL COMMENT AND RECOMMENDED MANAGEMENT. END OF PROBLEM 7.]

NOW DEVELOP RESPONSE 167 FOR ADDITIONAL INFORMATION AND INSTRUCTIONS

SECTION 7-H

YOU WOULD NOW RECOMMEND (CHOOSE ONLY ONE):

168 Spinal fusion

168 [The surgical procedure was uneventful. The patient's postoperative course was satisfactory and he was discharged home. You later hear that the patient's original pain recurred when the patient returned to his previous level of activity. TURN NOW TO SECTION 7-G, PAGE 83.]

169	Laminectomy and excision of intervertebral disc	**169**	[No evidence of protruded disc found at surgery. The patient's postoperative course was satisfactory and he was discharged home. However, you later hear that the patient's original pain recurred when the patient returned to previous preop level of activity. TURN NOW TO SECTION 7-G, PAGE 83.]
170	Combination of above	**170**	[No evidence of protruded disc found at surgery. The patient's postoperative course was satisfactory and he was discharged home. However, you later hear that the patient's original pain recurred when the patient returned to his previous level of activity. TURN NOW TO SECTION 7-G, PAGE 83.]
171	Exploratory surgical procedure on left hip	**171**	[No pathology found at surgery. The patient's postoperative course was satisfactory and he was discharged home. You later hear that the patient's original pain recurred when the patient returned to his previous level of activity. TURN NOW TO SECTION 7-G, PAGE 83.]
172	Exploratory sacroiliac joint surgery	**172**	[No pathology found at surgery. The patient's postoperative course was satisfactory and he was discharged home. You later hear that the patient's original pain recurred when the patient returned to his previous level of activity. TURN NOW TO SECTION 7-G, PAGE 83.]

173 Injection of disc with a collagenolytic enzyme (assume the Food and Drug Administration has a benign attitude toward this substance at this time)

173 [The procedure was uneventful. The patient's postoperative course was satisfactory and he was discharged home. You later hear that the patient's original pain recurred when the patient returned to his previous level of activity. TURN NOW TO SECTION 7-G, PAGE 83.]

174 Lumbar dorsal root anesthetic block

174 [The patient is discharged home. You later hear that the patient's original pain recurred when he returned to his previous level of activity. TURN NOW TO SECTION 7-G, PAGE 83.]

SECTION 7-I

On returning to his old level of activity, the patient has suffered a recurrence of his original symptoms. He calls you for advice.

YOU WOULD NOW (CHOOSE ONLY ONE):

175 Reassure the patient and advise he be treated with analgesics, and that serious consideration be given to changing his employment and the level of his daily activities

175 [TURN TO SECTION 7-G, PAGE 83.]

176 Readmit the patient to hospital for further diagnostic studies

176 [TURN TO SECTION 7-L, PAGE 94.]

177 Readmit the patient to hospital for an orthopedic surgical procedure

177 [TURN TO SECTION 7-H, PAGE 83.]

178 Readmit the patient for intensive nonsurgical treatment

178 [TURN TO SECTION 7-E, PAGE 76.]

SECTION 7-J

YOU WOULD NOW ORDER THE FOLLOWING DETERMINATIONS (SELECT AS MANY AS YOU CONSIDER INDICATED):

Blood

179	Red blood cell count	**179**	[4,300,000/mm³.]
180	Hemoglobin	**180**	[14.1 g/100 ml.]
181	Hematocrit	**181**	[42%.]
182	White blood cell count	**182**	[7,825/mm³.]
183	Differential	**183**	[neutrophils – 66%, eosinophils – 2%, basophils – 1%, lymphocytes – 26%, monocytes – 5%.]
184	Sedimentation rate	**184**	[5 mm/hour (Wintrobe).]

Urine

185	Specific gravity	**185**	[1.020.]
186	pH	**186**	[6.0.]
187	Protein	**187**	[None.]
188	Sugar	**188**	[None.]
189	Acetone	**189**	[None.]
190	Microscopic	**190**	[A few urate crystals, some epithelial cells and 5 white blood cells/hpf.]

Blood and Serum Studies

191	Sugar (fasting)	**191**	[105 mg/100 ml.]

192	Urea nitrogen	**192**	[12 mg/100 ml.]
193	Nonprotein nitrogen	**193**	[20 mg/100 ml.]
194	Calcium	**194**	[5.0 mEq/L.]
195	Chlorides	**195**	[105 mEq/L.]
196	Potassium	**196**	[4.1 mEq/L.]
197	Sodium	**197**	[142 mEq/L.]
198	Phosphorus	**198**	[1.5 mEq/L.]
199	Carbon dioxide	**199**	[27 mEq/L.]
200	Magnesium	**200**	[1.8 mEq/L.]
201	Creatine	**201**	[0.5 mg/100 ml.]
202	Creatinine	**202**	[0.9 mg/100 ml.]
203	Protein bound iodine	**203**	[5.8 μg/100 ml.]
204	Radioactive iodine (^{131}I) uptake/ 24 hours	**204**	[Uptake – 32%.]
205	Uric acid	**205**	[3.8 mg/100 ml.]
206	Acid phosphatase	**206**	[1.5 units (King-Armstrong).]
207	Alkaline phosphatase	**207**	[16 units (King-Armstrong).]
208	Bilirubin direct	**208**	[0.2 mg/100 ml.]
209	Bilirubin total	**209**	[0.6 mg/100 ml.]
210	Cholesterol	**210**	[520 mg/100 ml.]
211	Thymol turbidity	**211**	[1.0 units.]
212	Albumin	**212**	[3.1 g/100 ml.]

213	Globulin	**213**	[3.4 g/100 ml.]
214	Albumin/globulin ratio	**214**	[1:1.]
215	Amylase	**215**	[92 units/100 ml (Somogyi).]
216	Lipase	**216**	[0.8 ml (Cherry-Crandall).]
217	Adolase	**217**	[3 IU/L.]
218	Serum glutamic oxalacetic transaminase	**218**	[15 IU/L.]
219	Serum glutamic pyruvic transaminase	**219**	[12.5 IU/L.]
220	Creatine phosphokinase	**220**	[25 IU/L.]
221	Lactic dehydrogenase	**221**	[300 units/ml (Wroblewski).]
222	Clotting time	**222**	[8 minutes.]
223	Prothrombin consumption	**223**	[90% consumed in one hour.]
224	Prothrombin time	**224**	[12.0 seconds.]
225	Clot retraction (quantitative)	**225**	[75% (Didisheim).]
226	Serum iron and iron binding capacity	**226**	[Serum iron – 100 μg/100 ml; iron binding capacity – 300 μg/100 ml.]
227	Serum protein electrophoresis	**227**	[Albumin – 50%; $Alpha_1$ globulin – 4%; $Alpha_2$ – 9%; Beta – 12%; Gamma – 25%.]

Special Urine Studies

228	24 hour calcium excretion	**228**	[150 mg/24 hours.]
229	Lead	**229**	[50 μg/24 hours.]

230	Uroporphyrins	230	[5 μg/24 hours.]
231	Porphobilinogen	231	[0.8 mg/24 hours.]
232	Bence-Jones protein	232	[Negative.]
233	Creatine (24 hour)	233	[12 mg/24 hours.]
234	Creatinine (24 hour)	234	[1.1 g/24 hours.]
235	17–OH steroids	235	[7.5 mg/24 hours.]
236	17–Ketosteroids	236	[14.2 mg/24 hours.]

Stool Studies

237	Guaiac (occult blood)	237	[Negative.]
238	Parasite search	238	[Negative.]

Serology

239	STS	239	[Nonreactive.]
240	Fluorescent Treponemal Antibody Absorption test	240	[Nonreactive.]
241	Sheep cell agglutination titer	241	[Zero.]
242	Latex fixation titer	242	[Zero.]
243	C-Reactive protein	243	[Negative.]
244	Hetrophile antibody determination	244	[Negative.]
245	Antistreptolysin titer	245	[Zero.]

Bacteriology

246	Blood culture	246	[Three specimens — no growth.]
247	Sputum culture	247	[No growth.]
248	Sputum for TB	248	[No acid-fast bacilli seen; guinea pig innoculation and cultures started.]
249	24 hour urine for TB	249	[No acid-fast bacilli seen; guinea pig innoculation and cultures started.]

Special Tests and Procedures

250	Basal metabolic rate	250	[+9%.]
251	Electrocardiogram	251	[SEE FIGURE 2, PAGE 405; IF YOU REQUIRE INTERPRETATION OF THIS TRACING, DEVELOP RESPONSE 252 BELOW.]
		252	[ST and T wave abnormalities consistent with myocardial ischemia are noted; normal sinus rhythm.]
253	Electroencephalogram	253	[Normal tracing.]
254	Electromyogram	254	[Studies of gluteal and leg musculature bilaterally are normal with no evidence suggestive of myopathy or denervation.]
255	Nerve conduction time-sciatic nerve	255	[Normal.]
256	Bromsulphalein clearance	256	[3% retention at 45 minutes.]
257	Creatinine clearance	257	[98 cc per minute.]

258 Spinal tap

258 [Pressure 80 mm water; all electrolyte determinations within normal limits; color clear; microscopic shows no cells; Queckenstedt test is positive and normal.]

Radiologic Studies

259 Lumbosacral spine

259 [SEE FIGURES 53 AND 54, PAGE 421. IF YOU REQUIRE INTERPRETATION, DEVELOP RESPONSE 260 BELOW.]

260 [AP and lateral views show some narrowing of L5-S1 disc space and mild degenerative changes, but no evidence of fracture, neoplasm or other pathologic process. The complete lumbar spine was not visualized on these films. Repeat films were requested and showed no additional pathologic process.]

261 Lumbosacral spine-oblique views

261 [SEE FIGURES 55 AND 56, PAGE 421. IF YOU REQUIRE INTERPRETATION, DEVELOP RESPONSE 262 BELOW.]

262 [Oblique views of the lumbosacral spine show no evidence of spondylolisthesis or other congenital defects; both sacroiliac joints are normal.]

263 Cervical spine

263 [Some narrowing and slipping is noted at C5–C6–C7; there is no evidence of subluxation or destruction.]

264 Thoracic spine

264 [Normal thoracic spine.]

265	Skull	**265**	[Normal skull.]
266	Pelvis and both hips	**266**	[The pelvis is normal; the left hip shows mild early degenerative changes, with a little narrowing of the joint space, some sclerosis, and [illegible] normal.]
267	Abdomen, flat film	**267**	[The bowel markings are normal; there is no evidence of free air.]
268	Upper gastrointestinal series	**268**	[Upper gastrointestinal series including esophagus, stomach, and two-hour follow-up films — normal.]
269	Barium enema	**269**	[Barium studies including postevacuation film show a normal colon and sigmoid.]
270	Pneumoencephalogram	**270**	[Refused by patient.]
271	Myelogram	**271**	[Studies of the lumbar area show an essentially normal neural canal without evidence of intra- or extradural abnormalities.]
272	Discogram	**272**	[Studies of L4–L5 and L5–S1 discs are normal; neither disc would accept 1 cc of dye.]
273	Laminogram of lumbosacral spine	**273**	[Study including films at six levels in the AP plane shows no abnormalities.]
274	Left hip arthrogram	**274**	[Study following injection of 2 cc of contrast medium shows a normal joint with no evidence of loose bodies or other abnormalities.]

275	Intravenous pyelogram	**275**	[The kidneys are normal, as are both calyces; the ureters appear normal.]
276	Translumbar aortogram	**276**	[There is complete obliteration of the left internal iliac artery at its origin; the external iliac artery is moderately narrowed.]
277	Bronchogram	**277**	[Studies indicate a normal bronchial tree with no evidence of neoplasm.]

YOU WOULD NOW (CHOOSE ONLY ONE):

278	Take a history if you have not previously done so	**278**	[TURN TO SECTION 7-F, PAGE 77.]
279	Perform a physical examination if you have not previously done so	**279**	[TURN TO SECTION 7-C, PAGE [illegible].]
280	Seek consultation	**280**	[TURN TO SECTION 7-B, PAGE [illegible].]
281	Initiate definitive treatment	**281**	[TURN TO SECTION 7-D, PAGE [illegible].]

SECTION 7-K

YOU WOULD NOW ORDER (SELECT AS MANY AS YOU CONSIDER INDICATED):

282	Bed rest, pelvic traction, and analgesics as required	**282**	[Patient remains completely pain free during this period of treatment which is maintained for four days.]
283	Series of manipulations of the spine, carried out by yourself or the hospital physiatrist	**283**	[Patient remains pain free during this period.]

284	A period of physical therapy in the hospital department of Physical Therapy in the form of exercise and/or diathermy and/or intermittent traction	**284**	[Patient remains pain free during most of these procedures, although on occasion he complains of mild pain similar to his original complaint.]

YOU WOULD NOW (CHOOSE ONLY ONE):

285	Recommend an orthopedic surgical operation	**285**	[TURN TO SECTION 7-H, PAGE 83.]
286	Discharge the patient	**286**	[TURN TO SECTION 7-I, PAGE 85.]
287	Undertake further diagnostic studies	**287**	[CONTINUE WITH SECTION 7-L.]

SECTION 7-L

YOU WOULD NOW ORDER THE FOLLOWING DETERMINATIONS (SELECT AS MANY AS YOU CONSIDER INDICATED):

Blood

288	Red blood cell count	**288**	[4,300,000/mm^3.]
289	Hemoglobin	**289**	[14.1 g/100 ml.]
290	Hematocrit	**290**	[42%.]
291	White blood cell count	**291**	[7,825 per mm^3.]
292	Differential	**292**	[Neutrophils — 66%; eosinophils — 2%; basophils — 1%; lymphocytes — 26%; monocytes — 5%.]
293	Sedimentation rate	**293**	[5 mm/hour (Wintrobe).]

Urine

294	Specific gravity	**294**	[1.020.]
295	pH	**295**	[6.0.]
296	Protein	**296**	[None.]
297	Sugar	**297**	[None.]
298	Acetone	**298**	[None.]
299	Microscopic	**299**	[A few urate crystals, some epithelial cells, and 5 white blood cells/hpf.]

Blood and Serum Studies

300	Sugar (fasting)	**300**	[105 mg/100 ml.]
301	Urea nitrogen	**301**	[12 mg/100 ml.]
302	Nonprotein nitrogen	**302**	[20 mg/100 ml.]
303	Calcium	**303**	[5 mEq/L.]
304	Chlorides	**304**	[105 mEq/L.]
305	Potassium	**305**	[4.1 mEq/L.]
306	Sodium	**306**	[142 mEq/L.]
307	Phosphorus	**307**	[1.5 mEq/L.]
308	Carbon dioxide	**308**	[27 mEq/L.]
309	Magnesium	**309**	[1.8 mEq/L.]
310	Creatine	**310**	[0.5 mg/100 ml.]
311	Creatinine	**311**	[0.9 mg/100 ml.]

312	Protein bound iodine	312	[5.8 μg/100 ml.]
313	Radioactive iodine (^{131}I) uptake/ 24 hours	313	[Uptake → 32%.]
314	Uric acid	314	[3.8 mg/100 ml.]
315	Acid phosphatase	315	[1.5 units (King-Armstrong).]
316	Alkaline phosphatase	316	[16 units (King-Armstrong).]
317	Bilirubin direct	317	[0.2 mg/100 ml.]
318	Bilirubin total	318	[0.6 mg/100 ml.]
319	Cholesterol	319	[520 mg/100 ml.]
320	Thymol turbidity	320	[1.0 units.]
321	Albumin	321	[3.4 g/100 ml.]
322	Globulin	322	[3.4 g/100 ml.]
323	Albumin/globulin ration	323	[1:1.]
324	Amylase	324	[92 units/100 ml (Somogyi).]
325	Lipase	325	[0.8 ml (Cherry-Crandall).]
326	Aldolase	326	[3 IU/L.]
327	Serum glutamic oxalacetic transaminase	327	[15 IU/L.]
328	Serum glutamic pyruvic transaminase	328	[12.5 IU/L.]
329	Creatine phosphokinase	329	[25 IU/L.]
330	Lactic dehydrogenase	330	[300 units/ml (Wroblewski).]
331	Clotting time	331	[8 minutes.]

332 Prothrombin consumption — 332 [90% consumed in one hour.]

333 Prothrombin time — 333 [12.0 seconds.]

334 Clot retraction (quantitative) — 334 [75% (Di[illegible])]

335 Serum iron and iron binding capacity — 335 [Serum iron – [illegible] µg/100 ml; iron binding capacity – [illegible] µg/100 ml.]

336 Serum protein electrophoresis — 336 Albumin – [illegible]; Alpha globulin – 4%; Alpha – 9%; Beta – 12%; Gamma – [illegible]]

Special Urine Studies

337 24 hour calcium excretion — 337 [150 mg/24 hours.]

338 Lead — 338 [50 µg/24 hours.]

339 Uroporphyrins — 339 [5 µg/24 hours.]

340 Porphobilinogen — 340 [0.8 mg/24 hours.]

341 Bence-Jones protein — 341 [Negative.]

342 Creatine (24 hour) — 342 [12 mg/24 hours.]

343 Creatinine (24 hour) — 343 [1.1 g/24 hours.]

344 17–OH steroids — 344 [7.5 mg/24 hours.]

345 17–Ketosteroids — 345 [[illegible] mg/24 hours.]

Stool Studies

346 Guaiac (occult blood) — 346 [Negative.]

347 Parasite search — 347 [Negative.]

Serology

348	STS	**348**	[Nonreactive.]
349	Fluorescent Treponemal Antibody Absorption Test	**349**	[Nonreactive.]
350	Sheep cell agglutination titer	**350**	[Zero.]
351	Latex fixation titer	**351**	[Zero.]
352	C-Reactive protein	**352**	[Negative.]
353	Heterophile antibody determination	**353**	[Negative.]
354	Antistreptolysin titer	**354**	[Zero.]

Bacteriology

355	Blood culture	**355**	[Three specimens -- no growth.]
356	Sputum culture	**356**	[No growth.]
357	Sputum for TB	**357**	[No acid-fast bacilli seen; guinea pig innoculation and cultures started.]
358	24-hour urine for TB	**358**	[No acid-fast bacilli seen; guinea pig innoculation and cultures started.]

Special Tests and Procedures

359	Basal metabolic rate	**359**	[+9%.]
360	Electrocardiogram	**360**	[SEE FIGURE 2, PAGE 405. IF YOU REQUIRE INTERPRETATION OF THIS TRACING, DEVELOP RESPONSE 361 BELOW.]

		361	[ST and T wave abnormalities consistent with myocardial ischemia are noted; normal sinus rhythm.]
362	Electroencephalogram	362	[Normal tracing.]
363	Electromyogram	363	[Studies of gluteal and leg musculature bilaterally normal with no evidence suggestive of myopathy or denervation.]
364	Nerve conduction time-sciatic nerve	364	[Normal.]
365	Bromsulphalein clearance	365	[5% retention at 45 minutes.]
366	Creatinine clearance	366	[98 cc/minute.]
367	Spinal tap	367	[Pressure 80 mm water; all electrolyte determinations within normal limits; color clear, microscopic examination shows no cells; Queckenstedt Test is positive and normal.]

Radiologic Studies

368	Lumbosacral spine	368	[SEE FIGURES 53 AND 54, PAGE 321. IF YOU REQUIRE AN INTERPRETATION, DEVELOP RESPONSE 369 BELOW.]

		369	[AP and lateral views show some narrowing of L5–S1 disc space and mild degenerative changes, but no evidence of fracture, neoplasm or other pathologic process. The complete lumbar spine was not visualized on these [illegible] are re-quired [illegible] no addi-tional pathologic process.]
370	Lumbosacral spine – oblique views	370	[SEE FIGURES [illegible] AND [illegible], PAGE [illegible]. IF YOU REQUIRE AN INTERPRETATION, DEVELOP RESPONSE 371 BELOW.]
		371	[Oblique views of the lumbo-sacral spine show no evidence of spondylolisthesis or other con-genital defects; both sacroiliac joints are normal.]
372	Cervical spine	372	[Some narrowing and slipping is noted at C5–C6 – C7; there is no evidence of subluxation or destruction.]
373	Thoracic spine	373	[Normal thoracic spine.]
374	Skull	374	[Normal skull.]
375	Pelvis and both hips	375	[The pelvis is normal; the left hip shows mild early degenerative changes, with a little narrowing of the joint space, some sclerosis and minimal spurring.]
376	Abdomen, flat film	376	[The bowel markings are normal; there is no evidence of free air.]

Special Radiologic Studies

377	Upper gastrointestinal series	377	
378	Barium enema	378	
379	Pneumoencephalogram	379	
380	Myelogram	380	
381	Discogram	381	
382	Laminogram of lumbosacral spine	382	
383	Left hip arthrogram	383	
384	Intravenous pyelogram	384	
385	Translumbar aortogram	385	

386 Bronchogram

386 [Studies indicate normal bronchial tree, with no evidence of [illegible].]

YOU WOULD NOW REQUEST THE FOLLOWING CONSULTATIONS (SELECT AS MANY AS YOU CONSIDER INDICATED. IF YOU DO NOT WISH TO REQUEST ANY CONSULTATION SKIP 387 TO 402 AND CONTINUE WITH 403 TO 406, PAGE 106):

387 Allergist

387 [illegible] patient's other problems seem more pressing.]

388 Cardiologist

388 [This patient has a history of angina which is well controlled by the [illegible]; his electrocardiogram suggests moderate ischemia; he is not disabled by his symptoms and within reasonable limits, he should continue his work. His age and symptoms together with elevated cholesterol levels suggest generalized arterial disease.]

389 Dermatologist

389 [This patient has no dermatologic complaints other than mild seborrhea. His low back pain does not have the distribution of herpes zoster. Thank you for the consultation.]

390 Endocrinologist

390 [This patient has no apparent hormone imbalance on the basis of the history, physical examination or those investigations which have been done.]

391 Neurosurgeon

391 [This is an unusual problem and may represent an atypical disc syndrome. I would be happy to accept the patient on transfer with the thought that surgical management might be indicated after further investigation. IF YOU WISH TO TRANSFER THE PATIENT, DEVELOP RESPONSE 392 BELOW FOR INSTRUCTIONS. IF YOU DO NOT WISH TO TRANSFER THE PATIENT, SKIP 392 AND SIMPLY CONTINUE WITH THIS SECTION.]

392 [This patient has been transferred to the neurosurgical service and is lost to follow-up. DO NOT MAKE ANY MORE CHOICES IN THIS SECTION; INSTEAD, TURN NOW TO SECTION 7-G, PAGE 83.]

393 Ophthalmologist

393 [This patient has no acute eye problems; funduscopic examination suggests arteriosclerosis; no treatment recommended.]

394 Orthopedic surgeon

394 [This patient may represent one of those unusual situations where the pain is due to a protruding intervertebral disc without nerve root compression. It is interesting to note [illegible] [illegible] his work. I recommend that [illegible] be conservative, but surgery may eventually be required. IF YOU WISH TO TRANSFER THE PATIENT, DEVELOP RESPONSE 395 BELOW FOR INSTRUCTIONS; IF YOU DO NOT WISH TO TRANSFER THE PATIENT SKIP RESPONSE 395 AND SIMPLY CONTINUE WITH THIS SECTION.]

395 [This patient has been transferred to the orthopedic service and is lost to follow-up. DO NOT MAKE ANY MORE CHOICES IN THIS SECTION; INSTEAD TURN NOW TO SECTION 7-G, PAGE 83.]

396 Otolaryngologist

396 [The patient has no serious problem. He has a mild rhinitis with posterior nasal drip, but no other gross abnormalities. His larynx is normal.]

397 Psychiatrist

397 [This patient's symptoms may well be of psychiatric origin; he has marked conflicts in many areas. If you can find no organic explanation for the complaints, then I recommend transfer for psychiatric care. IF YOU WISH TO TRANSFER THE PATIENT, DEVELOP RESPONSE 398 BELOW FOR INSTRUCTIONS; IF YOU DO NOT WISH TO TRANSFER THE PATIENT, SKIP RESPONSE 398 AND SIMPLY CONTINUE WITH THIS SECTION.]

398 [This patient has been transferred to the psychiatric service and is lost to follow-up. DO NOT MAKE ANY MORE CHOICES IN THIS SECTION; INSTEAD TURN NOW TO SECTION 7-G, PAGE 83.]

399 Surgeon (general)

399 [The patient's symptoms are probably not originating in an abdominal viscus. I cannot explain them without further data. There may be a spine disorder, but other possibilities exist.]

400 Urologist

400 [This patient's complaints are probably not originating in the genitourinary system.]

401	Vascular surgeon	**401**	[The patient's complaints are related to obstruction of the [illegible] [illegible] WISH TO TRANSFER THE PATIENT, DEVELOP [illegible] BELOW FOR INSTRUCTIONS. IF YOU DO NOT [illegible] TRANSFER THE PATIENT, SKIP RESPONSE 402 AND SIMPLY CONTINUE WITH THIS SECTION.]
		402	[The patient has been transferred to the care of the vascular surgeon. You hear as a follow-up that the diagnosis has been confirmed and definitive treatment is being initiated. SEE APPENDIX N FOR ADDITIONAL COMMENTS AND RECOMMENDED MANAGEMENT. END OF PROBLEM 7.]

YOU WOULD NOW (CHOOSE ONLY ONE):

403	Discharge the patient	**403**	[Patient's symptoms recur. TURN TO SECTION 7-G, PAGE 83.]
404	Recommend an orthopedic surgical operation	**404**	[TURN TO SECTION 7-H, PAGE 83.]
405	Undertake a program of intensive nonsurgical treatment	**405**	[TURN TO SECTION 7-E, PAGE 76.]

PROBLEM 8

THE PREGNANT DIABETIC

On December 17, one of your patients, a 28-year-old woman whom you have not seen for five months, consults you, her family physician, to care for her first pregnancy. Your file contains a complete history and recent physical. Her menstrual periods have always been somewhat irregular, occurring at intervals of 28 to 40 days. Her last normal menstrual period was July 1.

The patient has diabetes and you have been giving her insulin for eight years. She presently takes 20 units of NPH insulin each morning and eats essentially "what I feel like I want." She checks a random urine sample with Clinitest® once or twice daily, usually late in the afternoon at which time it usually gives a 2 or 3 plus reaction. Her prepregnancy weight was 160 pounds and she is unsure as to whether she has gained any weight since she became pregnant. She wants to have the baby.

Her only complaint is that she sometimes loses urine when she coughs or sneezes. Except as noted above, the past history is unremarkable.

NOW CONTINUE WITH SECTION 8-A

SECTION 8-A

IN PERFORMING THE PHYSICAL EXAMINATION AT THIS VISIT, YOU WOULD BE PARTICULARLY INTERESTED TO CHECK (SELECT AS MANY AS YOU CONSIDER ESPECIALLY PERTINENT; YOU CAN RETURN TO THIS SECTION AT ANY TIME TO OBTAIN ANY ADDITIONAL INFORMATION YOU MAY REQUIRE ABOUT THE INITIAL PHYSICAL FINDINGS):

1	Cullen's sign (periumbilical darkening)	1	[Absent.]
2	Blood pressure	2	[122/75 mm Hg.]

3	Interspinous diameter	3	[Cannot be measured on physical examination.]
4	Auscultation of fetal heart	4	[Present in left lower quadrant at 140/minute.]
5	Uterus	5	[Symmetrically enlarged to two finger breadths above the umbilicus.]
6	Rinne test	6	[Positive bilaterally.]
7	Intertuberous diameter	7	[10.5 cm.]
8	Intercristal diameter	8	[42 cm.]
9	Optic fundi	9	[A few microaneurysms but no hemorrhages or exudates are present.]
10	Height and weight	10	[62 inches, 180 pounds.]
11	Diagonal conjugate	11	[Sacral promontory not reached.]
12	Deep tendon reflexes	12	[Equal and active bilaterally.]
13	Visual field determination	13	[Normal.]
14	Vaginal speculum examination	14	[Cervix bluish — no gross evidence of vaginitis.]
15	Hepatojugular reflux	15	[Not present.]

UNLESS OTHERWISE DIRECTED IN THE RESPONSE COLUMN CONTINUE WITH SECTION 8-B

SECTION 8-B

YOU WOULD NOW ORDER THE FOLLOWING DETERMINATIONS (SELECT AS MANY AS YOU CONSIDER INDICATED):

16	Blood glucose (random sample)	16	[220 mg/100 ml.]
17	Fasting blood glucose	17	[140 mg/100 ml.]
18	Pregnancy test	18	[Positive.]
19	Complete blood count	19	[Hct 38%; WBC 8600/mm^3; differential – normal.]
20	Electrocardiogram	20	[SEE FIGURE 1, PAGE 404.]
21	Indirect Coombs' test	21	[Negative.]
22	Urinary pregnanediol excretion	22	[24.6 mg/24 hours.]
23	Urinalysis and urine culture and sensitivity	23	[Specific gravity 1.022; albumin – negative; glucose 3+; 0-2 wbc/hpf; *E. coli* colony count $<10^4$/ml.]
24	Serologic test for syphilis	24	[Nonreactive.]
25	X-ray pelvimetry	25	[Inlet – 11.5 cm AP; 13 cm transverse. midplane – 12.5 cm AP; 10.8 cm transverse.]
26	Blood group and type	26	[Group A, Rh positive.]
27	Cholesterol	27	[185 mg/100 ml.]
28	Chest x-ray	28	[Lungs clear; heart size normal, hilar nodes not enlarged.]
29	Spectrophotometric analysis of amniotic fluid	29	[Normal curve.]
30	Serum glutamic oxalacetic transaminase	30	[22 IU/L.]
31	Thyroxine (Patee-Murphy)	31	[10.6 µg/100 ml.]

32	Abdominal x-ray for fetal maturity	32 [Skeleton of immature fetus seen.]
33	Ultrasonic determination of fetal head size	33 [Biparietal diameter [illegible] cm.]
34	Quantitative chorionic gonadotropin	34 [20 to [illegible] international rat units/[illegible].]
35	Intravenous pyelogram	35 [Mild hydronephrosis and hydroureter on right.]
36	Blood urea nitrogen	36 [18 mg/100 ml.]

YOU WOULD NOW ADVISE (CHOOSE ONLY ONE):

37	Patient return in four weeks for routine prenatal check-up	37 [TURN NOW TO SECTION 8-D, PAGE 114.]
38	Termination of pregnancy by surgical intervention	38 [The Abortion Committee is convened in accord with the rules of the hospital and your tentative recommendation is disapproved on the ground that medical indications are insufficient to justify termination of this pregnancy. NOW TURN TO SECTION 8-D, PAGE 114.]
39	NPH insulin increased to 25 units daily, keep record of fractional urines and return in two weeks	39 [TURN NOW TO SECTION 8-D, PAGE 114.]
40	Patient be hospitalized	40 [CONTINUE WITH SECTION 8-C, PAGE 111.]
41	1500 calorie diabetic diet, continue present insulin dosage, keep record of fractional urines, and return in one week for re-evaluation	41 [TURN NOW TO SECTION 8-D, PAGE 114.]

42 Therapeutic interruption of pregnancy by intrauterine injection of 50 cc 20% NaCl solution

42 [The Abortion Committee is convened in accord with the rules of the hospital and your tentative recommendation is disapproved on the ground that medical indications are insufficient to justify termination of this pregnancy. NOW TURN TO SECTION 8-D.]

SECTION 8-C

UPON ADMISSION TO THE HOSPITAL YOU WOULD ORDER (SELECT AS MANY AS YOU CONSIDER INDICATED):

43 Creatinine clearance

43 [Within normal limits for midtrimester pregnancy — will serve as baseline for follow-up studies.]

44 Renal scan

44 [No abnormal uptake found.]

45 Renal threshold for glucose

45 [Normal.]

46 Ultrasonic determination of size of fetal head

46 [Biparietal diameter 6 cm.]

47 X-ray determination of size of fetal head

47 [Radiologist suggests using ultrasonic method.]

48 Oxytocin challenge test

48 [Negative.]

YOUR ADMISSION ORDERS WOULD ALSO INCLUDE (CHOOSE ONLY ONE):

49 50 units of regular insulin given intravenously and 50 units in a rapid continuous infusion of of 0.9% saline solution

49 [Two hours after admission patient has a series of convulsions terminated by the intravenous injection of 50% glucose; make another choice from options 49-53.]

50	1500 calorie diabetic diet, NPH insulin 25 units each morning	**50**	[At the end of two weeks the diabetes has not been controlled even after upping insulin and diet. [illegible] MAKE AN-OTHER CHOICE FROM OP-TIONS [illegible].]
51	1500 calorie diabetic diet, NPH insulin 25 units every morning, and supplements of regular insulin four times daily according to urine spill	**51**	[At the end of one week the patient's fasting blood sugar has fallen to 130 mg/100 ml, her insulin requirement has stabilized at 35 units, she has lost approximately 10 pounds, and states that she feels quite well. NOW CONTINUE WITH OPTIONS 54-62.]
52	1500 calorie diabetic diet, NPH insulin 25 units every morning, regular insulin four times daily, plus 24 hour urine for total sugar	**52**	[At the end of one week the patient's fasting blood sugar has fallen to 130 mg/100 ml, her insulin requirement has stabilized at 35 units, she has lost approximately 10 pounds and states that she feels quite well. NOW CONTINUE WITH OPTIONS 54-62.]
53	1500 calorie diet, NPH insulin 25 units every morning, urine four times daily for sugar and acetone, supplements of regular insulin four times daily, according to urine spill, and 24 hour urine for sugar	**53**	[At the end of one week the patient's fasting blood sugar has fallen to 115 mg/100 ml, her insulin requirement has stabilized at 40 units, she has lost approximately 10 pounds and states that she feels quite well. NOW CONTINUE WITH OPTIONS 54-62.]

ON DISCHARGING THE PATIENT YOU WOULD NOW ADVISE (SELECT AS MANY AS YOU CONSIDER INDICATED):

54	Patient return in four weeks for routine prenatal check-up	**54**	[Patient agrees.]

55	Readmission and termination of pregnancy by surgical intervention	55	[The Abortion Committee is convened in accord with the rules of the hospital and your tentative recommendation is disapproved on the ground that medical indications are insufficient to justify termination of this pregnancy.]
56	Patient be offered an abortion	56	[Patient refuses.]
57	Patient continue present insulin dosage, keep records of fractional urines, and return in two weeks	57	[Patient agrees.]
58	1500 calorie diabetic diet, continue present insulin dosage and return in one week for reevaluation	58	[Patient agrees.]
59	Therapeutic interruption of pregnancy by intrauterine injection of 50 cc 20% NaCl solution	59	[The Abortion Committee is convened in accord with the rules of the hospital and your tentative recommendation is disapproved on the ground that medical indications are insufficient to justify termination of this pregnancy.]
60	Weekly urinary estriol determinations	60	[6 mg estriol/24 hours.]
61	Daily urinary estriol determinations	61	[Estriol ranges from 6 to 8 mg/24 hours.]
62	Weekly lecithin/sphingomyelin ratios obtained by amniocentesis	62	[1:1 L/S ratio reported on initial amniotic fluid sample.]

UNLESS OTHERWISE DIRECTED IN THE RESPONSE COLUMN CONTINUE WITH SECTION 8-D

SECTION 8-D

At her next visit a cytologic smear, taken from the cervix by the nurse at the time of the initial visit, is reported as Class III (Papanicolaou system). In addition, the cytologist comments that the atypical cells are squamous in nature and are accompanied by inflammatory cells. You are asked to repeat the test immediately. A subsequent report confirms Class III.

YOU WOULD NOW (CHOOSE ONLY ONE EACH TIME YOU ARE DIRECTED TO THIS SECTION):

63	Take a punch biopsy of the cervix directed by Schiller test	**63**	[SEE FIGURE 20, PAGE 413 AND THEN MAKE AN ADDITIONAL CHOICE IN THIS SECTION.]
64	Perform a total abdominal hysterectomy	**64**	[The Abortion Committee is convened in accord with the rules of the hospital. On the basis of the pathologist's report following cold knife conization of the cervix requested by Committee (SEE FIGURE 20, PAGE 413) your tentative recommendation is disapproved on the ground that medical indications are insufficient to justify proposed surgery. TURN NOW TO SECTION 8-F, PAGE 116.]
65	Do nothing further at this time, continue with regular office visits, and plan to reassess after delivery	**65**	[TURN NOW TO SECTION 8-F, PAGE 116.]
66	Perform a cold knife conization of the cervix	**66**	[Done. SEE FIGURE 20, PAGE 413 AND THEN CONTINUE WITH SECTION 8-E, PAGE 115.]
67	Perform a colposcopy and if squamocolumnar junction is well visualized, take biopsies of any suspicious area(s)	**67**	[Done. Colposcopically directed biopsies taken (SEE FIGURE 20, PAGE 413) — MAKE AN ADDITIONAL CHOICE IN THIS SECTION.]

SECTION 8-E

YOU WOULD NOW (CHOOSE ONLY ONE):

68	Terminate the pregnancy by abdominal hysterectomy and treat with external radiation and radium	**68**	[In discussing the case with chief of service, he feels that this is unwarranted treatment in this instance and refers case to Tumor Board which concurs with chief's recommendation. CONTINUE WITH SECTION 8-F, PAGE 116.]
69	Place radium against the cervix and plan to deliver the patient by cesarean section in four to six weeks	**69**	[On review of the pathologist's report, the radiologist advises that this course of action is contraindicated. The case is referred to the Tumor Board which concurs in the radiologist's recommendation. CONTINUE WITH SECTION 8-F, PAGE 116.]
70	Advise the patient that there is a change taking place in her cervix and that she should have routine Pap smears every six months	**70**	[CONTINUE WITH SECTION 8-F, PAGE 116.]
71	Begin external radiation therapy and subsequently insert radium	**71**	[On review of the pathologist's report, the radiologist advises that this course of action is contraindicated. The case is referred to the Tumor Board which concurs in the radiologist's recommendation, CONTINUE WITH SECTION 8-F, PAGE 116.]
72	Perform a radical abdominal hysterectomy (Wertheim) and pelvic lymphadenectomy	**72**	[In discussing the case with chief of service, he feels that this is unwarranted treatment in this instance and refers the case to Tumor Board which concurs with chief's recommendation. CONTINUE WITH SECTION 8-F, PAGE 116.]

73	Perform an abdominal total hysterectomy with ovarian conservation	**73**	[In discussing the case with chief of service, he feels that this is unwarranted treatment in this instance and refers case to Tumor Board which concurs with chief's recommendation. CONTINUE WITH SECTION 8-F, PAGE 116.]
74	Do nothing further at this time but advise the patient that she should have a vaginal hysterectomy six weeks postpartum	**74**	[CONTINUE WITH SECTION 8-F, PAGE 116.]
75	Administer Methotrexate 20 mg daily in five day courses until chorionic gonadotropin titer in urine is negative	**75**	[On February 10, patient goes into spontaneous labor and delivers 1000 g stillborn infant. The patient develops palatal ulceration, purpura and her white blood cell count is now 1300/ mm^3. TURN NOW TO SECTION 8-M, PAGE 128.]

SECTION 8-F

THE PATIENT IS SEEN IN THE OFFICE VISITS AT WEEKLY INTERVALS. AT ALL OF THESE PRENATAL VISITS YOU WOULD CHECK OR ORDER (SELECT AS MANY AS YOU CONSIDER INDICATED AT EACH VISIT):

76	Hematocrit	**76**	[Ranges from 35% to 38%.]
77	X-ray pelvimetry	**77**	[Inlet — 11.5 cm AP; 13 cm transverse; midplane — 12.5 cm AP; 10.8 cm transverse.]
78	Determination of weight and blood pressure	**78**	[Weight constant at 170 pounds; blood pressure at 110-120/70-80 mm Hg.]
79	Urinalysis	**79**	[Negative for protein; ranges from 0 to 2+ for sugar.]

80	Additional supplies of iron and vitamins	80	[Given.]
81	Serum cholesterol	81	[175 mg/100 ml.]
82	Abdominal palpation	82	[Uterus progressively enlarges.]
83	Review of home urine sugar chart	83	[Ranges from 0 to 2+ with positive findings usually during 6 and 10 p.m. tests.]
84	Fasting blood sugar	84	[Ranges from 80 to 120 mg/100 ml.]
85	Examination for presence of edema	85	[None present.]
86	Examination of eyegrounds	86	[Unchanged.]
87	Serum uric acid	87	[Ranges from 3.0 to 6.0 mg/100 ml.]
88	Serum electrolytes	88	[Na — 140 mEq/L; Cl — 96 mEq/L; K — 5 mEq/L.]
89	Vaginal smear for cornification	89	[20-25% cornified cells, 65-75% intermediate cells, 0-10% basal cells.]
90	Serum iron determination	90	[125-137 μg/100 ml.]
91	Hydroxyprogesterone caproate (Delalutin) 250 mg intramuscularly every two weeks until third trimester	91	[Given.]
92	Diethylstilbestrol given intramuscularly	92	[The clinical pharmacist points out a recent FDA warning about the possible delayed carcinogenic effect of this substance on female offspring.]

UNLESS OTHERWISE DIRECTED IN THE RESPONSE COLUMN CONTINUE WITH SECTION 8-G

SECTION 8-G

At a prenatal visit on March 1, you elect to readmit patient to OB ward for inpatient chronic fetal surveillance.

YOU WOULD NOW (SELECT AS MANY AS YOU CONSIDER INDICATED):

93 Ask the patient about fetal movements

93 [Felt some yesterday but none today.]

94 Terminate the pregnancy by abdominal hysterectomy

94 [At surgery, 1900 g infant is delivered. He is immediately placed in premature intensive care unit, but becomes apneic and expires six hours later. IGNORE INSTRUCTIONS AT END OF THIS SECTION; INSTEAD TURN NOW TO SECTION 8-N, PAGE 129.]

95 Order oxytocin challenge test weekly

95 [Negative results noted on strip chart recorder.]

96 Order estriol daily

96 [With daily variation of less than 25% there was a progressive rise from 16 to 28 mg/24 hours over the next four weeks.]

97 Induce labor with intramuscular Syntocinon

97 [Over next six hours labor supervenes with birth of 1900 g infant. He is immediately placed in premature intensive care unit, but becomes apneic and expires six hours later. IGNORE INSTRUCTIONS AT END OF THIS SECTION; INSTEAD TURN NOW TO SECTION 8-N, PAGE 129.]

98 Obtain B-scan ultrasound for fetal biparietal diameter approximately every week till delivery

98 [B scan biparietal diameter on admission to hospital was 8.4 cm.]

99	Obtain B-scan for placental localization	**99**	[Placenta noted to be anterior and fundal.]
100	Obtain serum fibrinogen	**100**	[575 mg/100 ml.]
101	Obtain abdominal x-ray	**101**	[Spalding's sign not present.]
102	Order bed rest and limited activity	**102**	[Order noted.]
103	Obtain Lee-White clotting time	**103**	[5 minutes, 30 seconds.]
104	Perform tourniquet test	**104**	[Negative.]
105	Obtain pregnancy test	**105**	[Positive.]
106	Order creatinine clearance	**106**	[No signs of renal function deterioration relative to previous baseline studies.]
107	Perform intrauterine transfusion with group O, Rh negative packed cells	**107**	[Pediatrician and obstetrician decline to perform this procedure without any indication of Rh *incompatibility*.]
108	Perform weekly amniocentesis for lecithin/sphingomyelin ratio and creatinine concentration	**108**	[Order noted.]

UNLESS OTHERWISE DIRECTED IN THE RESPONSE COLUMN CONTINUE WITH SECTION 8-H

SECTION 8-H

The patient has been in hospital for four weeks. On April 1, the patient's status is as follows: diabetes is under good control; blood pressure is 120/76 mm Hg, weight 180 pounds, no edema, uterine fundus 31 cm above symphysis (four fingerbreadths below xiphoid), lie uncertain, fetal heart sounds heard in right lower quadrant at 140 per minute. You are uncertain as to fetal size because of maternal obesity.

YOU CONSIDER THE FOLLOWING ADVISABLE AT THIS STAGE (SELECT AS MANY AS YOU CONSIDER INDICATED):

109	Estimated fetal weight	**109**	[Between 2800 and 3200 g.]
110	X-ray pelvimetry	**110**	[Inlet — 11.5 cm AP, 13 cm transverse; midplane — 12.5 cm AP, 10.9 cm transverse.]
111	Urinary pregnanediol excretion	**111**	[48.6 mg per 24 hours.]
112	Pregnancy test	**112**	[Positive.]
113	Abdominal x-ray	**113**	[SEE FIGURE 50, PAGE 420.]
114	Glucose tolerance test (100 g glucose orally)	**114**	[Fasting — 110 mg/100 ml; 1/2 hour — 180 mg/100 ml; 1 hour — 200 mg/100 ml; 2 hour — 180 mg/100 ml.]
115	Serum oxytocinase determination	**115**	[12 units/ml.]
116	Spectrophotometric analysis of amniotic fluid	**116**	[Optical density 0.12 at 450 nm.]
117	Amniocentesis for L/S ratio and amniotic fluid creatinine concentration	**117**	[L/S ratio 3; amniotic fluid creatinine concentration, 2.5 mg%.]
118	Vaginal examination for evaluation of cervix	**118**	[Os dilated 1 cm; cervix partially effaced and fixed in posterior position.]
119	Ultrasonic determination of fetal position and biparietal diameter	**119**	[Cephalic presentation — biparietal diameter of fetal head, 10.4 cm.]
120	Measure abdominal girth	**120**	[104 cm.]
121	Radioisotopic localization of placenta	**121**	[Placenta high in fundus and anterior.]

122	Enovid 10 mg daily, given orally for three days	**122**	[Given.]

BASED ON THE ABOVE INFORMATION YOU WOULD NOW (CHOOSE ONLY ONE):

123	Await spontaneous onset of labor	**123**	[On April 25, patient goes into spontaneous labor and gives birth to 3.2 kg macerated stillborn infant. TURN NOW TO SECTION 8-O, PAGE 129.]
124	Perform low cervical cesarean section under continuous epidural anesthesia	**124**	[Done. CONTINUE WITH SECTION 8-I, PAGE 122.]
125	Induce labor with intrauterine injection of hypertonic saline	**125**	[Over next 72 hours labor supervenes with birth of 3.0 kg macerated stillborn infant. TURN NOW TO SECTION 8-O, PAGE 129.]
126	Perform internal podalic version and extraction under spinal anesthesia	**126**	[This obstetrical maneuver results in breech extraction of a markedly depressed 3.0 kg male. At one minute, the Apgar score is 3; despite appropriate resuscitative attempts (including endotracheal intubation) the Apgar at 5 minutes is only 6. Baby expires on 2nd day; autopsy findings confirm massive cerebral hemorrhage. TURN NOW TO SECTION 8-P, PAGE 129.]
127	Perform classical cesarean section under local anesthesia	**127**	[CONTINUE WITH SECTION 8-I, PAGE 122.]
128	Reexamine in one week and induce with oxytocin if the cervix has ripened	**128**	[On April 7, patient goes into spontaneous labor and gives birth to 3.0 kg macerated stillborn infant. TURN NOW TO SECTION 8-O, PAGE 129.]

129 Call in obstetrical consultant **129** [Consultant induces labor by amniotomy and dilute intravenous oxytocin, utilizes continuous epidural anesthesia throughout the active phase of labor, provides for electronic surveillance of fetal heart rate and uterine activity throughout labor and delivery, and orders fetal scalp blood sample(s) for pH as a complementary test indicating possible hypoxemia. NOW CONTINUE WITH SECTION 8-I, PAGE 122.]

SECTION 8-I

After delivery the infant has a one minute Apgar score of 5. Resuscitation with only mask and bag ventilation is instituted with adequate response of vital signs. At five minutes, the Apgar score is 7. After seven minutes, the infant cries lustily. At this time, his heart rate is 150 per minute; breath sounds are heard throughout both lung fields. The liver is 3 cm below the right costal margin. No other masses are felt. Silver nitrate solution is placed in both eyes.

His birth weight was 3.0 kg; his length 48 cm. Blood was obtained from the placental vessels and saved for the pediatrician. Three blood vessels are seen in the umbilical cord and this information is recorded on the chart.

YOU RECOMMEND THAT THE INFANT NOW BE ADMITTED TO (CHOOSE ONLY ONE):

130 Regular Nursery **130** [Transferred to pediatric Intensive Care Unit at one hour of age.]

131 Pediatric Intensive Care Unit **131** [Placed in heated incubator.]

132 Pediatric Infant's Ward **132** [Placed in heated incubator.]

YOU WOULD ORDER IMMEDIATELY (SELECT AS MANY AS YOU CONSIDER INDICATED):

133	Incubator heated to 85F	**133**	[Infant's temperature remains at 94F.]
134	Oxygen, not to exceed 40% concentration	**134**	[Given.]
135	15 cc dextrose in water every three hours for four feedings, then formula	**135**	[Infant gags and vomits.]
136	Nothing by mouth	**136**	[Ordered.]
137	As infant's condition stabilizes initiate feedings with 10% glucose in H_2O at approximately three hours of age	**137**	[Done.]
138	Portable x-ray of chest	**138**	[Heart moderately enlarged with mild reticulogranular pattern to lung fields.]
139	Complete blood count	**139**	[Hgb — 20.5 g/100 ml.; WBC total — 12,000/mm^3. Differential: polys — 62%, lymphs — 30%, monos — 8% nucleated RBC's are seen.]
140	Cord blood sent for carbon dioxide, chloride, sodium, and magnesium determinations	**140**	[Na — 140 mEq/L; Cl — 100 mEq/L; Mg — to be done; CO_2 — 17 mEq/L.]
141	Electrocardiogram	**141**	[Right axis deviation, mild right-sided hypertrophy.]
142	Warmed (heel-stick) blood for gases and acid-based parameters	**142**	[Results: pH — 7.26, Pco_2 — 50 mm Hg, Base excess — 9 mEq/L, Po_2 — 40 mm Hg.]
143	Urinalysis	**143**	[The infant is anuric for 24 hours.]

144	Procaine penicillin G 60,000 μ and streptomycin 50 mg every 12 hours	**144**	[Given.]
145	Serum bilirubin level	**145**	[2.5 mg/100 ml.]
146	Electroencephalogram	**146**	[Mostly 2-4 cycles per second activity in all leads; not abnormal for patient's age.]
147	Vital signs every 30 minutes	**147**	[Respirations 65/minute at one hour; 70/minute at two hours; 60/minute at three hours; heart rate 130-150/minute.]
148	Lumbar puncture	**148**	[Bloody tap after two tries.]
149	Procaine penicillin G 60,000 μ and kanamycin 15 mg every 12 hours	**149**	[Given.]
150	Blood culture	**150**	[No growth at 48 hours.]
151	Skull x-ray	**151**	[Within normal limits.]
152	Blood sent for calcium, glucose, blood urea nitrogen, and sodium determinations	**152**	[Ca – 4.2 mEq/L; Glucose – 35 mg/100 ml; BUN – 9 mg/100 ml; Na – 140 mEq/L.]
153	Infant placed on critical list	**153**	[Done and proper authorities notified.]

UNLESS OTHERWISE DIRECTED IN THE RESPONSE COLUMN CONTINUE WITH SECTION 8-J

SECTION 8-J

Over the next three hours, the infant's respirations increase to 80 per minute, an expiratory grunt is audible, cyanosis is apparent in spite of administration of 60% O_2. Intercostal and subcostal retractions are moderate with flaring of the nasal alae. The arterial blood gas and pH studies suggest acidosis.

YOUR THERAPEUTIC ORDERS AT THIS STAGE INCLUDE (SELECT AS MANY AS YOU CONSIDER INDICATED):

154	THAM buffer stat	**154**	[Infant becomes apneic and dies. IGNORE INSTRUCTIONS AT END OF THIS SECTION; INSTEAD TURN NOW TO SECTION 8-Q, PAGE 130.]
155	Repeat blood gases stat	**155**	[With infant breathing 80% O_2: pH — 7.23, P_{CO_2} — 50 mm Hg, Base excess — 12 mEq/L, P_{O_2} — 35 mm Hg.]
156	Intravenous glucose, saline, and sodium lactate	**156**	[Given; condition deteriorates.]
157	Repeat glucose stat	**157**	[Glucose 25 mg/100 ml.]
158	Digitalize – with 1/2 total dose, stat	**158**	[Given, no change in condition.]
159	Intravenous glucose (20%) 120-150 cc per kilo, per 24 hours	**159**	[Edema, heart failure, and death in 48 hours. IGNORE INSTRUCTIONS AT END OF THIS SECTION; INSTEAD TURN NOW TO SECTION 8-Q, PAGE 130.]
160	Repeat stat portable chest film with bilateral air bronchograms	**160**	[Poor aeration of lungs.]
161	Intravenous 10% glucose 65 cc per kilo, per 24 hours	**161**	[Given, some improvement.]
162	Continuous positive airway pressure breathing (CPAP)	**162**	[Initiated with infant status reflecting improvement in respiratory distress syndrome.]
163	Oxygen 100%	**163**	[Given.]
164	Intravenous $NaHCO_3$ administered in doses of 2 to 3 mEq per kg	**164**	[Given by slow push. No marked change in condition.]
165	Oxygen not to exceed 40%	**165**	[Infant still cyanotic.]

166 Oxygen, in concentrations necessary to prevent cyanosis — 166 [Given.]

UNLESS OTHERWISE DIRECTED IN THE RESPONSE COLUMN CONTINUE WITH SECTION 8-K

SECTION 8-K

Therapy is modified as required and the infant improves slowly over the next two to three days. After 72 hours, he is taking formula well. At age 36 hours he is noted to be jaundiced and the icterus increases.

IN YOUR WORK-UP AND TREATMENT OF THE INFANT OVER THE NEXT 48 HOURS YOUR ORDERS WOULD INCLUDE (SELECT AS MANY AS YOU CONSIDER INDICATED):

167 Blood type of baby and mother — **167** [Baby — Type O, Rh+; mother — Type A, Rh+.]

168 Coombs' test — **168** [Negative.]

169 Blood culture — **169** [No growth.]

170 Transfusion of whole blood — **170** [Develops fever.]

171 Urinalysis — **171** [pH — 6.0, albumin — 1+, sugar — trace, acetone — negative.]

172 Red cell assay for galactose-1-phosphate uridyl transferase — **172** [Normal.]

173 Bilirubin levels every 12 hours — **173**

Hours	Total mg/100 ml	Indirect mg/100 ml
36	12.0	11.0
48	16.0	13.0
60	18.0	16.0
72	17.0	14.0

174	Exchange transfusion	**174**	[Infant has apnea and cardiac arrest after 200 ml of blood has been exchanged. IGNORE INSTRUCTIONS AT END OF THIS SECTION. INSTEAD TURN NOW TO SECTION 8-[illegible], PAGE 1[illegible]0.]
175	Phototherapy	**175**	[Bilirubin continues to drop. Child's icterus improves.]
176	Phenobarbital 7 1/2 mg twice a day	**176**	[Bilirubin continues to drop. Child's icterus improves.]
177	Complete blood count	**177**	[Hb — [illegible] g/100 ml; WBC — 8200/mm³; differential: Polys 52%, lymphs — 44%, monos — 4%.]
178	Intravenous pyelogram	**178**	[Within normal limits.]
179	Intravenous administration of sodium glucuronide	**179**	[Given.]
180	Stool guaiac	**180**	[Negative.]

UNLESS OTHERWISE DIRECTED IN THE RESPONSE COLUMN CONTINUE NOW WITH SECTION 8-L

SECTION 8-L

After 7 days of age the infant appears to be doing well and is discharged after a blood sample is obtained for a phenylalanine level determination. The blood phenylalanine value was 3.2 mg/100 ml.

At 14 days of age, the infant is brought to the Emergency Room with bilateral purulent conjunctivitis, the pus is creamy yellow, and eyes are swollen and red.

IN VIEW OF THE HISTORY AND PREVIOUS THERAPY, THIS EYE PROBLEM COULD BE DUE TO (CHOOSE ONE OR MORE):

181 *Staphylococcus aureus*

181 [The diagnosis was made by a smear and culture of the pus. The conjunctivitis responded to specific therapy.]

182 Gonococcus

182 [Culture from the lesion failed to demonstrate gonococci.]

183 *E. Coli*

183 [The diagnosis was made by a smear and culture of the pus. The conjunctivitis responded to specific therapy.]

184 Silver nitrate

184 [The diagnosis was subsequently made by a smear and culture of the pus. The conjunctivius responded to specific therapy.]

185 A virus

185 [The diagnosis was made by a smear and culture of the pus on blood agar. The conjunctivitis responded to specific therapy.]

UNLESS OTHERWISE DIRECTED IN THE RESPONSE COLUMN TURN TO SECTION 8-R WHEN YOU HAVE COMPLETED THIS SECTION

SECTION 8-M

186 Record cause of death in the space below:

____

____

____

____

____

____

186 [Autopsy revealed a premature, somewhat jaundiced infant with early hepatocellular destruction and multiple gastrointestinal ulcerations and hemorrhage. The placenta had many hemorrhagic areas with little inflammation. See Appendix G for additional comment and recommended management. END OF PROBLEM 8.]

NOW DEVELOP RESPONSE 186 OPPOSITE FOR ADDITIONAL INFORMATION AND INSTRUCTIONS

SECTION 8-N

187 Record cause of death in the space provided below:

____

187 [Autopsy showed a premature infant with bilateral pneumonitis, pulmonary microemboli, and partial atelectasis bilaterally. See Appendix G for additional comment and recommended management. END OF PROBLEM 8.]

NOW DEVELOP RESPONSE 187 OPPOSITE FOR ADDITIONAL INFORMATION AND INSTRUCTIONS

SECTION 8-0

188 Record cause of death in the space provided below:

____

188 [Autopsy showed a macerated full term infant, the skin was meconium stained; small intracerebral hemorrhagic ulcerations of the small and large bowel and stomach were present. Focal hemorrhages of both kidneys and adrenal cortex were also found. See Appendix G for additional comment and recommended management. END OF PROBLEM 8.]

NOW DEVELOP RESPONSE 188 OPPOSITE FOR ADDITIONAL INFORMATION AND INSTRUCTIONS

SECTION 8-P

189 Record cause of death in the space below:

____

189 [Autopsy showed a massive intracerebral and subdural hemorrhage. See Appendix G for additional comment and recommended management. END OF PROBLEM 8.]

NOW DEVELOP RESPONSE 189 OPPOSITE FOR ADDITIONAL INFORMATION AND INSTRUCTIONS

SECTION 8-Q

190 Record cause of death in the space below:

____

____

____

190 [The chart showed cause of death to be hyaline membrane disease. See Appendix G for additional comment and recommended management. END OF PROBLEM 8.]

NOW DEVELOP RESPONSE 190 OPPOSITE FOR ADDITIONAL INFORMATION AND INSTRUCTIONS

SECTION 8-R

191 Record your diagnostic impressions in the space below:

____

____

____

____

191 [Culture from the pus revealed *Staphylococcus aureus* coagulase positive, sensitive to penicillin and chloromycetin. See Appendix G for additional comment and recommended management. END OF PROBLEM 8.]

NOW DEVELOP RESPONSE 191 OPPOSITE FOR ADDITIONAL INFORMATION AND INSTRUCTIONS

PROBLEM 9

THE UNRELIABLE PATIENT, SHORT OF BREATH

You are called to the Emergency Room at 1:30 A.M. to see a 66-year-old saleswoman brought there by a cab driver because of her acute shortness of breath. She is moderately obese, cyanotic, and sitting on the edge of the bed with markedly labored respirations. Coarse bubbling rales are easily audible without a stethoscope. The patient is so acutely ill you have difficulty obtaining the history.

NOW CONTINUE WITH SECTION 9-A

SECTION 9-A

BEFORE INITIATING THERAPY YOU WOULD (SELECT AS MANY AS YOU CONSIDER AS ESPECIALLY PERTINENT):

1	Inquire into family history of allergy	1	[Mother had hay fever.]
2	Inquire into precipitating factors of this episode	2	[No unusual activities.]
3	Obtain history of medication	3	[Has been taking small white pills, nature unknown.]
4	Obtain information about cardiac background	4	[Gradually increasing dyspnea; no known hypertension.]
5	Inquire into allergic history	5	[Allergy to ragweed, no asthma.]

6	Determine patient's emotional status	6	[Patient extremely apprehensive and restless.]
7	Inquire about presence of chest pain	7	[No pain with this episode.]
8	Determine history of hemoptysis	8	[Never coughed up blood.]
9	Inquire into history of night sweats	9	[No night sweats.]
10	Determine history of similar episodes	10	[Three milder episodes during past two weeks.]
11	Determine blood pressure, pulse, respirations and temperature	11	[Blood pressure — 138/90 mm Hg; pulse — 116 per minute; respirations — 32 per minute; temperature 98.6F (oral).]
12	Examine neck	12	[No neck vein distension.]
13	Examine the chest	13	[Chest barrel-shaped; coarse bubbling rales heard at both bases up to scapulae; prolonged expiratory phase.]
14	Perform complete neurologic examination	14	[No abnormalities detected.]
15	Examine the heart	15	[Point of maximum impulse 3 cm lateral to midclavicular line; heart tones obscured by presence of rales.]
16	Dilate pupils and examine optic fundi	16	[Moderate increase in light reflex
17	Examine for adenopathy	17	[No significant lymphadenopathy
18	Perform auscultation of the abdomen	18	[Unsatisfactory examination; patient unable to lie flat.]
19	Examine extremities	19	[Nail beds cyanotic; no clubbing or edema.]

20	Perform Rinne test of auditory function	20	[Air conduction twice that of bone conduction.]

UNLESS OTHERWISE DIRECTED IN THE RESPONSE COLUMN CONTINUE WITH SECTION 9-B

SECTION 9-B

HAVING COMPLETED THE PRELIMINARY HISTORY AND PHYSICAL EXAMINATION YOU WOULD NOW (SELECT AS MANY AS YOU CONSIDER INDICATED):

21	Arrange return appointment in one week and defer treatment until drug history is known	21	[Patient collapses at hospital door and expires 10 minutes later. DO NOT MAKE ANY MORE CHOICES IN THIS SECTION: TURN NOW TO SECTION 9-H, PAGE 140.]
22	Order oxygen	22	[Oxygen mask applied.]
23	Perform phlebotomy	23	[500 cc blood removed.]
24	Apply tourniquets	24	[Rotating tourniquets applied.]
25	Administer morphine sulfate 15 mg subcutaneously	25	[Given.]
26	Administer 0.4 cc of 1:1000 aqueous adrenalin hydrochloride subcutaneously	26	[Patient's condition deteriorates. DO NOT MAKE ANY MORE CHOICES IN THIS SECTION; TURN NOW TO SECTION 9-H, PAGE 140.]
27	Administer 0.8 mg digitoxin intravenously	27	[Medication given.]
28	Administer 0.8 mg lanatoside C (Cedilanid) intravenously	28	[Medication given.]
29	Administer 600,000 units of procaine penicillin G intramuscularly	29	[Medication given; no change in patient's condition.]

30	Administer 200 cc of 3% sodium chloride intravenously	30	[Condition of patient deteriorates: DO NOT MAKE ANY MORE CHOICES IN THIS SECTION; TURN NOW TO SECTION 9-H, PAGE 140.]
31	Administer 0.5 g aminophyllin intravenously	31	[Medication given.]
32	Administer furosemide 40 mg intravenously	32	[Medication given.]
33	Order electrocardiogram	33	[SEE FIGURE 3, PAGE 406 for TRACING MADE TWO HOURS AFTER ADMISSION.]

UNLESS OTHERWISE DIRECTED IN THE RESPONSE COLUMN CONTINUE WITH SECTION 9-C

SECTION 9-C

The patient is moved to a hospital room. You see her there six hours later and she is more comfortable, no longer cyanotic.

TO COMPLETE YOUR EVALUATION YOU WOULD NOW (SELECT AS MANY AS YOU CONSIDER AS ESPECIALLY PERTINENT):

34	Inquire about previous electrocardiograms	34	[Electrocardiogram reported to have been "normal" one year ago.]
35	Obtain family history	35	[Mother had diabetes, controlled by diet.]
36	Perform ophthalmoscopic examination	36	[Moderate increase in light reflex.]
37	Perform auscultation of the lungs	37	[Rales now heard only at the right base.]
38	Examine the heart	38	[Heart sounds distant and regular; no murmur detected.]

39	Examine the abdomen	39	[Liver edge at right costal margin on inspiration.]
40	Determine blood pressure, pulse, respirations and temperature	40	[Blood pressure – 120/80 mm Hg; pulse – 80 per minute, regular, respirations – 18 per minute; temperature – 98.8F (oral).]
41	Digitalize the patient	41	[Done.]
42	Advise that the patient may walk	42	[Patient too weak to walk.]
43	Seek history of angina pectoris	43	[Present for six months; no recent change in pattern of pain.]

UNLESS OTHERWISE DIRECTED IN THE RESPONSE COLUMN CONTINUE WITH SECTION 9-D

SECTION 9-D

IN ADDITION YOU WOULD NOW ORDER THE FOLLOWING DETERMINATIONS (SELECT AS MANY AS YOU CONSIDER INDICATED):

44	No further laboratory evaluation at this time	44	[DO NOT MAKE ANY MORE CHOICES IN THIS SECTION; TURN NOW TO SECTION 9-E, PAGE 136.]
45	Serum glutamic oxalacetic transaminase determinations daily for three days	45	[38 IU/L on Day 1, 42 IU/L on Day 2, 50 IU/L on Day 3.]
46	Master's two-step test	46	[Patient unable to perform the test.]
47	Basal metabolism	47	[+ 15%; + 25%.]
48	Serum cholesterol	48	[240 mg/100 ml.]
49	Upper gastrointestinal tract series	49	[Patient too weak for adequate examination.]

50	Serum sodium, potassium, chloride	50	[Na – 140 mEq/L; K – 4.0 mEq/L; Cl – 98 mEq/L.]
51	Sputum culture	51	[Normal flora.]
52	Stool for blood	52	[Negative.]
53	Nasal smear for eosinophils	53	[Normal smear, no eosinophils.]
54	Two-hour postprandial blood sugar	54	[110 mg/100 ml.]
55	Marrow puncture, stain for iron pigment	55	[Normal smear without excess iron pigment.]
56	Chest x-ray	56	[SEE FIGURE 42, PAGE 418.]
57	Circulation time (arm to tongue)	57	[22 seconds.]
58	Electrocardiogram	58	[SEE FIGURE 6, PAGE 406.]
59	Scratch skin testing for allergens	59	[Positive for ragweed, alternaria, and tomatoes.]

UNLESS OTHERWISE DIRECTED IN THE RESPONSE COLUMN CONTINUE WITH SECTION 9-E

SECTION 9-E

The patient has now recovered from the acute episode and you have arrived at a definite diagnosis.

IN ADDITION TO PERIODIC VISITS AT YOUR OFFICE YOUR LONG-TERM MANAGEMENT OF THE PATIENT WOULD NOW INCLUDE (SELECT AS MANY AS YOU CONSIDER INDICATED):

60	400 mg sodium diet	60	[Diet discussed with patient.]
61	2000 mg sodium diet	61	[Diet discussed with patient.]
62	No dietary restriction	62	[Patient so informed.]
63	Continuation of digitalis	63	[Program outlined to patient.]

64	Discontinuation of digitalis	**64**	[Digitalis discontinued. Patient's condition deteriorates. A colleague reinstitutes digitalis.]
65	Desensitization to allergens	**65**	[Regimen of desensitization outlined.]
66	Hydrochlorothiazide 50 mg per day, four days out of seven	**66**	[Ordered.]
67	Diuretics to be given for weight gain	**67**	[Patient advised to call you if weight increases by 4 pounds or if edema occurs.]
68	Use of elastic stockings at night	**68**	[Ordered.]

UNLESS OTHERWISE DIRECTED IN THE RESPONSE COLUMN CONTINUE WITH SECTION 9-F

SECTION 9-F

The patient's condition has stabilized. She returns to work, but fails to continue her medication or to keep appointments with you. You next see her four months after discharge at which time she is complaining of increasing fatigue, weight gain, orthopnea, and swelling of the ankles. She is dyspneic, the neck veins are distended, moist rales are present over the lower half of each lung, the apical pulse is felt at the anterior axillary line, and 3+ pitting edema of the ankles is present.

YOU ARRANGE HOSPITALIZATION; YOUR INITIAL ORDERS WOULD NOW INCLUDE (SELECT AS MANY AS YOU CONSIDER INDICATED):

69	White blood cell count and differential	**69**	[WBC – 9500/mm^3; Differential: neutrophils – 68%; lymphocytes – 26%; monocytes – 6%.]
70	Record temperature every four hours	**70**	[Order noted.]
71	Record weights daily	**71**	[Order noted.]
72	Vital capacity	**72**	[2500 cc.]

73	Electrocardiogram	73	[SEE FIGURE 8, PAGE 406.]
74	Master's two-step test	74	[Dyspnea prevents completion of test.]
75	Digitalization	75	[Patient rapidly digitalized and placed on maintenance dose beginning second day.]
76	Chest x-ray	76	[SHOWN IN FIGURE 42, PAGE 418.]
77	Blood culture	77	[No growth.]
78	400 mg sodium diet	78	[Patient objects but accepts diet.]
79	Furosemide 40 mg intravenously	79	[Good diuresis within first 24 hours.]
80	Bronchoscopy	80	[Consultation ordered.]

UNLESS OTHERWISE DIRECTED IN THE RESPONSE COLUMN CONTINUE WITH SECTION 9-G

SECTION 9-G

Initially the patient shows symptomatic improvement. During the first week she loses 7 pounds and she shows clinical improvement. At this point you are called out of town. When you return at the end of two weeks you find the following progress note, entered the previous day by your associate who has been caring for the patient in your absence: "Despite earlier success with diuretics, edema and orthopnea have recurred. The patient has become increasingly anorexic and somnolent." You examine the patient, confirm these findings and detect cyanosis of lips and nail beds.

YOU WOULD NOW (SELECT AS MANY AS YOU CONSIDER INDICATED):

81	Increase digitalis preparation	81	[No significant improvement.]

82 Order 300 cc of 3% sodium chloride by slow intravenous drip 82

83 Institute tetracycline therapy 83

84 Search for signs of thromboembolic disease 84

85 Order electrocardiogram 85

86 Order chest x-ray 86

87 Order serum sodium, potassium, chloride, carbon dioxide determinations 87

88 Obtain blood cultures 88

89 Administer oxygen 89

90 Order white blood cell count and differential 90

91 Record daily weights 91

92 Arrange for cardiac catheterization 92

IN VIEW OF THE INFORMATION AVAILABLE YOU WOULD NOW ORDER (SELECT AS MANY AS YOU CONSIDER INDICATED):

93 Fluid restriction to 1000 cc per day 93

94	Parenteral mercurial furosemide and ammonium chloride, 6 g per day by mouth	**94**	[Considerable improvement.]
95	Parenteral mercurial furosemide and potassium chloride, 3 g per day by mouth	**95**	[Considerable improvement.]
96	Parenteral furosemide	**96**	[Improvement.]
97	Chloramphenicol (Chloromycetin) added to regimen	**97**	[No change in condition; patient later develops agranulocytosis.]
98	Lanatoside C (Cedilanid) 0.4 mg intravenously	**98**	[Bigeminal pulse develops.]
99	200 cc of 3% sodium chloride	**99**	[Patient deteriorates rapidly and dies. DO NOT MAKE ANY MORE CHOICES IN THIS SECTION; CONTINUE NOW WITH SECTION 9-H.]
100	Thoracentesis	**100**	[Little clinical change.]
101	Peritoneal dialysis against hypertonic bath	**101**	[Patient improves.]

UNLESS OTHERWISE DIRECTED IN THE RESPONSE COLUMN CONTINUE WITH SECTION 9-H

SECTION 9-H

102	Record your diagnoses below: ____________________ ____________________ ____________________ ____________________	**102**	[The complete diagnosis as recorded on the patient's chart was severe congestive cardiac failure. SEE APPENDIX I FOR ADDITIONAL COMMENT AND RECOMMENDED MANAGEMENT. END OF PROBLEM 9.]

NOW DEVELOP RESPONSE 102 FOR ADDITIONAL INFORMATION AND INSTRUCTIONS

PROBLEM 10

A COMPLICATED ABDOMINAL PROBLEM

Mr. J. C., a 65-year-old factory worker, comes to you complaining of pain in the epigastrium present for 12 months. He states that the pain is disturbing him so much at night that he is unable to sleep and is losing weight. He also complains of increasing tiredness over this period and some swelling of his feet in the last six months.

NOW CONTINUE WITH SECTION 10-A

SECTION 10-A

YOU WOULD FIRST (CHOOSE ONLY ONE):

1	Perform physical examination	**1**	[CONTINUE WITH SECTION 10-B.]
2	Admit the patient to hospital for further evaluation	**2**	[TURN TO SECTION 10-C, PAGE 148.]
3	Take further history	**3**	[TURN TO SECTION 10-D, PAGE 149.]
4	Order laboratory investigation on an outpatient basis	**4**	[TURN TO SECTION 10-E, PAGE 154.]
5	Give patient medication for his gastrointestinal complaints	**5**	[TURN TO SECTION 10-F, PAGE 161.]

6	Arrange for patient to see surgical consultant	6	[Consultant states patient appears to have a surgical problem and indicates he would be willing to accept management of the patient. [illegible]]

SECTION 10-B

Nurse records patient's weight at 142 pounds, height 5′ 6″.

IN PERFORMING THE PHYSICAL EXAMINATION YOU WOULD BE PARTICULARLY INTERESTED TO CHECK (SELECT AS MANY AS YOU CONSIDER ESPECIALLY PERTINENT; YOU CAN RETURN TO THIS SECTION AT ANY TIME TO OBTAIN ANY ADDITIONAL INFORMATION YOU MAY REQUIRE ABOUT INITIAL PHYSICAL FINDINGS):

General Examination

7	General appearance	7	[Asthenic individual of sallow complexion. Some recent truncal weight loss is evident and he appears tired and unhappy.]
8	Race	8	[Caucasian.]
9	Posture	9	[Normal.]
10	Gait	10	[Patient walks with a little difficulty, but has a normal gait.]
11	Mentation	11	[Normal for the patient's age. The patient is intelligent and cooperative.]
12	Obvious physical deformities	12	[None seen.]

Head, Scalp, and Neck

13	Hair	13	[Brown-grey, balding.]

14	Scalp	14
15	Skull shape	15
16	Auscultation of skull	16
17	Neck palpation	17
18	Conjunctivae	18

Ear, Nose, and Throat

19	External ears	19
20	Mastoid area	20
21	Otoscopic examination	21
22	Funduscopic examination	22
23	Pupils and corneae	23
24	Nasal cavities	24
25	Tongue	25
26	Teeth	26
27	Oral cavity	27
28	Laryngeal visualization (mirror)	28

Upper Limbs

29	Color of hands	**29**	[Pale.]
30	Skin texture	**30**	[Thin, dry and a little scaly.]
31	Nail beds	**31**	[Pale; no visual pulsations.]
32	Radial pulses	**32**	[Normal and symmetrically equal.]
33	Radial pulses with arms in various positions	**33**	[No change.]

Chest and Cardiovascular Systems

34	Pulse	**34**	[98 per minute, regular.]
35	Blood pressure (right arm)	**35**	[180/120 mm Hg.]
36	Examination of jugular vein	**36**	[Jugular vein pulsations visible 2 cm above clavicle with patient sitting up.]
37	Hepatojugular reflux	**37**	[Absent.]
38	Chest palpation	**38**	[No abnormality detected.]
39	Percussion of cardiac outline	**39**	[Heart is enlarged, lateral border at anterior axillary line.]
40	Auscultation of heart	**40**	[Heart sounds normal.]
41	Auscultation of chest	**41**	[Bilateral moist basal sounds heard posteriorly.]
42	Position of trachea	**42**	[Midline.]
43	Chest percussion	**43**	[Resonant throughout.]

Alimentary System

44	Examination of tongue	**44**	[Coated.]
45	Palpation of neck	**45**	[No abnormality detected.]
46	Inspection of abdomen	**46**	[Appears normal.]
47	Palpation of abdomen	**47**	[Liver is enlarged 4 cm – firm and nontender. Epigastrium moderately tender to deep pressure. Spleen not palpable; no other masses or tenderness.]
48	Percussion of abdomen	**48**	[No abnormality detected.]
49	Auscultation of abdomen	**49**	[Bowel sounds heard in all areas at four-to six-minute intervals.]
50	Inguinal region	**50**	[No abnormality detected.]
51	Genitalia	**51**	[Small left hydrocele – testes normal.]
52	Rectal examination	**52**	[Grade II firm, nontender, prostatic enlargement; watery brown offensive stool on glove.]
53	Sigmoidoscopic examination	**53**	[Examination is stopped by the patient who complains of chest pain.]
54	Cullen's sign (periumbilical darkening)	**54**	[Negative.]
55	McBurney's point tenderness	**55**	[None elicited.]
56	Rovsing's sign (pressure applied to descending colon)	**56**	[No pain elicited in area of cecum.]
57	Psoas and obturator signs	**57**	[Negative.]
58	Palpation of umbilicus	**58**	[No abnormality detected.]

Lower Limbs

59	Inspection of limbs	59
60	Palpation of ankles	60
61	Palpation of calves	61
62	Skin color	62
63	Homan's sign	63
64	Veins	64
65	Femoral pulses	65
66	Distal pulses	66
67	Auscultation in femoral triangles	67
68	Size and nutrition of limbs	68

Neurologic Examination

69	Cranial nerves I, II, VII, VIII, IX, XI, XII	69
70	Sensory system – upper limbs	70
71	Sensory system – lower limbs	71
72	Reflexes – upper limbs	72
73	Reflexes – lower limbs	73
74	Motor system	74

75	Position sense	**75**	[Good.]
76	Heat and cold sensation	**76**	[Present.]
77	Vibration sense	**77**	[Present and normal.]
78	Cranial nerves III, IV, V, VI	**78**	[Normal eye movements and corneal sensitivity.]
79	Neck movements	**79**	[Full neck mobility is present.]
80	Upper limb joints	**80**	[No limitation of movement.]
81	Lower limb joints	**81**	[No limitation of movement.]
82	Straight leg raising	**82**	[No pain elicited.]
83	Trendelenburg test	**83**	[Negative.]

YOU WOULD NOW (CHOOSE ONLY ONE):

84	Admit the patient to hospital for investigation if you have not already done so	**84**	[CONTINUE WITH SECTION 10-C.]
85	Initiate laboratory investigation on an outpatient basis if you have not already done so	**85**	[TURN TO SECTION 10-E, PAGE 154.]
86	Obtain further history if you have not already done so	**86**	[TURN TO SECTION 10-D, PAGE 149.]
87	Initiate medical management if you have not already done so	**87**	[TURN TO SECTION 10-F, PAGE 161.]
88	Modify or extend therapeutic program initiated earlier	**88**	[TURN TO SECTION 10-G, PAGE 163.]
89	Prepare patient for surgery	**89**	[TURN TO SECTION 10-G, PAGE 163.]

90 Request a surgical consultation **90** [Consultant states that patient appears to have a surgical problem and indicates that he would be willing to accept management of the patient. TURN TO SECTION 10-I, PAGE 167.]

SECTION 10-C

YOU WOULD NOW (CHOOSE ONLY ONE):

91 Arrange for a surgical consultant to see the patient **91** [Consultant states that patient appears to have a surgical problem and indicates that he would be willing to accept management of patient. TURN TO SECTION 10-I, PAGE 167.]

92 Obtain further history if you have not already done so **92** [CONTINUE WITH SECTION 10-D.]

93 Order appropriate laboratory tests if you have not already done so **93** [TURN TO SECTION 10-E, PAGE 158.]

94 Perform physical examination if you have not already done so **94** [TURN TO SECTION 10-B, PAGE 142.]

95 Initiate medical management if you have not already done so **95** [TURN TO SECTION 10-F, PAGE 161.]

96 Modify or extend therapeutic program initiated earlier **96** [TURN TO SECTION 10-G, PAGE 163.]

97 Prepare patient for surgery **97** [TURN TO SECTION 10-G, PAGE 163.]

SECTION 10-D

IN TAKING FURTHER HISTORY YOU WOULD BE PARTICULARLY INTERESTED TO INQUIRE ABOUT (SELECT AS MANY AS YOU CONSIDER ESPECIALLY PERTINENT; YOU CAN RETURN TO THIS SECTION AT ANY TIME TO OBTAIN ANY ADDITIONAL HISTORICAL INFORMATION YOU MAY REQUIRE):

98	Nature of the abdominal pain	**98**
99	What makes pain worse	**99**
100	What makes pain better	**100**
101	Exact location of pain	**101**
102	Effect of coughing on pain	**102**
103	Nature of bowel movements	**103**
104	Color of bowel movement	**104**
105	Appetite	**105**
106	Nausea	**106**
107	Vomiting	**107**
108	Vomiting of blood	**108**
109	Blood in stools	**109**
110	Black stools	**110**

111	Recent changes in weight	111	[8-pound loss in last four months, but I have regained some of this since my legs have become swollen.]
112	Foods that are upsetting	112	[Yes — onions and fatty foods.]
113	Peculiar tastes in the mouth	113	[Sometimes when I wake up in the morning I have a bad taste.]
114	Difficulty in swallowing	114	[None.]

General Health and Family History

115	Previous surgery	115	[Appendectomy 20 years ago.]
116	Serious illnesses	116	[None.]
117	Health of mother and father	117	[Mother died at 72 of a heart attack and father at 66 of bowel cancer.]
118	Brothers and sisters	118	[None.]
119	Nature of job	119	[I am a foreman of a section that puts baffle plates in car batteries.]
120	Smoking habits	120	[About a pack and a half a day.]
121	Alcohol intake	121	[About half a bottle of whiskey a day.]
122	Recent changes in level of activity and energy	122	[I've been very tired recently.]

Ear, Nose, and Throat

123	Hearing	123	[Normal.]
124	Ear infections	124	[None.]

125	Chronic cough	125	[Yes, especially in the mornings.]
126	Head colds	126	[Rarely.]
127	Nasal discharge	127	[Only with a cold.]
128	Ulcers and sores in the mouth	128	[None.]
129	Bleeding gums	129	[Sometimes, when I eat an apple.]

Respiratory and Cardiovascular Systems

130	Recent changes in breathing	130	[Yes, I'm more breathless recently.]
131	Shortness of breath	131	[Yes, I get out of breath easily.]
132	Short of breath at night	132	[I don't think so, at least it never wakes me.]
133	Coughing up blood	133	[Never.]
134	Changes in ability to perform physical activities	134	[Yes, I can't climb stairs very easily any more.]
135	Number of pillows for sleeping	135	[Two.]
136	Leg pain	136	[Sometimes I get cramps in my legs at night.]
137	Chest pain	137	[Yes, especially when I do heavy work.]
138	Arm pain	138	[Yes, the chest pain sometimes goes down into my left arm.]
139	Feeling of heart racing or beating unevenly	139	[Occasionally.]
140	Leg pain at night	140	[Sometimes I get cramps in my legs at night.]

141	Swelling of ankles	**141**	[Yes, toward the end of the day.]
142	Sputum	**142**	[About half a cup of greyish sputum most mornings.]

Genitourinary System

143	Urination	**143**	[No problems.]
144	Difficulty in starting stream	**144**	[Sometimes it is difficult to start.]
145	Burning on urination	**145**	[None.]
146	Frequency of urination at night	**146**	[Twice a night.]
147	Sores or discharge from genitals	**147**	[None.]

Other Systems

148	Dizziness, headaches, or visual disturbances	**148**	[Occasional headaches only.]
149	Feelings of nervousness or anxiety	**149**	[None.]
150	Kind of weather preferred	**150**	[Warm weather.]
151	Difficulty in walking	**151**	[None.]
152	Joint pains	**152**	[None.]
153	Swelling in abdomen	**153**	[None.]
154	Allergies	**154**	[None.]
155	Attacks of weakness	**155**	[Nothing other than what I have told you.]
156	Nose bleeds	**156**	[None.]
157	Recent changes in skin color	**157**	[Yes, it is paler and more like the color of wax.]

158	Sleeping habits	**158**	[I don't sleep too well; I often awake at night with a pain in my stomach.]
159	Belching	**159**	[That happens a lot.]
160	Present medications	**160**	[Nothing regular, just something for the pain once in a while.]
161	Bruising	**161**	[I don't bruise easily.]
162	Night sweats	**162**	[Only on hot nights.]

YOU WOULD NOW (CHOOSE ONLY ONE):

163	Arrange for laboratory investigation on an outpatient basis if you have not already done so	**163**	[CONTINUE WITH SECTION 10-E.]
164	Admit to hospital for investigation if patient is not already in hospital	**164**	[TURN TO SECTION 10-C, PAGE 148.]
165	Perform physical examination if you have not already done so	**165**	[TURN TO SECTION 10-B, PAGE 142.]
166	Initiate medical management if you have not already done so	**166**	[TURN TO SECTION 10-F, PAGE 161.]
167	Modify or extend therapeutic program initiated earlier	**167**	[TURN TO SECTION 10-G, PAGE 165.]
168	Prepare patient for surgery	**168**	[TURN TO SECTION 10-G, PAGE 165.]
169	Have surgical consultant see patient if you have not already done so	**169**	[Consultant states that patient appears to have a surgical problem and indicates that he would be willing to accept management of patient. TURN TO SECTION 10-J, PAGE 168.]

SECTION 10-E

YOU WOULD NOW ORDER THE FOLLOWING DETERMINATIONS (SELECT AS MANY AS YOU CONSIDER INDICATED):

Blood and Serum Studies

170	Red blood cell count	**170**	[RBC – 4.8 million/mm^3.]
171	Hemoglobin, hematocrit, white blood cell count, and differential	**171**	[Hb – 11.0 g/100 ml; Hct – 35%; WBC – 8500/mm^3; Differential: neutrophils – 75%, lymphocytes – 22%, monocytes – 3%.]
172	Sedimentation rate	**172**	[35 mm in the first hour (Wintrobe).]
173	Fasting blood sugar	**173**	[90 mg/100 ml.]
174	Blood urea nitrogen	**174**	[10 mg/100 ml.]
175	Blood sodium and potassium	**175**	[Na – 140 mEqL; K – 5 mEq/L.]
176	Calcium	**176**	[5 mEq/L.]
177	Chlorides	**177**	[103 mEq/L.]
178	Carbon dioxide combining power	**178**	[30 mEq/L.]
179	Magnesium	**179**	[2.0 mEq/L.]
180	Lead	**180**	[20 μg/100 ml.]
181	Creatinine	**181**	[1.2 mg/100 ml.]
182	Protein-bound iodine	**182**	[4 μg/100 ml.]
183	Uric acid	**183**	[5.9 mg/100 ml.]
184	Acid phosphatase	**184**	[4 units (King-Armstrong).]

185	Alkaline phosphatase	185	[14 units (King-Armstrong).]
186	Bilirubin (total)	186	[1.1 mg/100 ml.]
187	Cholesterol (total)	187	[200 mg/100 ml.]
188	Thymol turbidity	188	[2 units.]
189	Serum albumin	189	[5.0 g/100 ml.]
190	Serum globulin	190	[3.8 g/100 ml.]
191	Albumin globulin ratio	191	[3.2.]
192	Zinc turbidity	192	[10 units.]
193	Amylase	193	[102 units/100 ml (Somogyi).]
194	Lipase	194	[1.5 ml. (Cherry-Crandell).]
195	Aldolase	195	[30 IU/L.]
196	Serum glutamic oxalacetic transaminase	196	[36 IU/L.]
197	Serum glutamic pyruvic transaminase	197	[26 IU/L.]
198	Lactic dehydrogenase	198	[240 units/ml (Wroblewski).]
199	Bleeding time	199	[3 minutes (Ivy).]
200	Prothrombin time	200	[12.0 seconds (control – 13.0 seconds).]
201	Clot retraction (quantitative)	201	[70% (Didisheim).]
202	Serum iron	202	[120 μg/100 ml.]
203	Iron-binding capacity (unsaturated)	203	[200 μg/100 ml.]

204	Protein electrophoresis	**204**	[Albumin – 66%; Alpha$_1$ globulin – 4%; Alpha$_2$ – 7%; Beta – 8% Gamma – 15%.]

Serology

205	STS	**205**	[Nonreactive.]
206	Sheep cell agglutination	**206**	[Negative.]
207	Latex fixation titer	**207**	[Nonreactive.]
208	C-reactive protein	**208**	[Negative.]
209	Antistreptolysin titer	**209**	["0".]

Urine Studies

210	Specific gravity	**210**	[1.020.]
211	pH	**211**	[7.8.]
212	Protein	**212**	[Negative.]
213	Glucose	**213**	[Trace.]
214	Acetone	**214**	[Negative.]
215	Urobilinogen	**215**	[1.0 mg/24 hours.]
216	24-hour calcium	**216**	[200 mg/24 hours.]
217	Microscopic	**217**	[0 – 2 RBC, 0 – 3 WBC/hpf; no casts.]
218	Lead	**218**	[Negative.]
219	Porphobilinogen	**219**	[Negative (Watson-Schwartz Test).]
220	Bence-Jones protein	**220**	[Not present.]

221	Creatine	221	[100 mg/24 hours.]
222	Creatinine	222	[1.4 g/24 hours (70 kg man).]
223	17 – hydroxycorticoids and 17 ketosteroids	223	[17-Hydroxycorticoids — 15.0 mg/24 hours; 17-ketosteroids — 8 mg/24 hours.]

Stool Studies

224	Guaiac	224	[Negative.]
225	Parasite search	225	[Negative.]
226	Chemical fat analysis of feces	226	[Fecal fat 32% of dry weight; 6.5 g/24 hours.]
227	Radioactive fat analysis	227	[Fecal fat 32% of dry weight; 6.5 g/24 hours.]
228	D-Xylose absorption test	228	[15% of ingested dose excreted in urine in following five hours.]

Bacteriology

229	Blood culture	229	[Negative for bacteria and fungi.]
230	Sputum culture	230	[Negative for bacteria and fungi.]
231	Sputum for acid-fast bacilli	231	[No growth.]
232	24-hour urine for acid-fast bacilli	232	[No growth.]
233	Urine culture	233	[No growth of bacteria or fungi.]

Radiologic Studies

234	Cervical spine	234	[Interpreted as normal.]
235	Lumbosacral spine	235	[Moderate osteoarthritic changes.]

236	Dorsal spine	**236**	[Interpreted as normal.]
237	Skull	**237**	[Interpreted as normal.]
238	Pelvis	**238**	[Interpreted as normal.]
239	Chest	**239**	[Slight cardiomegaly, mild bilateral basal congestion.]
240	Abdomen (upright)	**240**	[No abnormality detected.]
241	Flat plate of abdomen (supine)	**241**	[No abnormality detected.]
242	Upper gastrointestinal series	**242**	[Stomach and duodenum within normal limits.]
243	Barium enema	**243**	[Within normal limits.]
244	Intravenous pyelogram	**244**	[No abnormality detected.]
245	Graham-Cole test (oral cholecystogram)	**245**	[Gallbladder visualizes moderately well; six nonopaque stones are seen in the fundus of the gallbladder.]
246	Intravenous cholecystogram	**246**	[No abnormality detected in the bile duct system.]
247	Aortogram	**247**	[No aneurysm or block demonstrated.]
248	Presacral pneumogram	**248**	[No abnormal mass detected.]
249	Myelogram	**249**	[No mass or occlusion demonstrated.]
250	Discogram	**250**	[Patient refuses the investigation.]
251	Bronchogram	**251**	[Normal bronchi.]
252	Tomograms of stomach	**252**	[No abnormal mass or defect seen in the stomach wall.]

Other Studies

253	Tomograms of gallbladder	253	[Multiple stones are seen in the gallbladder.]
254	Radioactive iodine (^{131}I) uptake	254	[Uptake — 30% of administered dose in 24 hours.]
255	Electrocardiogram	255	[Moderate left ventricular hypertrophy and S-T depression.]
256	Electroencephalogram	256	[Normal tracing.]
257	Nerve conduction time	257	[Normal.]
258	Bromsulphalein clearance	258	[14% retention in 45 minutes.]
259	Creatinine clearance	259	[100 cc/minute.]
260	Spinal tap	260	[CSF — protein 50 mg/100 ml, no cells.]
261	Pancreozymin-secretin test	261	[Low bicarbonate and low protein (moderate pancreatic deficiency).]
262	Glucose tolerance test	262	[Fasting blood glucose; 100 mg/100 ml; 170 mg/100 ml at one hour; 180 mg/100 ml at two hours; 110 mg/100 ml at three hours; urine consistently negative for glucose.]
263	Tri-iodothyronine uptake (Resin)	263	[Uptake — 30%.]
264	Liver biopsy	264	[Moderate hepatic fibrosis and fatty infiltration.]
265	Liver scan	265	[No defect seen. There is uniform uptake. The liver appears enlarged.]

266	Phenolsulfonphthalein excretion	266	[60% excreted in two hours.]
267	Gastroscopy	267	[Gastric mucosa hyperemic and bleeds easily; no ulcer or neoplasm visualized.]
268	Gastric acid analysis	268	[Gastric acidity normal.]
269	Gastric aspirate for malignant cells	269	[No abnormal cells seen.]
270	Biopsy of barely palpable supraclavicular node	270	[Normal.]
271	Biopsy of small moveable axillary node	271	[Normal lymph node.]
272	Skin biopsy	272	[Dermatologist requests you localize the area to be biopsied and state an indication for the biopsy.]
273	Muscle biopsy	273	[Surgeon reluctantly biopsies gastrocnemius muscle; pathologist reports normal muscle.]
274	Venous pressure	274	[Technical difficulties prevent accurate measurement, probably slightly raised.]
275	Circulation time (arm to tongue)	275	[18 seconds.]
276	Blood volume	276	[8.6% of body weight.]

YOU WOULD NOW (CHOOSE ONLY ONE):

277	Admit patient to hospital if you have not already done so	277	[TURN TO SECTION 10-C, PAGE 148.]
278	Initiate medical management if you have not already done so	278	[CONTINUE WITH SECTION 10-F.]

279	Modify or extend therapeutic program initiated earlier	**279**	[TURN TO SECTION 10-G, PAGE 163.]
280	Perform physical examination if you have not already done so	**280**	[TURN TO SECTION 10-C, PAGE 142.]
281	Arrange for surgical consultant to see patient	**281**	[Consultant states that patient appears to have a surgical problem and indicates that he would be willing to accept management of the patient. TURN TO SECTION 10-I, PAGE 167.]
282	Take further history if you have not already done so	**282**	[TURN TO SECTION 10-D, PAGE 149.]
283	Prepare patient for surgery	**283**	[TURN TO SECTION 10-G, PAGE 163.]

SECTION 10-F

IN YOUR INITIAL MANAGEMENT OF THIS PATIENT YOU WOULD ORDER (SELECT AS MANY AS YOU CONSIDER INDICATED):

284	Low-fat diet and pancreatic enzymes	**284**	[Diarrhea improves but general condition and pain remain the same.]
285	High-protein diet	**285**	[Symptoms do not improve.]
286	Bed rest at home	**286**	[Symptoms become worse.]
287	Antacid mixtures	**287**	[Pain is not relieved.]
288	Antispasmodic drugs	**288**	[Pain is not relieved.]
289	Ephedrine mixtures for cough	**289**	[Patient develops urinary retention and has to be catheterized.]

290	Digoxin and low-salt diet	**290**	[Pulse rate decreases, rales disappear, 6-pound weight loss, peripheral edema disappears.]
291	Diuretics	**291**	[Edema disappears.]
292	Stilbesterol	**292**	[Urinary symptoms are not improved and patient becomes nauseated.]
293	Dietary regime for peptic ulcer	**293**	[Pain becomes worse.]
294	Cessation of smoking	**294**	[Cough improves and morning nausea improves.]
295	Phenobarbital	**295**	[Symptoms remain the same.]
296	Aspirin or codeine compounds	**296**	[Pain is slightly relieved.]
297	Hydrochlorothiazide 50 mg, four days per week, guanethidine 10 mg, three times per day	**297**	[Blood pressure stabilizes at 140/100 mm Hg in two weeks; patient reports episodes of dizziness on arising.]

YOU WOULD NOW (CHOOSE ONLY ONE):

298	Continue medication for two weeks and review again	**298**	[Patient is not improved; fails to keep subsequent appointments; lost to follow-up. TURN TO SECTION 10-J, PAGE 168.]
299	Have a surgical consultant see the patient if you have not already done so	**299**	[Consultant states that patient appears to have a surgical problem and indicates that he would be willing to accept management of the patient. TURN TO SECTION 10-I, PAGE 167.]
300	Admit patient to hospital for investigation if you have not already done so	**300**	[TURN TO SECTION 10-C, PAGE 148.]

301	Initiate laboratory investigation on an outpatient basis if you have not already done so	**301**	[TURN TO SECTION 10-E, PAGE 154.]
302	Obtain further history if you have not already done so	**302**	[TURN TO SECTION 10-D, PAGE 149.]
303	Perform physical examination if you have not already done so	**303**	[TURN TO SECTION 10-B, PAGE 142.]
304	Modify or extend therapeutic program	**304**	[CONTINUE WITH SECTION 10-G.]
305	Prepare patient for surgery	**305**	[CONTINUE WITH SECTION 10-G.]

SECTION 10-G

YOUR WORKING DIAGNOSIS FOR THIS PATIENT INCLUDES (SELECT AS MANY AS YOU CONSIDER RELEVANT):

306	Gastritis	**306**	[Reconsider available data.]
307	Hiatus hernia	**307**	[Reconsider available data.]
308	Duodenal ulcer	**308**	[Reconsider available data.]
309	Indigestion	**309**	[Reconsider available data.]
310	Duodenitis	**310**	[Reconsider available data.]
311	Psychoneurosis	**311**	[Reconsider available data.]
312	Benign prostatic hypertophy	**312**	[Noted.]
313	Carcinoma of stomach	**313**	[Reconsider available data.]
314	Thoracolumbar back strain	**314**	[Reconsider available data.]
315	Herniated intervertebral disc	**315**	[Reconsider available data.]

316	Herpes zoster	316	[Reconsider available data.]
317	Carcinoma of pancreas	317	[Reconsider available data.]
318	Renal failure	318	[Reconsider available data.]
319	Phlebothrombosis	319	[Reconsider available data.]
320	Myocardial ischemia	320	[Noted.]
321	Carcinoma of lung	321	[Reconsider available data.]
322	Cardiac failure	322	[Noted.]
323	Carcinoma of prostate	323	[Reconsider available data.]
324	Cholelithiasis	324	[Noted.]
325	Carcinoma of gallbladder	325	[Reconsider available data.]
326	Chronic pancreatitis	326	[Noted.]
327	Lead poisoning	327	[Reconsider available data.]
328	Infectious diarrhea	328	[Reconsider available data.]
329	Gastric ulcer	329	[Reconsider available data.]
330	Hepatitis	330	[Reconsider available data.]
331	Primary hepatoma	331	[Reconsider available data.]
332	Pancreatic pseudocyst	332	[Reconsider available data.]
333	Perigastric abscess	333	[Reconsider available data.]

UNLESS OTHERWISE INSTRUCTED IN THE RESPONSE COLUMN, CONTINUE WITH SECTION 10-H

SECTION 10-H

IN THE MANAGEMENT OF THE PATIENT AT THIS STAGE YOU WOULD RECOMMEND (SELECT AS MANY AS YOU CONSIDER INDICATED):

334	High-protein diet	**334**	[Symptoms do not improve.]
335	Antacid mixtures	**335**	[Symptoms do not improve.]
336	Antispasmodic drugs	**336**	[Symptoms do not improve.]
337	Ephedrine	**337**	[Patient develops urinary retention and has to be catheterized.]
338	Digitalization	**338**	[Pulse rate decreases, rales disappear, 5-pound weight loss, peripheral edema decreases.]
339	Diuretics	**339**	[Edema disappears.]
340	Stilbesterol	**340**	[Urinary symptoms do not improve and nausea develops.]
341	Hydrochlorothiazide 50 mg, four days per week; guanethidine 10 mg three times per day	**341**	[Blood pressure stabilizes at 140/100 mm Hg in two weeks; patient reports episodes of dizziness on arising.]
342	Cessation of smoking	**342**	[Cough improves and morning nausea is less.]
343	Low-fat diet and pancreatic enzymes	**343**	[Diarrhea improves markedly.]
344	Aspirin or codeine compounds	**344**	[Pain is slightly improved.]
345	Radiation therapy	**345**	[Therapist states that condition would probably not be improved by radiation.]
346	Total gastrectomy	**346**	[IGNORE INSTRUCTIONS AT END OF THIS SECTION; INSTEAD TURN NOW TO SECTION 10-J, PAGE 168.]

347	Whipple's operation (pancreaticoduodenectomy)	347	[IGNORE INSTRUCTIONS AT END OF THIS SECTION; INSTEAD TURN NOW TO SECTION 10-J, PAGE 168.]
348	Pancreatectomy	348	[IGNORE INSTRUCTIONS AT END OF THIS SECTION; INSTEAD TURN NOW TO SECTION 10-J, PAGE 168.]
349	Cholecystectomy and exploration of common bile duct	349	[Stones are removed from the common duct and a diseased gallbladder is found; the pancreas is thickened and fibrotic.]
350	Retropubic prostatectomy	350	[IGNORE INSTRUCTIONS AT END OF THIS SECTION; INSTEAD TURN NOW TO SECTION 10-J, PAGE 168.]
351	Transurethral resection	351	[IGNORE INSTRUCTIONS AT END OF THIS SECTION; INSTEAD TURN NOW TO SECTION 10-J, PAGE 168.]
352	Mandelamine	352	[Symptoms remain as before.]
353	Prostatic biopsy	353	[Biopsy is negative and patient develops perineal abscess.]
354	Exploratory laparotomy	354	[A thickened fibrotic pancreas is discovered and stones are felt in the gallbladder.]
355	Gastrotomy	355	[Gastric mucosa is normal microscopically.]
356	Partial gastrectomy	356	[IGNORE INSTRUCTIONS AT END OF THIS SECTION; INSTEAD TURN NOW TO SECTION 10-J, PAGE 168.]

UNLESS OTHERWISE DIRECTED IN THE RESPONSE COLUMN TURN NOW TO SECTION 10-J

UNLESS OTHERWISE DIRECTED IN THE RESPONSE COLUMN TURN NOW TO SECTION 10-J

SECTION 10-I

IN LIGHT OF THE CONSULTANT'S REPORT, YOU WOULD NOW (CHOOSE ONLY ONE):

357	Transfer patient to consultant	**357**	[TURN TO SECTION 10-J, PAGE 168.]
358	Obtain further history if you have not already done so, prior to deciding on transfer	**358**	[TURN TO SECTION 10-D, PAGE 149.]
359	Perform physical examination if you have not already done so, prior to deciding on transfer	**359**	[TURN TO SECTION 10-B, PAGE 142.]
360	Order laboratory studies if you have not already done so, prior to deciding on transfer	**360**	[TURN TO SECTION 10-E, PAGE 154.]
361	Disregard consultant's advice and initiate appropriate medical management if you have not already done so	**361**	[TURN TO SECTION 10-F, PAGE 161.]
362	Modify or extend therapeutic program initiated earlier, in order to prepare patient for surgery	**362**	[TURN TO SECTION 10-G, PAGE 163.]

SECTION 10-J

363 Record your diagnoses below:

____
____
____
____
____
____

363 [The diagnosis on this patient's chart was recorded as: (i) cholethiasis with chronic pancreatitis, (ii) benign prostatic hypertrophy, (iii) congestive cardiac failure and myocardial ischemia probably due to arteriosclerosis. SEE APPENDIX F FOR ADDITIONAL COMMENTS AND RECOMMENDED MANAGEMENT. END OF PROBLEM 10.]

NOW DEVELOP RESPONSE 363 FOR ADDITIONAL INFORMATION AND INSTRUCTIONS

PROBLEM 11

A PALE, CONFUSED PATIENT

A young married woman brings her 57-year-old grey-haired mother to your office for a medical checkup. The daughter tells you that her mother's appetite, weight, strength, and well-being have progressively deteriorated over the last eight months. Lately she has become more confused and mildly disoriented and recently has exhibited slight memory loss. The patient added that for the past four weeks she has tired easily, especially when walking.

NOW CONTINUE WITH SECTION 11-A

SECTION 11-A

YOU WOULD NOW (CHOOSE ONLY ONE):

1	Defer investigation for the purpose of observation and ask the patient to return in three weeks	1	[CONTINUE WITH SECTION 11-B.]
2	Order chest, cervical spine, and skull films and ask patient to return in one week	2	[SEE FIGURES 33, 34, PAGE 416; 61, 62, AND 63, PAGE 423; THEN TURN TO SECTION 11-D; PAGE 176.]
3	Obtain further history and perform physical examination	3	[TURN TO SECTION 11-C, PAGE 170.]
4	Initiate therapy	4	[TURN TO SECTION 11-E, PAGE 177.]

SECTION 11-B

Over the period of observation, the patient's ability to walk has deteriorated.

YOU WOULD NOW (CHOOSE ONLY ONE EACH TIME YOU ARE DIRECTED TO THIS SECTION):

5	Request a neurosurgical consultation	**5**	[The neurosurgeon calls to tell you he feels the patient does not have a neurosurgical problem and that her daughter has informed him that she is going to another physician. TURN TO SECTION 11-K, PAGE 185.]
6	Arrange for laboratory evaluation on an inpatient basis	**6**	[TURN TO SECTION 11-F, PAGE 178.]
7	Arrange for laboratory tests on outpatient basis	**7**	[TURN TO SECTION 11-G, PAGE 180.]
8	Order chest, cervical spine, and skull films and ask the patient to return in one week	**8**	[SEE FIGURES 33, 34, PAGE 416; 61, 62 AND 63, PAGE 423; THEN TURN TO SECTION 11-D PAGE 176.]
9	Obtain further history and perform a physical examination	**9**	[CONTINUE WITH SECTION 11-C.]

SECTION 11-C

IN OBTAINING FURTHER HISTORY, YOU WOULD BE PARTICULARLY INTERESTED TO INQUIRE ABOUT (SELECT AS MANY AS YOU CONSIDER ESPECIALLY PERTINENT; YOU CAN RETURN TO THIS SECTION AT ANY TIME TO OBTAIN ANY ADDITIONAL HISTORICAL INFORMATION YOU MAY REQUIRE):

10	The family history	**10**	[No tuberculosis, diabetes, or hypertension.]
11	Episodes of febrile illness	**11**	[No recent febrile illness.]

12	Nausea and vomiting	12	[No history of nausea or vomiting.]
13	Frequency or urgency	13	[No history of frequency or urgency.]
14	Dietary intake	14	[Although her appetite has diminished somewhat, she has had an adequate and balanced diet.]
15	Food fads	15	[The patient has no known food fads.]
16	Soreness in mouth or tongue	16	[Her tongue has felt sore, especially the anterior half.]
17	Alcohol intake	17	[Occasional cocktail.]
18	History of diabetes mellitus	18	[None.]
19	History of hypertension	19	[No history of high blood pressure.]
20	History of heart disease	20	[No chest pain or palpitations.]
21	History of arthritis	21	[Occasional back stiffness on arising in the mornings for five years.]
22	Shortness of breath on exertion	22	[She can climb two flights of stairs but with marked dyspnea.]
23	Any abnormalities in sensation or changes in perception	23	[Numbness and tingling present in toes and feet for about one year; sees and hears well.]
24	Motor weakness	24	[For about three months has noted increasing weakness in walking and climbing stairs.]
25	Pain on urination	25	[None.]

26	Diarrhea	**26**	[Occasionally has had loose stool
27	Involuntary loss of urine	**27**	[None.]
28	Coordination	**28**	[Difficulty in maintaining her balance, holding utensils and buttoning clothes.]
29	Chest pain	**29**	[None.]
30	Cough	**30**	[None.]
31	Allergies	**31**	[None.]
32	Gait	**32**	[Awkward, with frequent staggering for past three months, especially at night.]
33	Changes in intellectual capacity	**33**	[Occasionally seemed confused in ordinary conversation during the last four months.]
34	Orientation to time, place, and people	**34**	[Would occasionally lose her way home from the neighborhood store.]
35	Uncontrollable crying and laughing	**35**	[None noted.]
36	Difficulty speaking	**36**	[None.]
37	Double vision	**37**	[None.]
38	Headaches	**38**	[Rare.]
39	Insomnia	**39**	[Restless sleep from time to time for about 10 years.]
40	Black stools	**40**	[None.]
41	Vaginal bleeding	**41**	[None.]

42 Leg pains 42

43 Dyspepsia 43

44 History of abdominal surgery 44

IN PERFORMING A PHYSICAL EXAMINATION, YOU WOULD BE PARTICULARLY INTERESTED TO CHECK (SELECT AS MANY AS YOU CONSIDER ESPECIALLY PERTINENT; YOU CAN RETURN TO THIS SECTION AT ANY TIME TO OBTAIN ANY ADDITIONAL INFORMATION ABOUT INITIAL PHYSICAL FINDINGS YOU MAY REQUIRE):

45 Extraocular movements 45

46 Fundi 46

47 Pupils 47

48 Mucosa and nail beds 48

49 Heart and lungs 49

50 Abdomen 50

51 Lymph nodes 51

52 Rectal 52

53 Pelvis 53

54	Sensory examination	54	[Diminished sensation to pin-prick and light touch from toes to knees; absent position sense in both great toes; diminished position sense in both ankles; vibration sense [illegible] diminished up to the knees; glovelike distribution of [illegible].]
55	Motor examination	55	[Moderate weakness at ankles, arms, and thighs; tone increased in legs but normal in arms.]
56	Deep tendon reflexes	56	[Hyperactive at ankles and knees; normal in arms.]
57	Babinski sign	57	[Positive bilaterally.]
58	Mental status	58	[Frequent mistakes in calculations; disoriented to time and place, but oriented to person; poor concentration and apathetic in appearance.]
59	Cerebellar system	59	[Very slight ataxia of heel to knee bilaterally; normal finger to nose and normal rapid alternating movements of hands.]
60	Romberg test	60	[Positive.]
61	Skin	61	[Pale, tallow color.]
62	Sclera	62	[Not icteric.]
63	Blood pressure, pulse, respirations, temperature	63	[Blood pressure, 130/85 mm Hg; pulse — 79 per minute; respirations — 16 per minute; temperature — 98.4F.]
64	Tongue	64	[Smooth and shiny, particularly at the tip and sides.]
65	Visual fields	65	[Normal to confrontation.]

66	Muscle atrophy	**66**	[No significant muscle atrophy.]
67	Breasts	**67**	[Pendulous; no palpable nodes or lumps.]
68	Tenderness over spine	**68**	[None.]

YOU WOULD NOW (CHOOSE ONLY ONE):

69	Initiate therapy	**69**	[TURN TO SECTION 11-E, PAGE 177.]
70	Arrange for an urgent psychiatric examination	**70**	[Psychiatrist reports that his evaluation reveals that the patient is somewhat confused and mildly disoriented, and that in his opinion these findings are attributable an organic disease involving the central nervous system. TURN TO SECTION 11-H, PAGE 182.]
71	Defer further investigation for observation, and ask patient to return in four weeks	**71**	[TURN TO SECTION 11-B, PAGE 170.]
72	Order chest, cervical spine, and skull films, and ask patient to return in one week	**72**	[SEE FIGURES 33, 34, PAGE 416; 61, 62, AND 63, PAGE 423; THEN CONTINUE WITH SECTION 11-D.]
73	Arrange for laboratory evaluation on an inpatient basis	**73**	[TURN TO SECTION 11-F, PAGE 178.]
74	Arrange for laboratory tests on an outpatient basis.	**74**	[TURN TO SECTION 11-G, PAGE 180.]

SECTION 11-D

YOU WOULD NOW (CHOOSE ONLY ONE):

75	Request a neurosurgical consultation	**75**	[The neurosurgeon calls to tell you he feels the patient does not have a neurosurgical problem, and that the daughter has informed him she is going to another physician. TURN TO SECTION 11-K, PAGE 185.]
76	Arrange for laboratory evaluation on an inpatient basis	**76**	[TURN TO SECTION 11-F, PAGE 178.]
77	Arrange for laboratory tests on an outpatient basis	**77**	[TURN TO SECTION 11-G, PAGE 180.]
78	Defer further investigation for the purpose of observation, and ask the patient to return in four weeks	**78**	[The patient's daughter calls after two and one-half weeks to tell you that her mother has grown worse and they have gone to another physician. TURN TO SECTION 11-K, PAGE 185.]
79	Initiate therapy	**79**	[CONTINUE WITH SECTION 11-E.]
80	Arrange for an urgent psychiatric evaluation	**80**	[Psychiatrist calls to tell you that his evaluation reveals that the patient is somewhat confused and mildly disoriented, and that in his opinion these findings are attributable to an organic disease involving the nervous system. TURN TO SECTION 11-H, PAGE 182.]

SECTION 11-E

YOU WOULD NOW PRESCRIBE (SELECT AS MANY AS YOU CONSIDER INDICATED):

81	Multivitamin capsules, one capsule three times a day	**81**	[The patient's daughter calls after two and one-half weeks to tell you that her mother has grown worse and they have gone to another physician.]
82	Aristocort, 4 mg twice a day	**82**	[The patient's daughter calls after two and one-half weeks to tell you that her mother has grown worse and they have gone to another physician.]
83	Vitamin B_{12}, 100 μg intramuscularly daily for several weeks, then once monthly	**83**	[Patient shows definite improvement.]
84	Folic acid 10 mg per day by mouth	**84**	[Patient shows some mild improvement.]
85	Physiotherapy	**85**	[The patient's daughter calls after two and one-half weeks to tell you that her mother has grown worse and they have gone to another physician.]
86	Iron	**86**	[No improvement; patient's hemoglobin continues to drop.]
87	Whole blood transfusion (3 units)	**87**	[Patient develops cardiac failure.]

UNLESS OTHERWISE DIRECTED IN THE RESPONSE COLUMN TURN NOW TO SECTION 11-K

SECTION 11-F

YOU WOULD NOW ORDER THE FOLLOWING DETERMINATIONS (SELECT AS MANY AS YOU CONSIDER INDICATED):

88	Hemoglobin, hematocrit, white blood cell count, differential	**88**	Hgb — 7.5 g/100 ml; Hct — 23%; WBC — 6500 mm[illegible]; differential segmented neutrophils — 60%, lymphocytes — [illegible], monocytes — 7%, eosinophils — [illegible]%.]
89	Urinalysis	**89**	[Glucose — 0, protein — trace, acetone — 0, specific gravity — 1.020, pH — 7.0, cells — 0 – 3 WBC/hpf.]
90	Tri-iodothyronine uptake	**90**	[Uptake 30%.]
91	Fasting blood sugar and two-hour postprandial blood sugar	**91**	[Fasting blood sugar, 80 mg/100 ml; two-hour postprandial, 90 mg/100 ml.]
92	Blood urea nitrogen	**92**	[14 mg/100 ml.]
93	Electrocardiogram	**93**	[SEE FIGURE 1, PAGE 404.]
94	Chest x-ray	**94**	[SEE FIGURES 33 AND 34, PAGE 416.]
95	Stools for occult blood	**95**	[Negative.]
96	Gastric analysis	**96**	[No free acid.]
97	Serum sodium, potassium, carbon dioxide, chloride	**97**	[Na — 138 mEq/L; K — 3.8 mEq/L; CO_2 — 26 mEq/L; Cl — 105 mEq/L.]
98	Skull x-ray	**98**	[SEE FIGURES 61 AND 62, PAGE 423.]
99	Bromsulphalein retention	**99**	[BSP — 5% retention in 45 minutes.]

100	Blood smear	100
101	Red cell indices	101
102	Sickle cell preparation	102
103	Lupus erythematosus cell preparation	103
104	Sedimentation rate	104
105	Serum creatinine	105
106	Serum uric acid	106
107	Serum total protein	107
108	STS	108
109	Stool for fat	109
110	Bone marrow	110

YOU WOULD NOW (CHOOSE ONLY ONE):

111	Initiate therapy	111
112	Arrange for further inpatient diagnostic procedures	112

113	Request a neurosurgical consultation	113	[Neurosurgeon calls to tell you he believes the patient does not have a neurosurgical problem and that the patient has informed him she is going to another physician. TURN TO SECTION 11-K, PAGE 185.]

SECTION 11-G

YOU WOULD NOW ORDER THE FOLLOWING DETERMINATIONS (SELECT AS MANY AS YOU CONSIDER INDICATED):

114	Hemoglobin, hematocrit, white blood count, differential	114	[Hgb – 6.5 g/100 ml; Hct – 19%, WBC – 6500/mm^3 with normal differential.]
115	Urinalysis	115	[Glucose – 0, acetone – 0, pH – 7.0, specific gravity: 1.020, protein – 0, cells 0 – 3 leukocytes.]
116	Tri-iodothyronine uptake (Resin)	116	[Uptake 30%.]
117	Fasting blood sugar and two-hour postprandial blood sugar	117	[Fasting blood sugar – 80 mg/100 ml; two-hour postprandial – 90 mg/100 ml.]
118	Blood urea nitrogen	118	[14 mg/100 ml.]
119	Electrocardiogram	119	[SEE FIGURE 1, PAGE 404.]
120	Chest x-ray	120	[SEE FIGURES 33 AND 34, PAGE 416.]
121	Stools for occult blood	121	[Negative.]
122	Gastric analysis	122	[No free acid.]
123	Serum sodium, potassium, carbon dioxide, chloride	123	[Na – 138 mEq/L; K – 3.8 mEq/L; CO_2 – 26 mEq/L; Cl – 105 mEq/L.]

124	Skull x-ray	**124**	[SEE FIGURES 61 AND 62, PAGE 423.]
125	Bromsulphalein retention	**125**	[BSP — 5% retention in 45 minutes.]
126	Blood smear	**126**	[Macrocytic red blood cells with occasional small irregular red blood cells, hypersegmented polymorphonuclear leukocytes also present.]
127	Red cell indices	**127**	[Mean corpuscular volume (MCV) 140 μ^3, mean corpuscular hemoglobin (MCH) 40 $\mu\mu$g; mean corpuscular hemoglobin concentration (MCHC) 35%.]
128	Sickle cell preparation	**128**	[Negative.]
129	Lupus erythematosus cell preparation	**129**	[Negative.]
130	Sedimentation rate	**130**	[13 mm/hr corrected (Wintrobe).]
131	Serum creatinine	**131**	[0.9 mg/100 ml.]
132	Serum uric acid	**132**	[4.0 mg/100 ml.]
133	Serum total protein	**133**	[6.0 g/100 ml.]
134	STS	**134**	[Nonreactive.]
135	Stool for fat	**135**	[17.5% of dry matter.]
136	Bone marrow	**136**	[There is increased cellularity of the bone
137	Serum barbiturates	**137**	[None found.]

138	Schilling test	**138**	[1% radioactive cobalt excreted in urine; 18% radioactive cobalt excreted in urine after administration of intrinsic factor.]
139	Serum B_{12} determination	**139**	[illegible]

YOU WOULD NOW (CHOOSE ONLY ONE):

140	Initiate therapy	**140**	[TURN TO SECTION 11-I, PAGE 183.]
141	Hospitalize the patient and arrange for further diagnostic procedures	**141**	[TURN TO SECTION 11-J, PAGE 184.]
142	Request a neurosurgical consultation	**142**	[The neurosurgeon calls to tell you he feels the patient does not have a neurosurgical problem and that she has informed him she is going to another physician. TURN TO SECTION 11-K, PAGE 185.]

SECTION 11-H

AFTER RECEIVING THIS REPORT, YOU WOULD NOW (CHOOSE ONLY ONE):

143	Initiate therapy	**143**	[TURN TO SECTION 11-E, PAGE 177.]
144	Arrange for laboratory evaluation on an inpatient basis	**144**	[TURN TO SECTION 11-F, PAGE 178.]
145	Arrange for laboratory tests on an outpatient basis	**145**	[TURN TO SECTION 11-G, PAGE 180.]

146	Request a neurosurgical consultation	**146**	[The neurosurgeon calls to tell you he feels the [illegible] does not have a neurosurgical problem, and that the daughter [illegible] informed him she is going to another physician. TURN TO SECTION 11-K, PAGE 185.]
147	Order chest, cervical spine and skull films and ask the patient to return in one week	**147**	[SEE FIGURES [illegible] 34, PAGE 416; 61, 62 AND 63, PAGE 423; THEN TURN TO SECTION 11-D, PAGE 176.]
148	Hospitalize patient in a mental institution	**148**	[TURN TO SECTION 11-K, PAGE 185.]

SECTION 11-I

YOU WOULD NOW PRESCRIBE (CHOOSE ONLY ONE):

149	Multivitamins, two tabs three times a day by mouth	**149**	[The patient's daughter calls after two and a half weeks to tell you that her mother has grown worse and they have gone to another physician. TURN TO SECTION 11-K, PAGE 18[illegible].]
150	Prednisone, 5 mg three times a day by mouth	**150**	[The patient's daughter calls after two and a half weeks to tell you that her mother has grown worse and they have gone to another physician. TURN TO SECTION 11-K, PAGE 18[illegible].]
151	Adrenocorticotropic hormone (ACTH) 30 units intravenous infusion	**151**	[Given, no improvement.]
152	Iron	**152**	[No improvement; patient's hemoglobin continues to drop.]
153	Vitamin B_{12} 100 μg intramuscularly daily for several weeks, then once monthly	**153**	[Patient's mood improves dramatically. Some objective improvement in neurologic status.]

154	Laminectomy for decompression of the spinal cord	**154**	[Spinal tap shows normal pressure. Neurosurgeon calls to tell you he believes the patient does not have a neurosurgical problem and that the daughter has informed him she is going to another physician. TURN TO SECTION 11-K, PAGE 185.]
155	Transfer patient to psychiatric ward	**155**	[Done. Patient continues to deteriorate; psychiatrist reports that his evaluation reveals that the patient is somewhat confused and mildly disoriented, and that in his opinion these findings are attributable to an organic disease involving the nervous system. TURN TO SECTION 11-H, PAGE 182!]
156	Whole blood transfusion (three units)	**156**	[Patient develo[illegible] cardiac fail[illegible]

UNLESS OTHERWISE DIRECTED IN THE RESPONSE COLUMN TURN NOW TO SECTION 11-K

SECTION 11-J

YOU WOULD NOW ORDER THE FOLLOWING DETERMINATIONS (SELECT AS MANY AS YOU CONSIDER INDICATED):

157	Lumbar puncture	**157**	[Cerebrospinal fluid clear, no cells; total protein 65 mg% and pressure is normal.]
158	Electroencephalogram	**158**	[Tracing interpreted as within normal limits.]
159	Bone marrow	**159**	[Cellular marrow with increased number of megaloblasts and much hemosiderin.]

160	Gastric analysis	**160**	[No free gastric acid.]
161	Serum calcium, phosphorus, alkaline phosphatase	**161**	[Ca – 5.0 mEq/L; P – 1.5 mEq/L; alkaline phosphatase – 10 units (King-Armstrong).]
162	Gastric analysis after subcutaneous histamine	**162**	[No free acid found.]
163	Serum B_{12}	**163**	[30 pg/ml.]
164	Myelogram	**164**	[Patient's family refuses to consent to procedure.]
165	Liver biopsy	**165**	[Pathologist reports normal liver tissue.]
166	Reticulocyte count	**166**	[2%.]
167	Schilling test	**167**	[1% radioactive cobalt excreted in urine; 18% radioactive cobalt excreted in urine after administration of intrinsic factor.]

UNLESS OTHERWISE DIRECTED IN THE RESPONSE COLUMN TURN NOW TO SECTION 11-I

SECTION 11-K

168	Record your diagnostic impressions below: ____________________ ____________________ ____________________ ____________________ ____________________ ____________________	**168**	[The diagnosis as recorded on the chart for this patient was (i) Vitamin B_{12} deficiency, subacute, combined degeneration of the posterolateral columns of the spinal cord; (ii) peripheral polyneuropathy; (iii) early dementia. SEE APPENDIX M FOR ADDITIONAL COMMENT AND RECOMMENDED MANAGEMENT. END OF PROBLEM 11.]

NOW DEVELOP RESPONSE 168 FOR ADDITIONAL INFORMATION AND INSTRUCTIONS

PROBLEM 12

WHAT IS WRONG WITH MY EAR?

A man, 35 years of age, presents himself with the following history: "I had a physical examination that is required before promotion in my company last week. The doctor said there was something wrong with my ear, the right ear. He said I had a perforated eardrum. That was the first I have ever heard of it, and I don't even know what it really means." The appearance of the right eardrum is shown in Figure 21, Page 413.

NOW CONTINUE WITH SECTION 12-A

SECTION 12-A

IN OBTAINING ADDITIONAL HISTORY YOU ARE PARTICULARLY INTERESTED TO INQUIRE ABOUT (SELECT AS MANY AS YOU CONSIDER ESPECIALLY PERTINENT; YOU CAN RETURN TO THIS SECTION AT ANY TIME TO OBTAIN ANY ADDITIONAL HISTORICAL INFORMATION YOU MAY REQUIRE):

1	Hearing loss with colds	**1**	[I don't think so.]
2	Hearing loss at any time	**2**	[I've never noticed any.]
3	Tinnitus	**3**	[I've done some hunting, and I have heard ringing after a day of shooting.]
4	Vertigo	**4**	[None.]
5	Runny ear	**5**	[One summer my ear ran after I went swimming, but it cleared up. I don't even remember which ear it was.]
6	Ear usually used in telephoning	**6**	[Left.]

7	Head injuries	7	[None.]
8	Earache in childhood	8	[I don't remember any.]
9	Any hearing differences between the two ears	9	[I don't think so. I've tried to see if I could notice any since I found out about this, but I can't be sure.]
10	History of tuberculosis	10	[None.]
11	History of scarlet fever	11	[None.]
12	Excessive sweating	12	[No.]
13	Can you hear a watch tick	13	[Yes.]
14	History of measles	14	[None.]
15	Any ear problems when flying	15	[No.]
16	Any skin problems	16	[Some acne when I was younger, but nothing else.]

UNLESS OTHERWISE DIRECTED IN THE RESPONSE COLUMN CONTINUE WITH SECTION 12-B

SECTION 12-B

On examination of the right ear, the skin lining of the external ear canal appears normal and dry. The appearance of the eardrum is shown in Figure 21, Page 413.

IN YOUR OPINION, THE MAJOR ABNORMALITY CAN BEST BE DESCRIBED AS (CHOOSE ONLY ONE):

17	A marginal perforation	17	[PLEASE RECONSIDER THE SITE OF THE PERFORATION IN FIGURE 21, PAGE 413.]
18	A central perforation	18	[Read instructions at end of this section.]

19	A globular foreign body	**19**	[No foreign body found.]
20	Perforation with atrophic scar	**20**	[Interpretation noted.]
21	Aural polyp	**21**	[No polyp found.]
22	Aural granuloma	**22**	[The lesion was found to be atrophic rather than granulomatous.]

UNLESS OTHERWISE DIRECTED IN THE RESPONSE COLUMN CONTINUE WITH SECTION 12-C

SECTION 12-C

IN ORDER TO CONFIRM YOUR DIAGNOSTIC IMPRESSION AND TO GUIDE YOUR MANAGEMENT OF THIS PATIENT YOU WOULD NOW PERFORM, OR ORDER (SELECT AS MANY AS YOU CONSIDER INDICATED):

23	Valsalva maneuver	**23**	[Drum does not move on right but does on left.]
24	Cold caloric test	**24**	[Not successfully carried [illegible]
25	Cold pressor test	**25**	[Blood pressure rises from 120/80 mm Hg to 180/90 mm Hg.]
26	Diagnostic myringotomy	**26**	[Patient becomes hypotensive and faints during intervention. Your efforts to revive the patient occupy the next 20 minutes.]
27	Politzer inflation	**27**	[Patient hears a click; hearing remains unchanged.]
28	Inspection with pneumatic otoscope	**28**	[Right drum does not move; left does.]
29	Stenger test	**29**	[No evidence of malingering.]

30	Schwabach test	**30** [Bone conduction equal to examiner's on left; longer than examiner's on right.]
31	Rinne test	**31** [Air conduction stronger than bone conduction on left, air conduction equal to bone conduction on right. Or stated in another way, + on left, ± on right.]
32	Gellé test	**32** [Vibrations of the fork are distinctly perceived bilaterally.]
33	Weber test	**33** [Lateralizes to right.]
34	Rotational testing	**34** [10 times to the right gives 1, 2, 3, degree nystagmus for 20 seconds; 10 times to the left gives same response.]
35	Audiometric testing	**35** RE[illegible]E 4[illegible]
36	Examination for postural vertigo	**36** [None found.]
37	Transillumination of sinuses	**37** [Frontals and maxillar[illegible] clear.]
38	X-ray of sinuses	**38** [All sinuses are normal on radiographic examination.]
39	Fistula symptom test	**39** [No nystagmus induced.]
40	Mastoid x-rays	**40** [SEE FIGURES 64 AND 65, PAGE 424.]
41	Eustachian tube inflation	**41** [Both are pat[illegible]]
42	Binaural loudness balance	**42** [No recruitment found.]
43	Laminograms of petrous pyramid	**43** [Done; no [illegible]ormalities discovered. For [illegible] mastoid SEE FIGURES [illegible] AND 65 [illegible]424[illegible]]

44	Cerebrospinal fluid test for syphilis	**44**	[Nonreactive]

UNLESS OTHERWISE DIRECTED IN THE RESPONSE COLUMN CONTINUE WITH SECTION 12-D

SECTION 12-D

ON THE BASIS OF THESE FINDINGS YOU CONCLUDE THAT (SELECT AS MANY AS YOU BELIEVE THE EVIDENCE SUPPORT AT THIS TIME):

45	The hearing is not equal in both	**45**	[Interpretation noted.]
46	The hearing is equal in both ears	**46**	[Review data and SEE FIGURE 7, PAGE 410.]
47	The right eardrum is not intact	**47**	[Interpretation noted.]
48	The right eardrum is intact	**48**	[Review data and SEE FIGURE 21, PAGE 413.]
49	There is demonstrable evidence of hearing loss	**49**	[Interpretation noted. Ignore instructions at end of this section; instead CONTINUE WITH SECTION 12-E.]
50	There is NO demonstrable hearing loss	**50**	[Review available data.]

UNLESS OTHERWISE DIRECTED IN THE RESPONSE COLUMN TURN NOW TO SECTION 12-F, PAGE 191

SECTION 12-E

THE HEARING LOSS YOU BELIEVE TO EXIST CAN BEST BE DESCRIBED AS (CHOOSE ONLY ONE):

51	Sensorineural, right	**51**	[Please reconsider findings from Schwabach and Rinne Tests (30 and 31, page 189).]
52	Sensorineural, left	**52**	[Please reconsider findings from Schwabach and Rinne tests (30 and 31, page 189).]

53	Conductive, right	53	[Interpretation noted.]
54	Conductive, left	54	[Please reconsider findings from Schwabach and Rinne tests (30 and 31, page 189) and audiometric tests (Figure 7, page 410.]
55	Mixed, right	55	[Please reconsider findings from Schwabach and Rinne tests (30 and 31, page 189) and audiometric tests (Figure 7, page 410.]
56	Mixed, left	56	[Please reconsider findings from Schwabach and Rinne tests (30 and 31, page 189) and audiometric tests (Figures 7, page 410.]
57	Some type other than those listed	57	[Please reconsider findings reported in Section 12-C above.]

UNLESS OTHERWISE DIRECTED IN THE RESPONSE COLUMN CONTINUE WITH SECTION 12-F

SECTION 12-F

YOU WOULD NOW RECOMMEND (CHOOSE ONLY ONE):

58	Surgical management	58	[CONTINUE WITH SECTION 12-G.]
59	Medical management	59	[TURN TO SECTION 12-H, PAGE 192.]
60	Prophylactic management	60	[TURN TO SECTION 12-I, PAGE 193.]
61	Referral to otolaryngologist	61	[Otolaryngologist informs you that he has advised the patient that only prophylaxis is now indicated. TURN TO SECTION 12-J, PAGE 193.]

SECTION 12-G

YOU WOULD NOW RECOMMEND (CHOOSE ONLY ONE):

62	Simple mastoidectomy	**62**	[Patient is reluctant to agree and requests consultation with otolaryngologist who advises that present management be limited to prophylactic treatment. TURN NOW TO SECTION 12-J, PAGE 193.]
63	Tympanoplasty	**63**	[Patient is reluctant to agree and requests consultation with otolaryngologist who advises that present management be limited to prophylactic treatment. TURN NOW TO SECTION 12-J, PAGE 193.]
64	Stapedectomy	**64**	[Patient is reluctant to agree and requests consultation with otolaryngologist who advises that present management be limited to prophylactic treatment. TURN NOW TO SECTION 12-J, PAGE 193.]

SECTION 12-H

YOU WOULD NOW PRESCRIBE (SELECT AS MANY AS YOU CONSIDER INDICATED):

65	Eardrops	**65**	[No change in condition.]
66	Antibiotics	**66**	[No change in condition.]
67	Antiseptic powder for application in middle ear	**67**	[No change in condition.]

UNLESS OTHERWISE DIRECTED IN THE RESPONSE COLUMN CONTINUE WITH SECTION 12-I

SECTION 12-I

YOU WOULD NOW ADVISE THE PATIENT (SELECT AS MANY AS YOU CONSIDER INDICATED):

68	To avoid getting water in the right ear	**68**	[Patient agrees to follow instructions.]
69	To return promptly to the office in case discharge from ear is noted	**69**	[Patient agrees to follow instructions.]
70	To return for a check-up every one to two years even if no further symptoms are noted	**70**	[Patient agrees to follow instructions.]
71	Clean ear daily with propylene glycol solution	**71**	[Patient agrees to follow instructions.]

UNLESS OTHERWISE DIRECTED IN THE RESPONSE COLUMN CONTINUE WITH SECTION 12-J

SECTION 12-J

72	Record your diagnoses below: ____________________ ____________________ ____________________ ____________________ ____________________	**72**	[The diagnosis recorded on the patient's chart was perforation of the right eardrum, patent central perforation, with surrounding atrophic scar. SEE APPENDIX K FOR ADDITIONAL COMMENT AND RECOMMENDED MANAGEMENT. END OF PROBLEM 12.]

NOW DEVELOP RESPONSE 72 FOR FURTHER INFORMATION AND INSTRUCTIONS

PROBLEM 13

THE SEVERELY TRAUMATIZED PATIENT

A 23-year-old man is brought to the hospital Emergency Room at 1:30 AM by the police. You are an intern on duty and quickly ascertain that the patient has a large laceration over the right eye and another over the occiput. There is also a gash over the anterior surface of the right leg, and gross deformity of the leg is still obvious despite the presence of a first aid splint applied to it by the police.

The patient is conscious but in some discomfort and appears confused and lethargic. He is pale and clammy. Blood pressure is 60/30 mm Hg; pulse 140 per minute, thready, decreased volume; respirations 40 per minute and shallow; temperature cool to touch.

NOW CONTINUE WITH SECTION 13-A

SECTION 13-A

BEFORE INSTITUTING EMERGENCY TREATMENT YOU WOULD (SELECT AS MANY AS YOU CONSIDER INDICATED):

1	Insert a large gauge needle or catheter into an arm vein, draw blood for type and crossmatch and start an IV drip	1	[Done.]
2	Ask the patient how thirsty he is	2	[Yes, he is very thirsty.]
3	Start intra-arterial fluids	3	[Done.]
4	Examine the circulation of the right leg and foot	4	[Right foot pulseless and cold.]

5 Take a brief history from the police officers who brought him in

5 [Patient was in a head-on automobile collision. Apparent fracture, right leg. First aid splint applied. Patient unconscious or partially conscious for 45 minutes after accident. Accident occured one hour and 10 minutes ago.]

6 Take a complete history from other occupants of the car

6 [They give a conflicting and confused story. Generally, they agree with the police report. The young man was sitting to the right of the driver and was loosely wearing a seat belt.]

7 Take a history of past health from the patient's mother who has arrived from home

7 [No significant family illness or past medical history.]

8 Examine the abdomen

8 [Not distended. Slight tenderness and some resistance is present in the right lower quadrant. Bowel sounds absent.]

9 Auscultate the chest

9 [Air enters both lung fields.]

10 Examine the eye grounds

10 [No papilledema.]

11 Remove splint and examine right leg

11 [Compound fracture of the bony structures of the lower part of the limb.]

12 Catheterize the patient's urinary bladder

12 [150 cc of clear urine obtained.]

13 Perform a rectal examination

13 [Done. Patient is restless. No gross or occult blood in stool.]

AT THIS TIME YOU WOULD (CHOOSE ONLY ONE):

14 Start immediate management of fracture(s)

14 [TURN TO SECTION 13-G, PAGE 209.]

15 Proceed to a systematic evaluation of the skeleton, gastrointestinal tract, liver, and central nervous system for further evidence of serious injury — 15 [TURN TO SECTION 13-[illegible], PAGE 20[illegible].]

16 Start immediate management of shock — 16 [TURN TO SECTION 13-[illegible], PAGE [illegible].]

17 Continue with pretreatment assessment — 17 [TURN TO SECTION 13[illegible], PAGE 20[illegible].]

18 Repair lacerations — 18 [TURN TO SECTION 13-[illegible], PAGE [illegible].]

SECTION 13-B

IN CARRYING OUT A SYSTEMATIC ASSESSMENT OF THE PATIENT'S NONSKELETAL INJURIES YOU WOULD (SELECT AS MANY AS YOU CONSIDER INDICATED):

19 Auscultate heart and lungs — 19 [Heart rate 100 per minute; no murmurs. Lungs clear.]

20 Auscultate the abdomen — 20 [No borborygmi heard. No bruits.]

21 Palpate the abdomen — 21 [Mobile, not distended. Some tenderness and resistance in right lower quadrant.]

22 Order examination of the stool for blood — 22 [Stool sent to lab.]

23 Obtain an electroencephalogram — 23 [EEG lab unable to do bedside recording at this time, patient cannot be transported to lab because of fractured leg.]

24	Obtain repeated electrocardiogram	24	[ECG done at bedside. Rate 100 per minute. No conduction abnormalities. No evidence of myocardial damage.]
25	Order serum glutamic oxalacetic transaminase determination	25	[30 IU/L.]
26	Order creatine phosphokinase determination	26	[70 U[illegible]]
27	Order blood urea nitrogen determination	27	[25 mg/100 ml.]
28	Order skull x-ray	28	[Patient has difficulty being positioned. No evidence of skull fracture.]
29	Order x-ray of the thorax (bony structures above the pelvis)	29	[No fractures seen.]
30	Order repeat chest x-ray	30	[No evidence of pneumothorax. No fluid levels seen. Normal chest film.]
31	Order x-ray of sinus	31	[Patient complains about positioning and cannot complete the procedure.]
32	Order flat plate of the abdomen	32	[There are multiple intracolonic and intrajejunal fluid levels. No air under the diaphragm.]
33	Order splenorenogram	33	[Radiologist questions the need for this procedure.]
34	Order barium swallow and follow through	34	[Patient cannot comply.]
35	Order barium enema	35	[Patient cannot comply.]
36	Order cerebral angiography	36	[Radiologist questions need for this procedure.]

37	Order myelography	**37**	[Patient unable to withstand procedure.]
38	Order intravenous pyelogram	**38**	[Patient cannot complete the procedure because of discomfort. Several films taken are normal.]
39	Examine the eyegrounds	**39**	[No papilledema seen.]
40	Perform a neurologic examination	**40**	[Normal except in right lower extremity where pain prohibits full evaluation.]
41	Request a neurosurgical consultation	**41**	[Neurosurgeon examines patient and finds no neurosurgical problems.]
42	Obtain spinal tap	**42**	[Pressure: 100 mm H_2O, cells: fewer than 3 WBC/mm^3 no RBCs, chloride: 125 mEq/L, glucose: 60 mg/100 ml, protein: 30 mg/100 ml; albumin – 58%, $alpha_1$ globulin – 5%, $alpha_2$ globulin – 14%, beta globulin – 10%, gamma globulin – 13%.]
43	Order pneumoencephalography	**43**	[Neurosurgeon refuses to perform one.]

AT THIS TIME YOU WOULD:

44	Complete the history, physical, and routine laboratory evaluation	**44**	[CONTINUE WITH SECTION 13-C, PAGE 199.]
45	Manage the skeletal injuries and lacerations if you have not already done so	**45**	[TURN TO SECTION 13-D, PAGE 203.]
46	Repair the lacerations if you have not already done so	**46**	[TURN TO SECTION 13-E, PAGE 205.]

47	Consider the urgent problems adequately dealt with and enter management of the recovery stage	47	[TURN TO SECTION 13-K PAGE 212.]

SECTION 13-C

IN COMPLETING THE HISTORY YOU WOULD BE PARTICULARLY INTERESTED TO INQUIRE ABOUT (SELECT AS MANY AS YOU CONSIDER ESPECIALLY PERTINENT):

48	Previous trauma history	48	[None significant.]
49	Previous hospitalizations	49	[In childhood for tonsilectomy and adenoidectomy.]
50	Previous surgery	50	[Tonsil and adenoidectomy in childhood; uneventful.]
51	Drug history	51	[Denies chronic use of any drug.]
52	Allergies	52	[Mild hay fever; no known drug allergies.]
53	Family history	53	[Unremarkable.]
54	Immunization history	54	[Patient not sure about those in childhood; had "boosters" five years ago while in the Army.]
55	Prenatal and perinatal history	55	["You'll have to ask my mother."]
56	Past medical history	56	[No significant illnesses.]
57	Bleeding tendency	57	[None evident.]
58	Previous headaches	58	[Only rare, mild headaches.]
59	History of seizures or "black-outs"	59	[None known.]
60	History of the accident	60	[Amnesic for the events.]

IN COMPLETING THE PHYSICAL EXAMINATION YOU WOULD BE PARTICULARLY INTERESTED TO CHECK (SELECT AS MANY AS YOU CONSIDER EXPECIALLY PERTINENT):

61	Blood pressure, pulse, respiration, and temperature	**61**	[Blood pressure — 104/68 mm Hg; pulse — 96 per minute; respirations — 20 per minute; temperature — 98F.]
62	Height and weight	**62**	[Nurse refuses to move patient for these data.]
63	Level of consciousness	**63**	[Awake and responsive; more comfortable than earlier.]
64	Fundi	**64**	[Normal discs; no evidence of papilledema or hemorrhages.]
65	Pupils	**65**	[Normal size; equal; equally reactive.]
66	Extraocular movements	**66**	[Full.]
67	Cranial nerves V, VII-XII	**67**	[All intact.]
68	Gait and station	**68**	[Patient refuses to cooperate.]
69	Strength	**69**	[Normal except in right lower extremity where pain prevents movements.]
70	Cerebellar function	**70**	[Unable to test except in upper extremities where it is normal.]
71	Sensation	**71**	[Grossly intact for all modalities; no spinal level evident, but subjective decrease in right leg.]
72	Deep tendon reflexes	**72**	[Intact and normal except in right lower extremity where the maneuver causes distress and poor cooperation.]
73	Head	**73**	[Previously described lacerations over right eye and occiput.]

74	Ears	**74**	[Normal; no blood evident.]
75	Neck	**75**	[Supple; [illegible] not palpable.]
76	Chest and lungs	**76**	[Normal [illegible]; no abnormal[illegible]es on auscultation; no pain on movement.]
77	Heart	**77**	[Normal [illegible] rhythm; no murmurs.]
78	Abdomen	**78**	[Mobile; not distended; slight tenderness in the right pelvic region; absent bowel sounds.]
79	Genitalia	**79**	[No abnormalities.]
80	Extremities	**80**	[Evident compound fracture of right leg with laceration over anterior surface of right leg; right foot cold and pulseless. Pain on movement of right hip.]
81	Range of motion of spine	**81**	[Difficult to evaluate. Patient complains of pain in pelvic area.]
82	Straight leg raising	**82**	[Markedly limited by pain on right.]

IN OBTAINING ADDITIONAL LABORATORY AND ROUTINE X-RAY STUDIES YOU WOULD NOW ORDER (SELECT AS MANY AS YOU CONSIDER INDICATED):

83	Complete blood count	**83**	[Hgb — 12.4 g/100 ml; Hct — 35; WBC — 7400 mm^3 normal differential.]
84	Urinalysis	**84**	[Specific gravity — 1.024, 0 protein, 0 acetone, 0 glucose, 8-10 RBC, 1-3 WBC per hpf. No casts.]
85	Serum calcium and phosphorus	**85**	[Ca, 4.5 mEq/L; P, 1.0 mEq/L.]

86	Blood urea nitrogen	**86**	[24 mg/100 ml.]
87	Blood sugar	**87**	[100 mg/100 ml.]
88	Sedimentation rate	**88**	[37 mm/one hour (Wintrobe).]
89	Circulating blood volume	**89**	[Normal for patient's size.]
90	Electrocardiogram	**90**	[Normal.]
91	Electroencephalogram	**91**	[Normal.]
92	Chest x-ray	**92**	[Normal.]
93	Skull x-ray	**93**	[Normal; no fractures seen.]
94	Sinuses	**94**	[Normal; no clouding or fractures.]

YOU WOULD NOW (CHOOSE ONLY ONE):

95	Proceed to a systematic evaluation of the skeleton, gastrointestinal tract, liver, and central nervous system for further evidence of serious injury	**95**	[TURN TO SECTION 13-B, PAGE 196.]
96	Manage the skeletal injuries and lacerations if you have not already done so	**96**	[TURN TO SECTION 13-D, PAGE 203.]
97	Deal with the lacerations if you have not already done so	**97**	[TURN TO SECTION 13-E, PAGE 205.]
98	Consider the urgent problems adequately dealt with and enter management of the recovery stage	**98**	[TURN TO SECTION 13-K, PAGE 212.]

SECTION 13-D

IN MANAGING THE PATIENT'S SKELETAL INJURIES AND LACERATIONS YOU WOULD (SELECT AS MANY AS YOU CONSIDER INDICATED):

99	Palpate the bony structures from head to toe	**99**	[Patient complains of pain in the right side of the pelvis in the right hip.]
100	Gently attempt to assess passive movement of all joints but the right leg	**100**	[Right hip movement is very painful.]
101	Obtain radiographs of all the pelvic structures and the right leg	**101**	[TURN NOW TO SECTION J, PAGE 211.]
102	Obtain radiographs of both arms	**102**	[No abnormalities are seen in the skeletal structure; there are no fractures.]

IN TREATING THE FRACTURED STRUCTURES, YOU WOULD RECOMMEND (SELECT AS MANY AS YOU CONSIDER INDICATED):

103	Surgical approach and traction be avoided, physical therapy to be initiated later.	**103**	[Fractures do not heal. Leg suppurates and gangrene supervenes.]
104	Reduction and treatment by continuous traction after giving Demerol	**104**	[Fractures eventually heal but do not remain stable and result in deformity of the leg.]
105	General anesthesia	**105**	[Given.]
106	Spinal or epidural anesthesia	**106**	[Given.]
107	Local anesthesia	**107**	[Area of compound fracture infiltrated.]
108	Reduction of deformity of the fractured limb by longitudinal traction, no cast applied	**108**	[Fractures do not heal. Leg suppurates and gangrene supervenes.]

109	Temporary management in traction, then surgery	**109**	[Traction applied; surgery scheduled.]
110	Surgical resection of the loose bone fragment from the region of the sciatic nerve	**110**	[Bone removed. At operation the nerve appeared intact.]
111	Fixation with screws	**111**	[Done.]
112	Surgical treatment be deferred for six months until patient is rehabilitated from other injuries	**112**	[Leg fractures do not heal and amputation becomes necessary.]
113	Hip pinning	**113**	[REVIEW FIGURE 46, PAGE 419.]
114	Manipulative reduction and cast immobilization	**114**	[Fractures eventually heal but do not remain stable and result in deformity of the leg.]
115	Pelvic sling suspension	**115**	[Leg fractures do not heal and amputation becomes necessary.]
116	Immobilization in a cast	**116**	[Done.]
117	Internal fixation with plate and screws	**117**	[Tibia fixed.]
118	Maintenance of reduction by skeletal traction, through the os calcis	**118**	[Done.]

IN TREATING THE LACERATIONS YOU WOULD (SELECT AS MANY AS YOU CONSIDER INDICATED):

119	Carefully debride the wounds	**119**	[Done.]
120	Undermine the scalp and close the lacerations	**120**	[Done.]
121	Close all the wounds with sutures	**121**	[Done.]

122	Leave the leg laceration open	**122**	[Area suppurates. Eventually heals with massive scar. Osteomyelitis, however, develops under wound.]

AT THIS TIME YOU WOULD (CHOOSE ONLY ONE):

123	Proceed to a systematic evaluation of the skelton, gastrointestinal tract, liver, and central nervous system for further evidence of serious injury if you have not already done so	**123**	[TURN TO SECTION 13-B, PAGE 196.]
124	Complete the history, physical, and routine laboratory evaluation if you have not already done so	**124**	[TURN TO SECTION 13-C, PAGE 199.]
125	Consider the urgent problems adequately dealt with and enter management of the recovery stage	**125**	[TURN TO SECTION 13-K, PAGE 212.]

SECTION 13-E

IN REPAIRING THE PATIENT'S LACERATIONS YOU WOULD (SELECT AS MANY AS YOU CONSIDER INDICATED):

126	Expose the pretibial wound, irrigate and cover immediately with sterile dressing	**126**	[Done.]
127	Administer general anesthesia	**127**	[Done.]
128	Use local anesthetic	**128**	[Area of compound fracture infiltrated.]
129	Use topical anesthetic	**129**	[Xylocaine jelly applied.]

130	Use a regional block; use spinal or epidural anesthesia; suture the leg wound	**130**	[Done.]
131	Surgically explore the posterior tibial artery of the right leg as an emergency procedure	**131**	[Artery found to be contused and compressed. Injury repaired.]
132	On second thought delay management of the lacerations for two weeks	**132**	[Lesion suppurates.]
133	Suture the scalp lacerations	**133**	[Done.]
134	Debride the wounds and then suture them	**134**	[Done.]
135	Ask a plastic surgeon to assist in the scalp laceration repairs	**135**	[He is glad to help. Laceration repaired.]

UNLESS OTHERWISE INSTRUCTED IN THE RESPONSE COLUMN TURN NOW TO SECTION 13-K

SECTION 13-F

IN MANAGING THE PATIENT'S SHOCK YOU WOULD (SELECT AS MANY AS YOU CONSIDER INDICATED):

136	Elevate patient's legs while maintaining the patient supine	**136**	[Patient has much pain.]
137	Raise foot of the stretcher (Trendelenburg position)	**137**	[No change.]
138	Raise the head of the stretcher	**138**	[Patient becomes dizzy.]
139	Keep the patient supine and flat	**139**	[Done.]
140	Pass a nasogastric tube	**140**	[Patient gags but the tube is passed.]
141	Administer oxygen by mask	**141**	[Done.]

142	Monitor heart and respiratory rate by indwelling catheter	**142**	[Catheter placed.]
143	Monitor central venous pressure by indwelling catheter	**143**	[Catheter placed.]
144	Monitor pulmonary artery pressure by Swan-Ganz catheter	**144**	[Catheter placed.]
145	Continue to monitor urine output	**145**	[Catheter in place. 130 cc of clear urine excreted.]
146	Measure forced expiratory volume	**146**	[Patient cannot comply with request.]
147	Monitor tidal volume, minute volume, sigh volume, and compliance by respirometer	**147**	[Values remain within normal limits.]
148	Measure blood volume	**148**	[6% of body weight (20% decrease).]
149	Determine total extracellular fluid	**149**	[Determination cannot be made at your hosptial.]
150	Monitor blood pH five times a day	**150**	[7.29 to 7.30.]
151	Monitor P_{O_2}, P_{CO_2} five times a day	**151**	[P_{O_2} — 75 mm Hg; P_{CO_2} — 50 mm Hg.]
152	Order chest film stat	**152**	[Heart size normal, lung fields clear.]
153	Determine cardiac output by dye dilution method	**153**	[Small decrease in cardiac output.]
154	Determine cardiac output by determining A-V O_2 difference	**154**	[Small decrease in cardiac output.]
155	Order hematocrit and hemoglobin	**155**	[Hgb — 12.4 g/100 ml; Hct — 35%.]

156	Order complete blood count	156	[WBC – 7000/ mm^3; differential: segmented neutrophils – 73%, lymphocytes – 22%, monocytes – 3%, eosinophils – 2%.]
157	Order electrolyte determination	157	[Na – 150 mEq/L; K – 5.8 mEq/L; Cl – 112 mEq/L.]
158	Order blood glucose stat	158	[130 mg/100 ml.]
159	Administer oxygen by naso-pharyngeal tube	159	[Patient gags, oxygen started, gives rise to sharp abdominal pain.]
160	Start IV with dextrose and water as well as 2 cc of levarterenol and wait for blood to arrive	160	[Given. Blood pressure rises a little but fluctuates.]
161	Start IV with Ringer's lactate	161	[Temporary improvement in vital signs. IGNORE INSTRUCTIONS AT THE END OF THIS SECTION; INSTEAD TURN TO SECTION 13-H PAGE 210 AS SOON AS YOU HAVE COMPLETED THIS SECTION.]
162	Start IV therapy with lactated Ringer's solution and a balanced salt solution	162	[Temporary improvement in vital signs. IGNORE INSTRUCTIONS AT THE END OF THIS SECTION; INSTEAD TURN TO SECTION 13-H PAGE 210 AS SOON AS YOU HAVE COMPLETED THIS SECTION.]
163	Administer Ringer's lactate and salt solution and proceed to dextran	163	[Continued improvement in vital signs. IGNORE INSTRUCTIONS AT THE END OF THIS SECTION; INSTEAD TURN TO SECTION 13-H PAGE 210 AS SOON AS YOU HAVE COMPLETED THIS SECTION.]

164	Administer Ringer's lactate, dextran and whole blood as it arrives	**164**	[Rapid improvement in vital signs. IGNORE INSTRUCTIONS AT THE END OF THIS SECTION; SECTION 13-H PAGE 210 AS SOON AS YOU HAVE COMPLETED THIS SECTION.]
165	Determine quantity of fluid to be administered by changes in the hematocrit	**165**	[Hct — 48%; seems not to reflect clinical status.]
166	Administer antibiotics parenterally	**166**	[Given.]
167	Administer steroids in the IV or by IV push	**167**	[Given. No change.]
168	Administer digitalis	**168**	[Given. No change.]
169	Produce hypothermia	**169**	[Patient's condition is not altered by this procedure.]
170	Administer epinephrine, levarterenol or isoproterenol	**170**	[Blood pressure rises temporarily.]
171	Prepare to administer dopamine if evidence of sharp drop in central venous pressure occurs	**171**	[IV prepared but central venous pressure does not fall significantly.]

UNLESS OTHERWISE DIRECTED IN THE RESPONSE COLUMN, TURN NOW TO SECTION 13-K

SECTION 13-G

AS YOU START TO WORK ON THIS ASPECT OF THE PATIENT'S PROBLEM, YOU NOTICE A SHARP DECLINE IN THE VITAL SIGNS. AT THIS TIME YOU WOULD (CHOOSE ONLY ONE):

172	Start immediate management of shock	**172**	[PROCEED TO SECTION 13-F, PAGE 206.]

173 Increase the rate of flow of the intravenous fluids

173 [Patient expires. END OF PROBLEM. TURN TO SECTION 13-K, PAGE 212.]

174 Call for assistance

174 [Surgeon arrives and relieves you of the problem. You are later told patient has done well. TURN TO SECTION 13-K, PAGE 212.]

SECTION 13-H

Vital Signs Are Now Stable

YOU WOULD NOW ORDER (CHOOSE ONLY ONE):

175 Morphine 15 mg or Demerol 75 mg IV

175 [Pain is relieved rapidly. IGNORE INSTRUCTIONS AT END OF THIS SECTION AND TURN NOW TO SECTION 13-J, PAGE 212.]

176 Demerol 100 mg by mouth every four hours

176 [Not much relief of pain.]

177 Darvon capsules one every four hours

177 [No relief of pain.]

178 Morphine 15 mg or Demerol 75 mg IM

178 [Pain is relieved in 20 minutes; IGNORE INSTRUCTIONS AT END OF THIS SECTION INSTEAD TURN NOW TO SECTION 13-J, PAGE 212.]

179 Morphine 40 mg or Demerol 150 mg IV

179 [Patient goes into acute respiratory failure; your efforts to restore breathing are unsuccessful. IGNORE INSTRUCTIONS AT END OF THIS SECTION AND TURN NOW TO SECTION 13-K, PAGE 212.]

UNLESS OTHERWISE DIRECTED IN THE RESPONSE COLUMN TURN NOW TO SECTION 13-K

SECTION 13-I

AT THIS TIME REVIEW FIGURES 45 AND 46, PAGE 419. THE FOLLOWING STRUCTURES APPEAR TO BE FRACTURED (SELECT AS MANY AS YOU CONSIDER ACCURATE):

180	The subtrochanteric part of the femoral shaft	**180**	[REVIEW FIGURE 46, PAGE 419.]
181	The trochanteric region of the right femur	**181**	[REVIEW FIGURE 46, PAGE 419.]
182	The right femoral neck	**182**	[REVIEW FIGURE 46, PAGE 419.]
183	A chondro-osseous fracture of the femoral head	**183**	[REVIEW FIGURE 46, PAGE 419.]
184	The posterior acetabular margin	**184**	[Radiologist concurs.]
185	The superior pubic ramus	**185**	[REVIEW FIGURE 46, PAGE 419.]
186	The inferior pubic ramus	**186**	[Radiologist concurs.]
187	The sacroiliac joint	**187**	[REVIEW FIGURE 46, PAGE 419.]
188	Central acetabulum	**188**	[Radiologist concurs.]
189	None of the above listed	**189**	[REVIEW FIGURE 46, PAGE 419.]
190	Compound fracture of the right tibia	**190**	[Radiologist concurs.]

RETURN TO SECTION 13-D AND COMPLETE IT FROM THE POINT AT WHICH YOU LEFT

SECTION 13-J

YOU WOULD NOW (CHOOSE ONLY ONE):

191 Proceed to a systematic evaluation of the skeleton, gastrointestinal tract, liver, and central nervous system for further evidence of serious injury

191 [TURN TO SECTION 13-B, PAGE 198.]

192 Complete the history, physical, and routine laboratory investigation if you have not already done so

192 [TURN TO SECTION 13-C, PAGE 199.]

193 Manage the skeletal injuries and lacerations if you have not already done so.

193 [TURN TO SECTION 13-D, PAGE 203.]

194 Deal with the lacerations if you have not already done so

194 [TURN TO SECTION 13-E, PAGE 203.]

SECTION 13-K

195 Record your diagnostic impressions below:

195 [The diagnoses as recorded on the patient's chart included (I) shock, (II) open fracture of right tibia, (III) fractures of posterior acetabular margin, the inferior pubic ramus and central acetabulum, (IV) multiple lacerations. SEE APPENDIX T FOR ADDITIONAL COMMENT AND RECOMMENDED MANAGEMENT. END OF PROBLEM 13.]

NOW DEVELOP RESPONSE 195 FOR ADDITIONAL INFORMATION AND INSTRUCTIONS

PROBLEM 14

A UTERINE CERVICAL LESION

The patient is a 42-year-old woman Para I. She has come to the clinic for evaluation of the lesion illustrated in Figure 23, page 413.

NOW CONTINUE WITH SECTION 14-A

SECTION 14-A

YOU WOULD RECOMMEND THAT THE FOLLOWING DIAGNOSTIC PROCEDURES BE ORDERED (SELECT AS MANY AS YOU CONSIDER INDICATED):

1	Pap smear	1	[Class 1]; negative for dyskaryotic cells.]
2	Biopsy of lesion	2	[The stratified squamous eipthelium shows no abnormality in cell morphology or maturation. Marked stromal infiltration by leukocytes and vascular hyperemia is noted.]
3	Conization of cervix	3	[The stratified squamous epithelium shows no abnormality in cell morphology or maturation. Marked stromal infiltration by leukocytes and vascular hyperemia is noted. No evidence of reserve cell hyperplasia is noted at the squamocolumnar junction.]
4	Dilatation and curettage	4	[Secretory endometrium.]

5	Wet smear, hanging drop preparation	5	[Many motile pear-shaped flagellates showing undulating membranes and appearing somewhat smaller than the adjacent vaginal squamous cells are seen.]
6	Wet smear, treated with 10% potassium hydroxide	6	[Much debris noted.]
7	Wet smear, treated with Gram's stain	7	[Many white blood cells and parabasal cells are seen; several pear-shaped forms showing flagellae, do[illegible] undulating membranes and a[illegible]yles are noted.]
8	Swab for culture on blood Agar 10% CO_2	8	[No growth in 72 hours.]
9	Swab for culture on simplified trypticase serum	9	[Active growth of trichomonads in 72 hours.]
10	Swab for culture on Nickerson's medium	10	[No growth in 72 hours.]
11	Swab for culture of bacterial pathogens	11	[No growth in 72 hours.]
12	Swab for guinea pig innoculation	12	[No growth in guinea pig.]
13	Scraping for dark field examination	13	[No *Treponema pallidum* seen.]
14	Scraping and stain for Donovan bodies	14	[None seen.]
15	Frei test	15	[A 2-mm area of erythema is noted at 48 hours.]
16	Purified protein derivative skin test	16	[Negative 1/1000 strength.]
17	STS	17	[Nonreactive.]

18	Fluorescent Treponema Antibody Absorption Test	**18**	[Nonreactive.]
19	Two-hour postprandial blood sugar	**19**	[94 mg/100 ml.]

UNLESS OTHERWISE DIRECTED IN THE RESPONSE COLUMN CONTINUE WITH SECTION 14-B

SECTION 14-B

YOU WOULD NOW RECOMMEND (CHOOSE ONLY ONE):

20	Close observation and reassurance without specific therapy at this time	**20**	[Two weeks later another physician requests your records on this patient who has consulted him about the same complaint. TURN TO SECTION 14-H, PAGE 218.]
21	Initiate treatment	**21**	[CONTINUE WITH SECTION 14-C.]

SECTION 14-C

YOU WOULD NOW RECOMMEND (CHOOSE ONLY ONE):

22	A treatment plan which includes medical management	**22**	[CONTINUE WITH SECTION 14-D, PAGE 216.]
23	A treatment plan which includes radiation therapy and/or surgical intervention but does not include medical management	**23**	[TURN TO SECTION 14-E, PAGE 217.]

SECTION 14-D

YOU WOULD NOW RECOMMEND (SELECT AS MANY AS YOU CONSIDER INDICATED):

24	Triple sulfa vaginal cream at bedtime for 10 days	**24**	[No improvement noted while the patient was on this therapy.]
25	Nystatin vaginal suppositories 100,000 units, one at bedtime for 15 days	**25**	[No improvement noted while the patient was on this therapy.]
26	Procaine penicillin G with 2% aluminum monosterate, 4.8 million units over 7-14 days	**26**	[No improvement noted; patient develops urticaria.]
27	Benzanthine penicillin G, 1.8 million units in a single injection	**27**	[No improvement; patient develops urticaria.]
28	Stilbesterol vaginal suppository, 0.5 mg, one at bedtime for 21 days	**28**	[No improvement noted while the patient was on this therapy.]
29	Metronidazole tablets (Flagyl), 250 mg by mouth three times a day for 10 days for patient and husband	**29**	[The patient's condition improves.]
30	Tetracycline, 500 mg by mouth every six hours for five days	**30**	[No improvement noted while the patient was on this therapy; patient becomes sun sensitive.]
31	(INH) Isoniazide hydrozide, 5 mg per kg body weight plus para-aminosalicylic acid (PAS) 3 gms four times a day	**31**	[No improvement noted; patient develops gastric distress and acneiform eruption.]
32	1500 calorie American Diabetic Association diet	**32**	[No improvement noted while the patient was on this therapy.]
33	6-Mercaptopurine 2.5 mg per kg per day	**33**	[No improvement noted; patient develops agranulocytosis.]

UNLESS OTHERWISE DIRECTED IN THE RESPONSE COLUMN CONTINUE WITH SECTION 14-E

SECTION 14-E

YOU WOULD NOW RECOMMEND (CHOOSE ONLY ONE):

34	A treatment plan which includes radiation therapy	**34**	[CONTINUE WITH SECTION 14-F, PAGE 217.]
35	A treatment plan which includes surgical therapy but not radiation therapy	**35**	[TURN TO SECTION 14-G, PAGE 217.]
36	No further treatment	**36**	[TURN TO SECTION 14-H, PAGE 218.]

SECTION 14-F

AS RADIATION THERAPY YOU WOULD NOW RECOMMEND (SELECT AS MANY AS YOU CONSIDER INDICATED):

37	External – 4000r to Point B intracavitary tandem and ovoids – 6000r to Point A	**37**	[A radiation reaction ensues; patient requests consultation and transfer to another physician.]
38	Intracavitary Heyman packing with Campbell applicators – 5000r to the uterus; ovoids to vaginal vault; 5000r to vaginal vault mucosa	**38**	[A radiation reaction ensues; patient threatens to consult her attorney, and requests transfer to another physician.]

UNLESS OTHERWISE DIRECTED IN THE RESPONSE COLUMN TURN TO SECTION 14-H

SECTION 14-G

YOU WOULD NOW RECOMMEND (SELECT AS MANY AS YOU CONSIDER INDICATED):

39	Local excision	**39**	[Done; pathology report: mild, nonspecific chronic inflamatory cervicitis. No improvement noted.]

40	Cold knife conization of cervix	**40**	[Done; chronic cervicitis; no improvement noted.]
41	Radial cautery of cervix	**41**	[Done; no improvement.]
42	Total hysterectomy	**42**	[Done; pathologist's report notes normal uterus, cervix, and ovaries. Tissue Committee asks you to appear before them.]
43	Radical hysterectomy and lymphadenectomy	**43**	[Done; pathologist's report notes normal uterus, cervix, adnexal tissue, ovaries, and nodes. Tissue Committee asks you to appear before them.]

UNLESS OTHERWISE DIRECTED IN THE RESPONSE COLUMN CONTINUE WITH SECTION 14-H

SECTION 14-H

44	Record your diagnoses below: ____________________ ____________________ ____________________ ____________________ ____________________	**44**	[The diagnosis as recorded on the chart for this patient is trichomonal infection of cervix. SEE APPENDIX O FOR ADDITIONAL COMMENT AND RECOMMENDED MANAGEMENT. END OF PROBLEM 14.]

NOW DEVELOP RESPONSE 44 FOR ADDITIONAL INFORMATION AND INSTRUCTIONS

PROBLEM 15

A UTERINE CERVICAL LESION

The patient is a 38-year-old woman Para IV. She has come to the clinic for postcoital spotting and evaluation of the cervical lesion illustrated in Figure 24, page 413.

NOW CONTINUE WITH SECTION 15-A

SECTION 15-A

AT THIS TIME, YOU WOULD RECOMMEND (SELECT AS MANY AS YOU CONSIDER INDICATED):

1	Pap smear	1	[Class IV.]
2	Punch biopsy of the lesion	2	[The stratified squamous epithelium of the specimens submitted shows disorderly proliferation of cells from basal layers to the surface. Many cells show large atypical nuclei in various stages of mitotic division. Giant nuclear forms containing course chromatin patterns and many nucleoli are also seen underlying the stroma which has been invaded by small nests of atypical cells.]
3	Tine test	3	[No erythema or induration at 72 hours.]

4	Dilatation and fractional curettage	**4**	[The uterus sounds to 6 cm. The endometrial cavity [illegible] contour. The cervical lesion [illegible] confined to the cervix. The [illegible] proliferative endometrium [illegible] significant abnormality [illegible] glandular [illegible] in the endocervical specimen [illegible]
5	Wet smear, hanging drop preparation	**5**	[Many red blood cells, white blood cells and bacteria are found.]
6	Wet smear, treated with 10% potassium hydroxide	**6**	[Much debris seen as well as cellular outlines; no yeast spores or hyphae identified.]
7	Wet smear, treated with Gram's stain	**7**	[Many red blood cells, white blood cells and tadpole cells seen.]
8	Swab for culture on blood Agar under 10% CO_2	**8**	[No growth in 72 hours.]
9	Swab for culture on simplified trypticase serum	**9**	[No growth in 72 hours.]
10	Swab for culture on Nickerson's medium	**10**	[No growth in 72 hours.]
11	Swab for culture of bacterial pathogens	**11**	[No growth of pathogenic organisms in 72 hours.]
12	Swab for guinea pig innoculation	**12**	[No growth in guinea pig.]
13	Scraping for dark field examination	**13**	[No *Treponema pallidum* seen.]
14	Scraping and stain for Donnovan bodies	**14**	[None seen.]

15	Total protein (serum)	**15**
16	Serum electrolytes	**16**
17	Frei test	**17**
18	Blood group and type	**18**
19	CO_2 combining power	**19**
20	STS	**20**
21	Protein-bound iodine	**21**
22	Fluorescent Treponema Antibody Absorption Test	**22**
23	Two-hour postprandial blood sugar	**23**
24	Blood urea nitrogen	**24**
25	Creatinine (serum)	**25**
26	Repeat speculum examination of the cervical lesion	**26**
27	Bimanual pelvic examination and rectal examination	**27**
28	Blood pressure	**28**
29	Intravenous pyelogram	**29**
30	Urinalysis	**30**

31	Sigmoidoscopic examination	31	[Normal rectal mucosa.]
32	Cystoscopic examination	32	[Normal urinary bladder.]
33	Electrocardiogram	33	[Normal.]
34	Complete blood count	34	[Hgb – 12 g/100 ml; WBC – 11,000/mm^3.]
35	Serum protein electrophoresis	35	[Normal electrophoretic pattern.]
36	Serum glutamic oxalacetic transaminase	36	[34 IU/L.]
37	Serum glutamic pyruvic transaminase	37	[28 IU/L.]
38	Radiologic survey of the skeleton	38	[Bones appear intact and of good density. There are no areas of radiolucency. Normal long bones, spine, skull, pelvis.]
39	Chest x-ray (PA and lateral)	39	[Lung fields show no evidence of congestion or consolidation. Diaphragm is smooth, costophrenic angles are clear, and the cardiac shadow is normal.]
40	Barium enema	40	[The colon, sigmoid and splenic flexures, hepatic flexures, and cecum are well visualized and fill without deformity. The mucosal pattern is normal.]

UNLESS OTHERWISE DIRECTED IN THE RESPONSE COLUMN CONTINUE WITH SECTION 15-B

SECTION 15-B

YOU WOULD NOW RECOMMEND (CHOOSE ONLY ONE):

41	Close observation and reassurance without specific therapy at this time	**41**	[Patient's symptoms become worse and she requests transfer to another physician for treatment. TURN TO SECTION 15-H, PAGE 227.]
42	Initiate treatment	**42**	[CONTINUE WITH SECTION 15-C.]

SECTION 15-C

YOU WOULD NOW RECOMMEND (CHOOSE ONLY ONE):

43	A treatment plan which includes medical management	**43**	[CONTINUE WITH SECTION 15-D.]
44	A treatment plan which includes radiation therapy or surgical intervention but does not include medical management	**44**	[TURN TO SECTION 15-E, PAGE 224.]

SECTION 15-D

YOU WOULD NOW RECOMMEND (SELECT AS MANY AS YOU CONSIDER INDICATED):

45	Triple sulfa vaginal cream at bedtime for 10 days	**45**	[No improvement noted while the patient was on this therapy.]
46	Nystatin vaginal suppositories 100,000 units, one at bedtime for 15 days	**46**	[No improvement in symptoms.]
47	Procaine penicillin G with 2% aluminum monosterate, 4.8 million units over 7-14 days	**47**	[No improvement in symptoms.]

48	Benzanthine penicillin G, 1.8 units in a single injection	**48**	[No improvement in symptoms.]
49	Stilbesterol vaginal suppository 0.5 mg, one at bedtime for 21 days	**49**	[No improvement. Postcoital bleeding becomes worse.]
50	Metronidazole tablets (Flagyl) 250 mg, by mouth three times a day for 10 days	**50**	[No improvement. Postcoital bleeding increases.]
51	Chlorambucil, 0.2 mg per kg per day	**51**	[No improvement. Patient becomes hyperpigmented. Agranulocytosis is noted in three weeks.]
52	(INH) Isoniazide hydrozide 5 mg per kg body weight plus paramino-salicylic acid (PAS) 3 grams four times a day daily	**52**	[No improvement. Patient complains about gastric distress.]
53	Premarin vaginal cream at bedtime for 10 days	**53**	[No improvement. Postcoital bleeding increases.]
54	6-Mercaptopurine, 2.5 mg per kg per day	**54**	[No improvement. Agranulocytosis noted in three weeks.]

UNLESS OTHERWISE DIRECTED IN THE RESPONSE COLUMN CONTINUE WITH SECTION 15-E

SECTION 15-E

YOU WOULD NOW RECOMMEND (CHOOSE ONLY ONE):

55	A treatment plan which includes radiation therapy	**55**	[CONTINUE WITH SECTION 15-F, PAGE 225.]
56	A treatment plan which includes surgical therapy but not radiation therapy	**56**	[TURN TO SECTION 15-G, PAGE 226.]

57	No further treatment	57	[TURN TO SECTION 15-H, PAGE 227.]
58	Combined radiation therapy and surgery	58	[Your suggestion is brought before the Tumor Board. Their view is that the complications (ie, a ureterovaginal fistula) exceed the possible benefits from the combined therapy. MAKE ANOTHER CHOICE IN THIS SECTION.]

SECTION 15-F

AS RADIATION THERAPY YOU WOULD NOW RECOMMEND (CHOOSE ONLY ONE):

59	External – 4000r to entire pelvis followed by intracavitary tandem and vaginal ovoids – 6000r in divided doses	59	[Tumor Board approves plan of management as adequate and appropriate for this stage of cervical lesion. CONTINUE WITH SECTION 15-G, PAGE 226.]
60	Intracavitary Heyman packing with Campbell applicators – 5000r to the serosal surface; ovoids to vaginal vault, 5000r to vaginal vault mucosa	60	[Tumor Board overrules this plan with comment that this therapy is both inappropriate and inadequate for this lesion. MAKE ANOTHER CHOICE IN THIS SECTION.]
61	Vaginal mold applied directly to lesion to a surface dose of 10,000r	61	[Tumor Board overrules this plan with comment that this is inadequate therapy for this lesion. MAKE ANOTHER CHOICE IN THIS SECTION.]

62	Radiation "strip therapy" to the entire abdomen with kidneys shielded	62	[Tumor Board overrules this plan with comment that this therapy is both inadequate and inappropriate for this lesion. MAKE ANOTHER CHOICE IN THIS SECTION.]

SECTION 15-G

YOU WOULD NOW RECOMMEND (SELECT AS MANY AS YOU CONSIDER INDICATED):

63	Local excision	63	[Done; lesion recurs in six months.]
64	Cryosurgery	64	[Done; lesion recurs in six months.]
65	Radial cautery of cervix	65	[Done; lesion recurs in six months.]
66	Total abdominal hysterectomy with salpingo-oophorectomy	66	[Chief of OB-GYN Department suggests this plan is inadequate for this stage of cervical lesion. MAKE ANOTHER CHOICE IN THIS SECTION.]
67	Radical hysterectomy and bilaterial pelvic lymphadenectomy	67	[Tumor Board agrees with this type of surgery. The surgery is performed. The patient returns six months later without evidence of recurrence.]
68	Vaginal hysterectomy	68	[Chief of OB-GYN Department comments that this is both inappropriate and inadequate therapy for this cervical leison. MAKE ANOTHER CHOICE IN THIS SECTION.]

UNLESS OTHERWISE DIRECTED IN THE RESPONSE COLUMN CONTINUE WITH SECTION 15-H

SECTION 15-H

69 Record your diagnosis and prognosis below:

____

____

____

____

____

69 [The diagnosis and prognosis as recorded on the chart for this patient was invasive squamous cell carcinoma of the cervix, international stage 1b. Prognosis – approximately 80% five-year survival, if properly managed with radical radiotherapy or radical surgery. SEE APPENDIX J FOR ADDITIONAL COMMENT AND RECOMMENDED MANAGEMENT; END OF PROBLEM 15.]

NOW DEVELOP RESPONSE 69 FOR ADDITIONAL INFORMATION AND INSTRUCTIONS

PROBLEM 16

THE SEVERELY BREATH-LIMITED PATIENT

You are called by your intern to see a comatose 53-year-old white man admitted to your service three hours ago via the hospital Emergency Room. The intern tells you that the patient was drowsy but conscious and oriented on admission and that he gave a history of increasing dyspnea on exertion and an increasingly productive cough for one month. One week prior to admission he developed malaise and recurring fever of 102F. Three days before admission his somnolence, periodic mental confusion, and cyanosis of the lips were noticed by his wife, which symptoms continued until admission.

The intern's physical examination revealed: temperature — 101F, blood pressure — 160/90 mm Hg, and pulse — 110 per minute. There was moderate cyanosis of the lips and finger tips and the latter were "slightly" clubbed. The anteroposterior diameter of the chest was increased, respiratory excursions were diminished, breath sounds were distant and faint over both lung fields, and diffuse expiratory wheezing and prolonged expiration were present. Crepitant rales were heard at the right base posteriorly. A gallop rhythm was heard at the lower left sternal border, and 1+ ankle edema was present.

Because of dyspnea and cyanosis the intern administered oxygen by face mask at the conclusion of his examination.

NOW CONTINUE WITH SECTION 16-A

SECTION 16-A

YOU WOULD FIRST (CHOOSE ONLY ONE):

1	Elicit further history from the patient's wife and daughter	1	[Patient's condition deteriorating rapidly; MAKE ANOTHER CHOICE IN THIS SECTION.]
2	Increase oxygen flow to mask	2	[Patient's condition deteriorating rapidly; MAKE ANOTHER CHOICE IN THIS SECTION.]
3	Order urgent laboratory tests and additional diagnostic procedures	3	[Patient's condition deteriorates rapidly; MAKE ANOTHER CHOICE IN THIS SECTION.]
4	Perform your own physical examination	4	[Patient unable to cooperate, condition deteriorating rapidly; MAKE ANOTHER CHOICE IN THIS SECTION.]
5	Remove oxygen mask	5	[Done; patient's color becomes more cyanotic but his respirations improve; TURN TO SECTION 16-F, PAGE 237.]
6	Order blood gas determinations	6	[Blood drawn and sent to lab; MAKE ANOTHER CHOICE IN THIS SECTION.]

SECTION 16-B

IN PERFORMING THE PHYSICAL EXAMINATION YOU WOULD BE PARTICULARLY INTERESTED TO CHECK (SELECT AS MANY AS YOU CONSIDER ESPECIALLY PERTINENT; YOU CAN RETURN TO THIS SECTION AT ANY TIME TO OBTAIN ANY ADDITIONAL INFORMATION YOU MAY REQUIRE ABOUT INITIAL PHYSICAL FINDINGS):

7	Pulse, respirations, blood pressure, and temperature	7	[Pulse — 110 per minute; respirations — 4 per minute, shallow and irregular; blood pressure — 200/100 mm Hg; temperature — 101F.]

8	Rectal examination	**8**	[Brown stool on glove, guaiac test negative.]
9	State of consciousness	**9**	[Semicomatose; responding only to painful stimuli.]
10	External genitalia	**10**	[1+ scrotal edema; penis normal; no varicosities.]
11	Color of lips and nail beds	**11**	[Cyanotic.]
12	Peripheral arterial pulses	**12**	[Full pulses — equal on right and left.]
13	Neck	**13**	[Veins distended to angle of jaw; prominent positive wave just preceding carotid systolic impulse.]
14	Ocular fundi	**14**	[Bilateral papilledema; arteries normal, veins distended.]
15	Neurologic examination	**15**	[Tendon reflexes hypoactive but symmetrically present; there is a flapping tremor of hands inconstantly elicited bilaterally; moves all four extremities in response to painful stimuli; plantar reflexes are flexor bilaterally.]
16	Heart	**16**	[Unchanged from findings noted by the intern.]
17	Lungs	**17**	[Unchanged from findings noted by the intern.]

YOU WOULD NOW (CHOOSE ONLY ONE):

18	Elicit further history if you have not already done so	**18**	[TURN TO SECTION 16-E, PAGE 235.]

19	Order immediate laboratory tests and additional diagnostic procedures if you have not already done so and/or review those previously obtained	19	[CONTINUE WITH SECTION 16-C.]
20	Carefully follow patient's clinical progress without further evaluation and therapy at this time	20	[Patient's condition begins to deteriorate; you are called by the intern at midnight and told that the patient has expired after a brief period of coma. TURN TO SECTION 16-H, PAGE 237.]
21	Initiate long-term management	21	[TURN TO SECTION 16-G, PAGE 238.]
22	Order extensive series of pulmonary function tests and await results	22	[Patient unable to complete studies. MAKE ANOTHER CHOICE IN THIS SECTION.]

SECTION 16-C

TO DIRECT YOUR CARE OF THE PATIENT OVER THE NEXT FEW HOURS YOU WOULD NOW ORDER THE FOLLOWING DETERMINATIONS (SELECT AS MANY AS YOU CONSIDER INDICATED):

23	Hemoglobin	23	[20 g/100 ml.]
24	Hematocrit	24	[57%.]
25	White blood cell count and differential	25	[WBC – 10,000/mm^3; differential: polymorphs – 80%; lymphocytes – 15%, eosinophils – 5%.]
26	Urinalysis	26	[Specific gravity – 1.018, sugar – 0, albumin – trace, acetone – 0, cells: 0 – 3 hpf.]
27	Thyroxine (Pattee-Murphy)	27	[5 μg/ml.]
28	Plasma sodium and potassium	28	[Na – 138 mEq/L; K – 4.6 mEq/L.]

29	Spinal fluid pressure, microscopic examination, and sugar	**29**	[Opening pressure: 200 mm H_2O; clear fluid; no cells; protein — 36 mg/100 ml; glucose — 68 mg/100 ml.]
30	Plasma chloride and bicarbonate	**30**	[Chlorides — 82 mEq/L; bicarbonate — 36 mEq/L.]
31	Smear and culture of sputum	**31**	[Smear: encapsulated gram-positive diplococci; culture: type 7 pneumococci.]
32	Electrocardiogram	**32**	[SEE FIGURE 4, PAGE 407.]
33	Chest x-ray	**33**	[SEE FIGURES 31 AND 32, PAGE 415.]
34	Arterial blood P_{CO_2}	**34**	[86 mm Hg.]
35	Venous pressure	**35**	[230 mm H_2O.]
36	Barium swallow	**36**	[Patient's condition makes test impossible to perform.]
37	Pulmonary function tests	**37**	[Consultation submitted. Patient deteriorates during attempted performance of vital capacity.]
38	Arterial blood pH	**38**	[7.16.]
39	Blood urea nitrogen	**39**	[24 mg/100 ml.]
40	Serum glutamic oxalacetic transaminase	**40**	[35 IU/L.]
41	Albumin/globulin ratio	**41**	[Albumin — 4.5 g, globulin — 3.0 g; A/G ratio — 1.5:1.]
42	Serum uric acid	**42**	[4.8 mg/100 ml.]
43	Serum bilirubin	**43**	[0.7 mg/100 ml.]
44	Alkaline phosphatase	**44**	[20 units (King-Armstrong).]

45 Arterial blood P_{O_2} — 45 [85 mm Hg.]

OU WOULD NOW (CHOOSE ONLY ONE):

46 Elicit further history if you have not already done so — 46 [TURN TO SECTION 16-E, PAGE 235.]

47 Perform your own physical examination if you have not already done so — 47 [TURN TO SECTION 16-B, PAGE 229.]

48 Initiate long-term management — 48 [TURN TO SECTION 16-G, PAGE 238.]

49 Carefully follow patient's clinical progress without further evaluation and therapy at this time — 49 [Patient's condition begins to deteriorate; you are called by the intern at midnight and told that the patient has expired after a brief period of coma. TURN TO SECTION 16-H, PAGE 239.]

50 Order extensive series of pulmonary function tests and await results — 50 [Patient unable to complete studies. MAKE ANOTHER CHOICE IN THIS SECTION.]

SECTION 16-D

S EMERGENCY TREATMENT YOU WOULD NOW ORDER (SELECT AS MANY AS YOU CONSIDER INDICATED):

51 Continous intravenous infusion of ethamivan (vanillic diethylamide) solution — 51 [No improvement.]

52 100% oxygen by nasal catheter at 6 liter per minute — 52 [The patient's respirations decrease; he becomes apneic and expires. TURN TO SECTION 16-H, PAGE 239.]

53 Tracheostomy and respirator — 53 [Done; patient slowly improves.]

54	A mixture of 90% oxygen and 10% CO_2	54	[Patient's condition deteriorates.]
55	Patient placed in a tank respirator	55	[Patient slowly improves.]
56	Direct mouth to mouth resuscitation	56	[After 30 minutes no change in patient's condition.]
57	Intermittent positive pressure using a Bennett respirator with 40% oxygen	57	[Patient improves slowly.]
58	Histamine 1: 1000 by aerosol	58	[The patient develops intense bronchoconstriction, becomes apneic and dies. TURN TO SECTION 16-H, PAGE 239.]
59	Insertion of a cuffed endotracheal tube	59	[Done.]
60	Pneumoperitoneum	60	[500 cc of air injected into peritoneum; respirations decrease; patient's condition deteriorates.]
61	Therapeutic bronchosocopy	61	[Much blood tinged, viscid, green mucus is aspirated; patient improves.]

YOU WOULD NOW (CHOOSE ONLY ONE):

62	Elicit further history	62	[CONTINUE WITH SECTION 16-E, PAGE 235.]
63	Perform your own physical examination	63	[TURN TO SECTION 16-B, PAGE 229.]
64	Order immediate laboratory tests and additional diagnostic procedures	64	[TURN TO SECTION 16-C, PAGE 231.]

65	Carefully follow patient's clinical progress without further evaluation and therapy at this time	65	Patient's condition begins to deteriorate; you are called by the intern at midnight and told that the patient has expired after a brief period of coma. TURN TO SECTION 16-H, PAGE 2[illegible]9.]
66	Initiate long-term management	66	[TURN TO SECTION 16-G, PAGE 238.]
67	Order extensive series of pulmonary function tests and await results	67	[Patient unable to complete studies: MAKE ANOTHER CHOICE IN THIS SECTION.]

SECTION 16-E

IN TAKING YOUR HISTORY, YOU ARE PARTICULARLY INTERESTED TO INQUIRE ABOUT (SELECT AS MANY AS YOU CONSIDER ESPECIALLY PERTINENT; YOU CAN RETURN TO THIS SECTION AT ANY TIME TO OBTAIN ANY ADDITIONAL HISTORICAL INFORMATION YOU MAY REQUIRE):

68	Psychosexual adjustments	68	[Wife says patient's libido has been very low for several years; asks how this information helps in his present condition.]
69	Joint symptoms	69	[Occasional mild stiffness and soreness in shoulders, knees and hips in recent years.]
70	Smoking habits	70	[One and one-half packs daily since age 15.]
71	Bowel habits	71	[Regular one per day; no recent change.]
72	Alcohol intake	72	[Occasional weekend drinker, rarely drinks heavily.]

73	Dyspnea	73	[Onset of chronic exertional dyspnea six years ago following an episode of pneumonia; slow progressive worsening since then.]
74	Recent abdominal surgery	74	[None.]
75	Past history of pneumonia	75	[Three episodes of pneumonia: nine, six, and two years ago.]
76	Family history of urinary lithiasis	76	[None known.]
77	Chronic cough	77	[Smoker's cough since age 40.]
78	Intermittent claudication	78	[No leg pain on exertion.]
79	Headache	79	[About once a month, relieved with aspirin.]
80	Amount and character of sputum	80	[Two to four tablespoonfuls of tenaceous and often yellowish sputum for past three years; small amounts of white sputum from age 40.]
81	Epigastric pain and heartburn	81	[Epigastric pain eight years ago, relieved by food; duodenal ulcer found on x-ray; responded to diet and antacids.]
82	Change in weight	82	[20-pound weight loss in past year associated with mild chronic anorexia.]
83	Exposure to industrial dust and fumes	83	[Worked as a soft coal miner from age 17 to 45.]
84	Hematuria	84	[None noticed.]

85	Wheezing	**85**	[Intermittent attacks of wheezing and shortness of breath for past six years; wheezes much of the time currently, especially during inclement weather.]

YOU WOULD NOW (CHOOSE ONLY ONE):

86	Perform your own physical examination if you have not already done so	**86**	[TURN TO SECTION 16-B, PAGE 229.]
87	Order immediate laboratory tests and additional diagnostic procedures if you have not already done so and/or review tests previously ordered	**87**	[TURN TO SECTION 16-C, PAGE 231.]
88	Carefully follow patient's clinical progress without further evaluation and therapy at this time	**88**	[Patient's condition begins to deteriorate; you are called by the intern at midnight and told that the patient has expired after a brief period of coma. TURN TO SECTION 16-H, PAGE 239.]
89	Initiate long-term management	**89**	[TURN TO SECTION 16-G, PAGE 238.]
90	Order extensive series of pulmonary function tests and await results	**90**	[Patient unable to complete tests. MAKE ANOTHER CHOICE IN THIS SECTION.]

SECTION 16-F

YOU WOULD NOW (CHOOSE ONLY ONE):

91	Elicit further history from wife and daughter	**91**	[Patient's condition rapidly deteriorating. MAKE ANOTHER CHOICE IN THIS SECTION.]

92	Perform your own physical examination	**92**	[Patient's condition rapidly deteriorating: MAKE ANOTHER CHOICE IN THIS SECTION.]
93	Initiate emergency treatment	**93**	[TURN TO SECTION 16-D, PAGE 233.]
94	Order immediate laboratory tests and additional diagnostic procedures	**94**	[Patient's condition deteriorating rapidly; make another choice in this section.]
95	Order blood gas determinations	**95**	[Blood drawn and sent to lab; make another choice in this section.]

SECTION 16-G

YOU WOULD NOW (SELECT AS MANY AS YOU CONSIDER INDICATED):

96	Refer the patient to a specialist in pulmonary diseases	**96**	[The patient's management is accepted by the physician to whom you refer the patient. DO NOT MAKE ANY MORE CHOICES IN THIS SECTION; TURN NOW TO SECTION 16-H, PAGE 239.]
97	Establish long-term therapy aimed at reducing infection, assisting ventilation and reducing bronchial obstruction	**97**	[The patient remains relatively well, but a slow decrease in ventilatory capacity continues.]
98	Discharge the patient after the acute episode has subsided	**98**	[You hear that the patient has died of CO_2 narcosis following recurrent bouts of pneumonia. DO NOT MAKE ANY MORE CHOICES IN THIS SECTION; TURN NOW TO SECTION 16-H, PAGE 239.]

99	Monitor blood gases periodically	99	[Done.]
100	Prescribe maintenance dose of ephedrine and aminopyline suppositories	100	[Temporary improvement in patient's condition is followed by CO_2 narcosis and death. DO NOT MAKE ANY MORE CHOICES IN THIS SECTION; TURN NOW TO SECTION 16-H, PAGE 239.]

UNLESS OTHERWISE DIRECTED IN THE RESPONSE COLUMN CONTINUE WITH SECTION 16-H

SECTION 16-H

101	Record your diagnoses below: ____________________ ____________________ ____________________ ____________________	101	[The complete diagnosis as recorded on the patient's chart was obstructive emphysema. SEE APPENDIX Q FOR ADDITIONAL COMMENT AND RECOMMENDED MANAGEMENT. END OF PROBLEM 16.]

NOW DEVELOP RESPONSE 101 FOR ADDITIONAL INFORMATION AND INSTRUCTIONS

PROBLEM 17

A URINARY PROBLEM IN A CHILD

As admitting doctor on the pediatric service you see a nine-year-old boy, A. A., who has been hospitalized because of pallor, lethargy of three week's duration, 3+ proteinuria, and hypertension (blood pressure 160/110 mm Hg recorded by his private physician on the day of admission).

NOW CONTINUE WITH SECTION 17-A

SECTION 17-A

YOU WOULD NOW (CHOOSE ONLY ONE):

1 Request a urologic consultation

1 [The consultant requests information about the history, performs a physical examination, and orders the following studies: intravenous pyelogram, serum creatinine and creatinine clearance determinations, and voided cystourethrogram before giving an opinion. IF YOU WISH TO COMPLETE THE WORK-UP YOURSELF, TURN NOW TO SECTION 17-G, PAGE 252; IF YOU WISH TO TRANSFER THE PATIENT TO THE UROLOGIST TURN NOW TO SECTION 17-H, PAGE 252.]

2 Order appropriate laboratory tests — [TURN TO SECTION 17-C, PAGE 248.]

3 Start emergency therapy — [CONTINUE WITH SECTION 17-B.]

4 Obtain further history of present and past illnesses — [TURN TO SECTION 17-F, PAGE 249.]

5 Perform a thorough physical examination — [TURN TO SECTION 17-D, PAGE 245.]

SECTION 17-B

YOUR IMMEDIATE THERAPEUTIC PROGRAM WOULD NOW INCLUDE (SELECT AS MANY AS YOU CONSIDER INDICATED):

6 Peritoneal dialysis

7 Blood transfusion – one unit

8 Calcium supplement

9 Extracorporeal hemodialysis

10 Hydralazine and reserpine

11 Hydralazine and apresoline

6 [Patient's condition deteriorates.]

7 [Hemoglobin increased 0.5 g/100 ml, patient has a chill. General condition unchanged.]

8 [Calcium gluconate 1 g three times a day given. No change in condition.]

9 [You are informed that the patient must wait to enter the dialysis unit because of a long waiting list.]

10 [Blood pressure decreases, mild orthostatic hypotension, and decrease in urine volume ensues.]

11 [Nurse questions order as recorded.]

12	Renal transplant	**12**	[The tissue typing has been done. The surgical consultant feels that the case has not been adequately studied and recommends further work-up before this procedure is given serious consideration.]
13	Low-protein diet	**13**	[No change in condition.]
14	Penicillin for 10 days	**14**	[*Proteus* cleared from urine.]
15	Sodium bicarbonate supplementation	**15**	[0.6 g three times a day ordered; no overt change in patient's condition.]
16	Dietary iron supplement	**16**	[Given, patient continues to deteriorate.]
17	Urologic consultation	**17**	[The consultant requests information about the history, does a physical examination and orders the following studies: intravenous pyelogram, serum creatinine and creatinine clearance determinations, and voided cystourethrogram before giving an opinion. IF YOU WISH TO TRANSFER THE PATIENT TO THE UROLOGIST, TURN NOW TO SECTION 17-H, PAGE 252; IF NOT TURN TO SECTION 17-I, PAGE 252 WHEN YOU HAVE COMPLETED THIS SECTION.]

UNLESS OTHERWISE DIRECTED IN THE RESPONSE COLUMN, TURN NOW TO SECTION 17-I, PAGE 252

SECTION 17-C

YOU WOULD NOW ORDER THE FOLLOWING DETERMINATIONS (SELECT AS MANY AS YOU CONSIDER INDICATED):

18	Hemoglobin and hematocrit	**18**	[Hgb – 7.0 g/100 ml, Hct – 20%.]
19	White blood cell count	**19**	[10,000/mm^3.]
20	Differential	**20**	[Polymorphonuclear leukocytes – 50%, lymphocytes – 35%, monocytes – 10%, eosinophils – 5%.]
21	Blood smear	**21**	[Red blood cells – normocytic, normochromic; platelets – adequate; WBC – no immature cells seen.]
22	Urinalysis	**22**	[Specific gravity 1.009; pH – 6.0; protein – 3+, sugar – 0, acetone – 0, cells: 2-3 RBC, 30-40 WBC, 1-3 hyaline and granular casts per hpf.]
23	Serum carbon dioxide	**23**	[12 mEq/L.]
24	Serum glutamic oxalacetic transaminase	**24**	[20 IU/L.]
25	Blood urea nitrogen	**25**	[162 mg/100 ml.]
26	Serum iron and unsaturated iron-binding capacity	**26**	[Fe: 90 μg/100 ml: iron-binding capacity: 325 μg/100 ml.]
27	Intravenous pyelogram	**27**	[Bilateral dilated tortuous ureters, dilated pelvices and delayed excretion.]
28	Phenolsulfonphthalein test	**28**	[10% excretion at the end of 90 minutes.]

29	X-ray of long bones	29	[Examination of the long bones fails to reveal any asymmetry, reactive bone formation, lytic lesion or fractures; normal [illegible] skeletal structures.]
30	Serum calcium and inorganic phosphorus	30	[Ca: 5.0 mEq/L; P: [illegible].0 mEq/L.]
31	Serum sodium	31	[135 mEq/L.]
32	Serum potassium	32	[5.2 mEq/L.]
33	Blood glucose	33	[84 mg/100 ml.]
34	Sedimentation rate	34	[24 mm/hour (Wintrobe).]
35	Electrocardiogram	35	[The QRS complexes suggest left ventricular hypertrophy.]
36	Clean, voided, midstream urine culture	36	[4.3×10^{6} colonies/cc of proteu mirabilis.]
37	Antistreptolysin titer	37	[125 units (Todd).]
38	Urine concentration test	38	[After 12 hours' water deprivation, specific gravity of urine: 1.010.]
39	Chest x-ray	39	[SEE FIGURE 30, PAGE 415.]
40	Bone marrow aspiration	40	[Bone marrow without evidence of blast cell formation, increased or decreased erythropoiesis.]
41	Lupus erythematosus cell preparation	41	[Negative.]
42	Serum creatinine	42	[8.5 mg/100 ml.]
43	Serum cholesterol	43	[196 mg/100 ml.]

44 Serum proteins and electrophoresis 44

YOU WOULD NOW (CHOOSE ONLY ONE):

45 Obtain additional history from the mother if you have not already done so 45

46 Perform physical examination if you have not already done so 46

47 Obtain additional laboratory studies 47

48 Initiate therapy 48

SECTION 17-D

Admission data were recorded as follows: weight – 45 pounds; respirations – 26 per minute; pulse – 112 per minute; oral temperature – 98.4F. The patient is responsive but lethargic. He is breathing deeply and is well hydrated.

IN THE PHYSICAL EXAMINATION, YOU WOULD BE PARTICULARLY INTERESTED TO CHECK (SELECT AS MANY AS YOU CONSIDER ESPECIALLY PERTINENT; YOU CAN RETURN TO THIS SECTION AT ANY TIME TO OBTAIN ANY ADDITIONAL INFORMATION YOU MAY REQUIRE ABOUT THE INITIAL PHYSICAL FINDINGS):

49 Ears 49

50	Optic fundi	**50**	[Arterial narrowing with prominent arteriovenous nicking.]
51	Facial nerve	**51**	[No facial weakness; Chvostek's sign — negative.]
52	Cervical nodes	**52**	[No nodes palpable.]
53	Blood pressure	**53**	[184/112 mm Hg in both upper extremities; 200/114 mm Hg in legs.]
54	Lungs	**54**	[Clea[illegible]n and auscultation[illegible]
55	Heart	**55**	[Heart sounds: grade II/III short systolic apical murmur. Rhythm regular — 78 per minute.]
56	Palpation of the abdomen	**56**	[Abdomen distended, round intra-abdominal mass felt above pubis.]
57	Flanks	**57**	[Questionable right costovertebral angle tenderness.]
58	Percussion of the abdomen	**58**	[Area of dullness extending from the symphysis pubis almost to the umbilicus.]
59	Abdomen for fluid	**59**	[No fluid wave; no shifting dullness.]
60	Genitalia	**60**	[Testes in scrotum; circumcised; meatus normal.]
61	Urinary system	**61**	[Stream weak with dribbling.]
62	Joint mobility	**62**	[Full range of motion without pain — active and passive movements.]
63	Reflexes	**63**	[Symmetrically present.]

64	Extremities for metaphyseal flaring or bowing	**64**	[The metaphyses show no abnormal configuration.]
65	Peripheral edema	**65**	[None.]
66	Skin	**66**	[Pale; no petechiae, purpura or jaundice. There is no frost on the upper lip.]
67	Rectal examination	**67**	[Sphincter normal, prostate normal, and no abnormal masses felt.]

YOU WOULD NOW (CHOOSE ONLY ONE):

68	Obtain further history from the mother if you have not already done so	**68**	[TURN TO SECTION 17-F, PAGE 249.]
69	Initiate therapy	**69**	[TURN TO SECTION 17-B, PAGE 241.]
70	Initiate laboratory investigation if you have not already done so	**70**	[TURN TO SECTION 17-C, PAGE 243.]
71	Obtain additional laboratory studies	**71**	[During the first 24 hours after admission, the patient urinates only 160 ml although his hydration remains adequate. Other than appearing somewhat more lethargic his clinical status appears unchanged. NOW TURN TO SECTION 17-E, PAGE 248.]

72 Request urologic consultation **72** [The consultant requests information about the history, performs a physical examination and orders the following studies: intravenous pyelogram, serum creatinine and creatinine clearance determinations and voiding cystourethrogram before giving an opinion. IF YOU WISH TO COMPLETE THE WORK-UP YOURSELF, TURN NOW TO SECTION 17-G, PAGE 251. IF YOU WISH TO TRANSFER THE PATIENT TO THE UROLOGIST, TURN NOW TO SECTION 17-H, PAGE 252.]

SECTION 17-E

IN LIGHT OF THE INFORMATION YOU NOW HAVE, YOU WOULD ORDER THE FOLLOWING ADDITIONAL LABORATORY STUDIES (SELECT AS MANY AS YOU CONSIDER INDICATED):

73 Catheterization for residual urine volume **73** [Residual volume — 540 ml.]

74 Renal arteriogram **74** [The secondary renal arteries are fanned out. Arteriogram is essentially normal.]

75 Intravenous pyelogram **75** [Bilateral dilated tortuous ureters, dilated pelvices and delayed excretion.]

76 Renal biopsy, percutaneous **76** [Renal biopsy performed. There is a great amount of bleeding and patient becomes hypotensive.]

77 Renal biopsy, open **77** [Histopathologic examination shows dilated tubules and atrophy of renal parenchyma.]

78	Voiding cystourethrogram	**78**	[Bilateral ureteral reflux, hydroureter and hydronephrosis; large amount of dye retention on post voiding film.]
79	Radioactive isotope renogram	**79**	[Delayed renal uptake and delayed excretion of isotope.]
80	12-hour Addis count	**80**	[Increased RBC, WBC, and casts.]
81	Cystoscopy	**81**	[Urethral valves seen in the posterior urethra.]
82	Red blood cell survival time (radioactive Cr)	**82**	[^{51}Cr, T 1/2 – 28 days.]
83	Creatinine clearance	**83**	[40 ml per minute.]
84	Serum creatinine	**84**	[9 mg/100 ml.]
85	Glucose tolerance test	**85**	[Fasting – 96 mg/100 ml one-half hour – 140 mg/100 ml two hour – 120 mg/100 ml three hour – 80 mg/100 ml.]

UNLESS OTHERWISE DIRECTED IN THE RESPONSE COLUMN TURN TO SECTION 17-B, PAGE 241

SECTION 17-F

IN TAKING THE HISTORY YOU ARE PARTICULARLY INTERESTED TO INQUIRE ABOUT (SELECT AS MANY AS YOU CONSIDER ESPECIALLY PERTINENT; YOU CAN RETURN TO THIS SECTION AT ANY TIME TO OBTAIN ANY ADDITIONAL HISTORICAL INFORMATION YOU MAY REQUIRE):

86	Known urinary tract infections	**86**	[None.]
87	Diet	**87**	[No excess intake of milk or alkali.]
88	History of bronchial asthma	**88**	[None.]
89	Bloody urine	**89**	[None noticed.]

90	Family history of diabetes	[None.]
91	Character of urinary stream	[Stream weak and dribbling.]
92	Edema	[None noticed.]
93	Behavioral disturbances	[None.]
94	Recent sore throat	[Mild sore throat without fever two months before admission.]
95	Melena or tarry stools	[None.]
96	Urinary frequency	[No.]
97	Recent ataxia, lack of coordination	[No.]
98	Enuresis	[Once or twice weekly since infancy.]
99	Bone pain	[No.]
100	Dysuria	[No.]
101	Recent episodes of diarrhea	[No.]
102	Jaundice	[No.]
103	Dribbling following micturition	[Frequently.]
104	Skin eruptions	[Only the usual childhood viral diseases.]
105	Weight loss	[None.]

YOU WOULD NOW (CHOOSE ONLY ONE):

106	Initiate therapy	[TURN TO SECTION 17-B, PAGE 241.]
107	Perform physical examination if you have not already done so	[TURN TO SECTION 17-D, PAGE 245.]

108	Initiate laboratory evaluation if you have not already done so	**108**	[TURN TO SECTION 17-C, PAGE 243.]
109	Obtain additional laboratory studies	**109**	[During the first 24 hours after admission, the patient urinates only 160 ml although his hydration remains adequate. Other than appearing somewhat more lethargic his clinical status appears unchanged. NOW TURN TO SECTION 17-E, PAGE 248.]
110	Request urologic consultation	**110**	[The consultant requests information about the history, performs a physical examination and orders the following studies: Intravenous pyelogram, serum creatinine and creatinine clearance determinations, and voided cystourethrogram before giving an opinion. IF YOU WISH TO COMPLETE THE WORK-UP YOURSELF, TURN NOW TO SECTION 17-G, PAGE 251; IF YOU WISH TO TRANSFER THE PATIENT TO THE UROLOGIST, TURN NOW TO SECTION 17-H, PAGE 252.]

SECTION 17-G

ON THE BASIS OF THIS RECOMMENDATION YOU WOULD NOW (CHOOSE ONLY ONE):

111	Initiate laboratory evaluation	[TURN TO SECTION 17-C, PAGE 243.]
112	Start emergency therapy	[TURN TO SECTION 17-B, PAGE 241.]
113	Obtain additional history	[TURN TO SECTION 17-F, PAGE 249.]

114 Perform physical examination	**114**	[TURN TO SECTION 17-D, PAGE 245.]

SECTION 17-H

115 Transfer patient	**115**	[Urologist prescribes sodium bicarbonate and supplements penicillin, hydralazine, and reserpine; orders insertion of Foley catheter and report excision of urethral valves was successfully carried out one week later. CONTINUE NOW WITH SECTION 17-I.]

SECTION 17-I

116 Record your diagnoses below: ____________________ ____________________ ____________________ ____________________	**116**	[The diagnosis as recorded on the patient's chart was: Obstructive uropathy with bilateral hydroureteronephrosis. SEE APPENDIX S FOR ADDITIONAL COMMENT AND RECOMMENDED MANAGEMENT. END OF PROBLEM 17.]

NOW DEVELOP RESPONSE 116 FOR ADDITIONAL INFORMATION AND INSTRUCTIONS

PROBLEM 18

A SURGICAL ABDOMEN

Assume you are a young general practitioner, a member of the staff of your modern 300-bed community hospital. You are called by the intern at 10:30 P.M. to see a patient in the Emergency Room.

When you arrive, you find a 47-year-old man who complains of abdominal pain and vomiting. The pain began three weeks ago; the patient took Bromo-Seltzer with some relief. He continued to work until one week ago when he stopped working because of vomiting; the pain was not severe. After two days at home the pain began to subside, but he began to vomit small amounts. Similar, though more severe, episodes of pain have occurred off and on for the past three years.

NOW CONTINUE WITH SECTION 18-A

SECTION 18-A

YOU WOULD NOW (CHOOSE ONLY ONE EACH TIME YOU ARE DIRECTED TO THIS SECTION):

1	Admit patient to hospital	1	[The patient is admitted; on the way to his room from the Emergency Room, he again vomits, but his pain is markedly diminished. CONTINUE WITH SECTION 18-B.]

2	Start treatment, reassure the patient, send him home, and plan to see him at home early next morning	**2**	[You arrive early next morning to discover that the patient had become progressively worse through the night and is now comatose. As you enter his room, he vomits again and aspirates, becomes cyanotic and sustains a cardiac arrest. TURN TO SECTION 18-P, PAGE 283.]
3	Obtain laboratory or x-ray examinations	**3**	[TURN TO SECTION 18-C, PAGE 255.]
4	Obtain more history from the patient	**4**	[TURN TO SECTION 18-D, PAGE 259.]
5	Examine the patient	**5**	[TURN TO SECTION 18-E, PAGE 263.]

SECTION 18-B

YOU WOULD NOW (CHOOSE ONLY ONE):

6	Obtain laboratory and x-ray studies	**6**	[CONTINUE WITH SECTION 18-C.]
7	Call the operating room and schedule the patient for immediate surgery	**7**	[After surgery, the patient fails to recover from his anesthetic. Two hours later he aspirates (while on nasogastric suction) and sustains a cardiac arrest. TURN TO SECTION 18-P, PAGE 283.]
8	Obtain further history from the patient	**8**	[TURN TO SECTION 18-D, PAGE 259.]
9	Observe the patient closely for the next few hours	**9**	[TURN TO SECTION 18-I, PAGE 275.]

10	Decide that admission to the hospital was not necessary after all; start treatment, send the patient home, and plan to see him at home early next morning	**10**	[You arrive early next morning to discover that the patient had become progressively worse through the night and is now comatose. As you enter his room, he vomits again and aspirates, becomes cyanotic, and sustains a cardiac arrest. TURN TO SEC-TION 18-[illegible], PAGE 263.]

SECTION 18-C

YOU WOULD NOW ORDER (SELECT AS MANY AS YOU CONSIDER INDICATED):

11	Hemoglobin and hematocrit	**11**	[Hgb – 16.8 g/100 ml, Hct – 48%.]
12	White blood cell count	**12**	[12,300/mm^3.]
13	Red cell smear, morphology	**13**	[The red cells are normochromic and normocytic.]
14	Differential white count	**14**	[Bands – 3%, neutrophils – 70%, lymphocytes – 24%, monocytes – 3%.]
15	Urinalysis	**15**	[Patient unable to void. IF YOU WISH TO CATHETERIZE THE PATIENT DEVELOP RESPONSE 16 BELOW FOR REPORT ON THE CATHETERIZED URINE SAMPLES.]
		16	Color – deep yellow, specific gravity – 1.036, pH – 5.2, protein – trace, glucose – 4+, acetone – 4+, bile – negative, microscopic – normal.]

17	Urine culture	**17**	[Patient unable to void spontaneously; catheter specimen sent to the lab.]
18	Stool guaiac	**18**	[Positive 2+.]
19	Erythrocyte sedimentation rate	**19**	[32 mm in one hour (Wintrobe).]
20	Serum electrolytes	**20**	[Na – 129 mEq/L; K – 2.8 mEq/L; Cl – 80 mEq/L; CO_2 – 18 mEq/L.]
21	Arterial pH and P_{CO_2} determinations	**21**	[pH – 7.28; P_{CO_2} – 21 mm Hg.]
22	Venous pH	**22**	[7.12.]
23	Blood urea nitrogen	**23**	[24 mg/100 ml.]
24	Serum creatinine	**24**	[1.3 mg/100 ml.]
25	Total serum protein	**25**	[8.0 g/100 ml.]
26	Albumin/globulin ratio	**26**	[5:3.]
27	Serum protein electrophoresis	**27**	[Albumin – 60%, $Alpha_1$-globulin – 6%, $Alpha_2$-globulin – 99%, Beta – 10%, Gamma – 15%.]
28	Blood ammonia	**28**	[8.0 μg/100 ml.]
29	Total and direct bilirubin	**29**	[Total – 1.6 mg/100 ml; direct – 0.9 mg/100 ml.]
30	Cholesterol	**30**	[300 mg/100 ml.]
31	Bromsulphalein retention	**31**	[10% retention at 45 minutes.]
32	Cephalin flocculation	**32**	[2+.]
33	Thymol turbidity	**33**	[Four units.]

34	Serum glutamic oxalacetic transaminase	34	[33 IU/L.]
35	Alkaline phosphatase	35	[12 units (King-Armstrong).]
36	Lactic dehydrogenase	36	[400 units/ml (Wroblewski).]
37	Acid phosphatase	37	[One unit (King-Armstrong).]
38	Serum amylase	38	[176 units/100 ml (Somogyi).]
39	Urine amylase	39	[1600 units/24 hours (Somogyi) (catheter collection).]
40	Blood sugar	40	[340 mg/100 ml.]
41	Two-hour postprandial blood sugar	41	[Patient vomiting.]
42	Serum calcium and inorganic phosphorus	42	[Ca — 5.0 mEq/L; P — 1.5 mEq/L.]
43	STS	43	[Nonreactive.]
44	Urine electrolytes	44	[Patient unable to void. IF YOU WISH TO CATHETERIZE THE PATIENT DEVELOP RESPONSE 45 BELOW FOR REPORT ON CATHETERIZED URINE SAMPLE.]
		45	[Na — 160 mEq/L; K — 20 mEq/L.]
46	Purified protein derivative skin test	46	[Skin test done, to be read in 24 and 48 hours.]
47	Blood volume	47	[4073 ml ≐ 6% of body weight.]
48	Gastric analysis	48	[Specimens contaminated by partially digested food; no free acid.]

49	Chest x-ray	**49**	[SEE FIGURES 35 AND 36, PAGE 416.]
50	Upright film of abdomen	**50**	[Scattered gas in small and large bowel, no fluid levels; large amounts of air in left upper quadrant; psoas shadow readily outlined.]
51	Flat film of abdomen	**51**	[Scattered gas in small and large bowel, large gas bubble in left upper quadrant.]
52	Barium enema	**52**	[Completed with difficulty, patient's condition deteriorates, SEE FIGURE 43, PAGE 418.]
53	Upper gastrointestinal tract series	**53**	[Small amount of barium given, patient vomits it promptly; test repeated next day, SEE FIGURE 44, PAGE 418.]
54	Intravenous pyelogram	**54**	[SEE FIGURE 51, PAGE 420.]
55	Oral cholecystogram	**55**	[Patient vomits dye tablets.]
56	Intravenous cholangiogram	**56**	[SEE FIGURE 52, PAGE 420.]
57	Electrocardiogram	**57**	[SEE FIGURE 5, PAGE 408.]
58	Central venous pressure	**58**	[30 mm water.]
59	Pulmonary artery wedge pressure	**59**	[4 mm mercury.]
60	Circulation time (arm to tongue)	**60**	[Five seconds.]
61	Hourly urine output	**61**	[22 cc/hour.]

YOU WOULD NOW (CHOOSE ONLY ONE IN THIS SECTION):

62	Admit patient to the hospital if you have not already done so	**62**	[TURN TO SECTION 18-I, PAGE 275.]

63	Obtain further history	63	[CONTINUE WITH SECTION 18-D.]
64	Schedule patient for urgent surgery	64	[Postoperatively, the patient fails to recover from his anesthetic. Two hours later he aspirates (while on nasogastric suction) and sustains a cardiac arrest. TURN TO SECTION 18-P, PAGE 283.]
65	Send the patient home with appropriate treatment and plan to see him again first thing in the morning	65	[You arrive early next morning to discover that the patient had become progressively worse through the night and is now comatose. As you enter his room, he vomits again and aspirates, becomes cyanotic, and sustains a cardiac arrest. TURN TO SECTION 18-P, PAGE 283.]
66	Examine the patient	66	[TURN TO SECTION 18-E, PAGE 263.]

SECTION 18-D

IN TAKING THE HISTORY YOU WOULD BE PARTICULARLY INTERESTED TO INQUIRE ABOUT (SELECT AS MANY AS YOU CONSIDER ESPECIALLY PERTINENT; YOU CAN RETURN TO THIS SECTION AT ANY TIME TO OBTAIN ANY ADDITIONAL HISTORICAL INFORMATION YOU MAY REQUIRE):

67	Headache	67	[Occasional headache relieved by aspirin.]
68	Epistaxis	68	[None.]
69	Hemoptysis	69	[None.]
70	Chest pain	70	[None.]
71	Cough	71	[None.]

72	Previous hypertension	72	[Two years ago blood pressure 140/90 mm Hg.]
73	Appetite	73	[Good until present illness; continued to eat until four days ago.]
74	Dysphagia	74	[None.]
75	Nausea and vomiting	75	[Nausea has not been excessive until today; vomiting began five days ago.]
76	Bowel habits	76	[One bowel movement per day.]
77	Type of pain	77	[Initially burning in character, now more aching.]
78	Location of pain	78	[Initially mild pain in epigastrium; for past three days has been more diffuse, still in epigastrium, but with radiation straight through to the back.]
79	Nature of vomiting	79	[Initially small volume, partially digested food; volume has steadily increased and now vomits all that he eats.]
80	Nature of stools	80	[Frequently hard, "normal" in color; have become darker during past week.]
81	Nature of diet	81	[Cabbage, fatty foods cause belching; otherwise eats all food; drinks "a lot" of water.]
82	Weight loss	82	[15 pounds in past three weeks; normal weight 155 pounds.]
83	Alcohol intake	83	[Admits to a "few beers"; wife says he gets drunk every Saturday night.]

84 Jaundice in past

85 Bleeding tendency

86 Belching

87 Radiation of pain

88 Chills and fever

89 Pruritis

90 Steatorrhea

91 Hematemesis

92 Food intolerance

93 Fatigue

94 Dizziness, vertigo, fainting

95 Character of urine

96 Family history

97 Angina

98 Dyspnea

99 Dysuria

84 [None.]

85 [None.]

86 [After fatty foods, cabbage.]

87 [For the past three days, straight through to the back from the epigastrium.]

88 [Had a chill two days ago.]

89 [Yes, generalized for one year.]

90 [None.]

91 [Small amount during similar, but less severe, episode two years ago.]

92 [Fatty foods and cabbage cause belching.]

93 [Has felt tired for two weeks.]

94 [Today has felt "light-headed" when sitting.]

95 [Usually voids a lot of light yellow urine but has not yet voided today.]

96 [Thinks his mother, who died some years ago in Mississippi, had "sugar diabetes."]

97 [None.]

98 [None.]

99 [None.]

100 Edema

100 [None.]

101 Allergies

101 [None.]

102 Drug history

102 [Takes Tums or Bromo-Seltzer intermittently for epigastric distress; two years ago was placed on bland diet, Probanthine and Maalox by physician; took these medications as directed for six weeks, but then stopped them.]

103 Smoking history

103 [Half pack a day for 30 years.]

104 Previous hospitalization

104 [None.]

105 Previous operations

105 [None.]

106 Previous x-ray studies

106 [Upper gastrointestinal series done two years ago showed duodenal bulb deformity and irritability.]

107 Trauma history

107 [None pertinent or significant.]

YOU WOULD NOW (CHOOSE ONLY ONE):

108 Perform physical examination if you have not already done so

108 [CONTINUE WITH SECTION 18-E.]

109 Admit patient to the hospital if you have not already done so and obtain appropriate laboratory and x-ray tests

109 [TURN TO SECTION 18-F, PAGE 266.]

110 Admit patient to the hospital if you have not already done so and schedule him for immediate surgery

110 [Postoperatively the patient fails to recover from his anesthetic. Two hours later he aspirates (while on nasogastric suction) and sustains a cardiac arrest. TURN TO SECTION 18-P, PAGE 283.]

111	Admit patient to the hospital if you have not already done so for observation and evaluation	**111**	[TURN TO SECTION 18-O, PAGE 276.]
112	Start appropriate nonoperative treatment; send the patient home, and plan to see him again early next morning	**112**	[You arrive early next morning to discover that the patient had become progressively worse through the night and is now comatose. As you enter his room, he vomits again and aspirates, becomes cyanotic, and sustains a cardiac arrest. TURN TO SECTION 18-P, PAGE 283.]

SECTION 18-E

THE PATIENT IS LYING QUIETLY, FLAT ON HIS BACK. IN PERFORMING THE PHYSICAL EXAMINATION YOU WOULD BE PARTICULARLY INTERESTED TO CHECK (SELECT AS MANY AS YOU CONSIDER ESPECIALLY PERTINENT; YOU CAN RETURN TO THIS SECTION AT ANY TIME TO OBTAIN ANY ADDITIONAL INFORMATION YOU MAY REQUIRE ABOUT THE INITIAL PHYSICAL FINDINGS):

113	Pupils	**113**	[Equal, react equally to light and accommodation.]
114	Eyegrounds	**114**	[Discs normal, vascularity normal, no copper or silver-wire changes.]
115	External ear	**115**	[External ears — skin clear; tympanic membrane normal.]
116	Scalp	**116**	[Male pattern alopecia; no skin disease.]
117	Nose	**117**	[Normal mucosa; no septal deviation.]
118	Mouth	**118**	[Several caries; thick mucous mixed with old vomitus on hard palate; some tongue furrowing; strong, sweetish breath odor.]

119	Pharynx	**119**	[Thick mucous mixed with old vomitus, otherwise normal.]
120	Neck	**120**	[No masses or other abnormality seen.]
121	Chest and lungs	**121**	[Normal to inspection, percussion and auscultation.]
122	Breasts	**122**	[Normal male breasts.]
123	Peripheral pulses	**123**	[Symmetrically present in the popliteal, posterior tibial, and dorsal pedis arteries.]
124	Blood pressure	**124**	[110/80 mm Hg.]
125	Valsalva maneuver	**125**	[Performed without change in symptoms or signs.]
126	Pulse rate	**126**	[84 per minute, regular.]
127	Respiratory rate	**127**	[38 per minute, regular and profound.]
128	Temperature	**128**	[99.2F.]
129	Abdominal wall	**129**	[Slightly protuberant and tender in epigastrium; no muscle spasm.]
130	Bowel sounds	**130**	[Normal borborygmi heard.]
131	Liver	**131**	[Not enlarged, not tender.]
132	Spleen	**132**	[Not palpable.]
133	Abdominal mass	**133**	[None palpable.]
134	Abdominal tenderness	**134**	[Tender in epigastrium.]
135	Inguinal area	**135**	[No hernias.]
136	External genitalia	**136**	[Normal.]

137	Right lower quadrant tenderness to palpation	**137**	[Absent.]
138	Rebound tenderness	**138**	[Absent.]
139	Referred rebound	**139**	[Absent.]
140	Costovertebral angle	**140**	[No tenderness or bulging.]
141	Back tenderness	**141**	[None.]
142	Range of motion of spine	**142**	[Full and normal range of motion.]
143	Straight leg raising	**143**	[No limitation, causes no symptoms.]
144	Rectal examination	**144**	[Small external hemorrhoids, otherwise normal.]
145	Sigmoidoscopy	**145**	[Normal to 25 cm.]
146	Skin	**146**	[Dry. Old excoriations are seen; there is decreased turgor.]
147	Heel-to-knee test	**147**	[Normal.]
148	Serial sevens	**148**	[Performed adequately.]
149	General appearance of patient	**149**	[Lethargic, tachypneic, well-developed, appears acutely ill, eyeballs soft, skin dry and shows decreased turgor.]
150	Chvostek's sign	**150**	[Absent.]
151	Axilla	**151**	[Dry; no palpable nodes; normal amount of hair.]
152	Visible peristalsis	**152**	[None seen after watching for five minutes.]

YOU WOULD NOW (CHOOSE ONLY ONE):

153	Obtain further history (if you have not already done so)	**153**	[TURN TO SECTION 18-D, PAGE 259.]
154	Admit patient to the hospital (if not admitted previously) and obtain appropriate laboratory and x-ray tests	**154**	[CONTINUE WITH SECTION 18-F.]
155	Admit patient to the hospital if you have not already done so, and schedule him for immediate surgery	**155**	[Postoperatively, the patient fails to recover from his anesthetic; two hours later he aspirates (while on nasogastric suction) and sustains a cardiac arrest. TURN TO SECTION 18-P, PAGE 283.]
156	Admit patient to the hospital (if not admitted previously) for observation and evaluation	**156**	[TURN TO SECTION 18-J, PAGE 276.]
157	Give antispasmodics, analgesics, antacids; send the patient home; and plan to see him again early next morning	**157**	[You arrive early next morning to discover that the patient had become progressively worse through the night and is now comatose. As you enter his room, he vomits again and aspirates, becomes cyanotic, and sustains a cardiac arrest. TURN TO SECTION 18-P, PAGE 283.]

SECTION 18-F

YOU WOULD NOW ORDER (SELECT AS MANY AS YOU CONSIDER INDICATED):

158	Hemoglobin and hematocrit	**158**	[Hgb = 16.8 g/100 ml; Hct = 48%.]
159	White blood cell count	**159**	[12,300/mm^3.]
160	Red cell smear, morphology	**160**	[Normochromic and normocytic.]

161	Differential white count	**161**	[Bands — 3%, neutrophils — 70%, lymphocytes — 24%, monocytes — 3%.]
162	Urinalysis	**162**	[Patient unable to void. IF YOU WISH TO CATHETERIZE THE PATIENT DEVELOP RESPONSE 163 BELOW FOR REPORT ON THE CATHETERIZED URINE SAMPLES.]
		163	[Color — deep yellow, specific gravity — 1.036, pH — 5.2, protein — trace, glucose — 4+, acetone — 4+, bile — negative, microscopic — normal.]
164	Urine culture	**164**	[Patient unable to void spontaneously; catheter specimen sent to the lab.]
165	Stool guaiac	**165**	[Positive 2+.]
166	Erythrocyte sedimentation rate	**166**	[32 mm in one hour (Wintrobe).]
167	Serum electrolytes	**167**	[Na — 129 mEq/L, K — 2.8 mEq/L, Cl — 80 mEq/L, CO_2 — 16 mEq/L.]
168	Arterial pH and P_{CO_2} determinations	**168**	[pH — 7.28; P_{CO_2} — 21 mm Hg.]
169	Venous pH	**169**	[7.12.]
170	Blood urea nitrogen	**170**	[24 mg/100 ml.]
171	Creatinine	**171**	[1.3 mg/100 ml.]
172	Total protein	**172**	[8.0 g/100 ml.]
173	Albumin/globulin ratio	**173**	[5:3.]

174	Serum protein electrophoresis	**174**	[Albumin — 60%, $Alpha_1$ — globulin — 6%, $Alpha_2$ — 9%, Beta — 10%, Gamma — 15%.]
175	Blood ammonia	**175**	[80 μg/100 ml.]
176	Total and direct bilirubin	**176**	[Total 1.6 mg/100 ml, direct 0.9 mg/100 ml.]
177	Cholesterol	**177**	[300 mg/100 ml.]
178	Bromsulphalein retention	**178**	[10% retention at 45 minutes.]
179	Cephalin flocculation	**179**	[2+.]
180	Thymol turbidity	**180**	[Four units.]
181	Serum glutamic oxalacetic transaminase	**181**	[33 IU/L.]
182	Alkaline phosphatase	**182**	[12 units (King-Armstrong).]
183	Lactic dehydrogenase	**183**	[400 units/ml (Wroblewski).]
184	Acid phosphatase	**184**	[One unit (King-Armstrong).]
185	Serum amylase	**185**	[176 units/100 ml (Somogyi) (Catheter specimen).]
186	Urine amylase	**186**	[600 units/24 hours.]
187	Fasting blood sugar	**187**	[340 mg/100 ml.]
188	Two-hour postprandial blood sugar	**188**	[Patient vomiting.]
189	Serum calcium and inorganic phosphorus	**189**	[Ca — 5 mEq/L, P — 1.5 mEq/L.]
190	STS	**190**	[Nonreactive.]

191	Urine electrolytes	**191**	[Patient unable to void. IF YOU WISH TO CATHETERIZE THE PATIENT DEVELOP RESPONSE 192 BELOW FOR REPORT ON CATHETERIZED URINE SAMPLE.]
		192	[Na – 160 mEq/L; K – 10 mEq/L.]
193	Purified protein derivative skin test	**193**	[Skin test done, to be read in 24 and 48 hours.]
194	Blood volume	**194**	[4073 ml = 6% of body weight.]
195	Gastric analysis, histamine	**195**	[Specimen contaminated by partially digested food; no free acid.]
196	Chest x-ray	**196**	[SEE FIGURES 35 AND 36, PAGE 416.]
197	Upright film of abdomen	**197**	[Scattered gas in small and large bowel, no fluid levels, large amounts of air in left upper quadrant, psoas shadow readily outlined.]
198	Flat film of abdomen	**198**	[Scattered gas in small and large bowel, large gas bubble in left upper quadrant.]
199	Barium enema	**199**	[Completed with difficulty, patient's condition deteriorates; SEE FIGURE 43, PAGE 418.]
200	Upper gastrointestinal tract series	**200**	[Small amount of barium given, patient vomits it promptly; test repeated next day, SEE FIGURE 44, PAGE 418.]
201	Intravenous pyelogram	**201**	[SEE FIGURE 51, PAGE 420.]

202	Oral cholecystogram	**202**	[Patient vomits dye tablets.]
203	Intravenous cholangiogram	**203**	[SEE FIGURE 52, PAGE 420.]
204	Electrocardiogram	**204**	[SEE FIGURE 5, PAGE 408.]
205	Central venous pressure	**205**	[20 mm water.]
206	Pulmonary artery wedge pressure	**206**	[5 mm mercury.]
207	Circulation time (arm to tongue)	**207**	[Five seconds.]
208	Hourly urine output	**208**	[22 cc/hour.]

UNLESS OTHERWISE DIRECTED IN THE RESPONSE COLUMN CONTINUE WITH SECTION 18-G

SECTION 18-G

YOU WOULD NOW ORDER (SELECT AS MANY AS YOU CONSIDER INDICATED):

209	Nothing by mouth	**209**	[Ordered.]
210	Clear liquid diet	**210**	[Patient vomits.]
211	Bland, low-residue diet	**211**	[Patient vomits.]
212	Force fluids	**212**	[Patient vomits.]
213	Nasogastric suction	**213**	[Tube passed, connected to suction; returns partially digested food, then plugs up.]
214	Long intestinal tube for suction	**214**	[Tube passed into stomach.]
215	Gastric lavage	**215**	[Returns large amount of partially digested food.]
216	Tap water enema	**216**	[Given; patient develops hypotension.]

217 Magnesium sulfate 15 g by mouth — **217** [Given; patient vomits.]

218 Catheterized urine for urinalysis — **218** [Color — Deep yellow, specific gravity — 1.036, pH — 5.2, protein — trace, glucose — 4+, acetone — 4+, bile — negative, microscopic — normal.]

219 Pyloric balance study — **219** [250 cc dextrose in water introduced into stomach; 350 cc fluid aspirated in one hour.]

220 Record intake and output — **220** [Patient not voiding at this time and cannot ingest food.]

221 Record urine output every two hours — **221** [Patient not voiding at this time.]

222 Pulmonary function studies — **222** [Scheduled for next morning.]

223 Maalox, 30 ml every hour — **223** [Patient vomits.]

224 Arterial pH, Po_2 and Pco_2 determinations — **224** [pH — 7.28, P_{O_2} — 78 mm Hg, Pco_2 — 24 mm Hg.]

225 Type and crossmatch 1500 cc whole blood — **225** [Blood sent to lab.]

226 Oxygen by nasal catheter at 6 liters per minute flow — **226** [Started.]

227 Irrigate nasogastric tube every hour — **227** [Done.]

228 Oxygen tent with high humidity — **228** [Patient placed in tent.]

229 Atropine 0.4 mg intravenously — **229** [Given.]

230 Morphine 5 mg intramuscularly — **230** [Given; some relief of pain.]

231 Meperidine 100 mg intramuscularly every four hours — **231** [Given; patient becomes semicomatose.]

232	Neomycin by mouth in therapeutic doses	**232**	[Patient vomits.]
233	Procaine penicillin G in therapeutic doses	**233**	[Given, no change in condition.]
234	Ampicillin in therapeutic doses	**234**	[Given, no change in condition.]
235	Kanamycin and penicillin in therapeutic doses	**235**	[Given, no change in condition.]
236	Chloramphenicol and penicillin in therapeutic doses	**236**	[Given, no change in condition.]
237	Lanatoside C 0.5 mg by mouth	**237**	[No change in patient's condition.]
238	Digitoxin 0.4 mg intravenously	**238**	[Auriculoventricular conduction defect develops.]
239	Methylprednisone intravenously	**239**	[Patient continues to vomit; condition deteriorates.]
240	NPH insulin 40 units subcutaneously	**240**	[No immediate change in patient' condition.]
241	Protamine zinc insulin 80 units subcutaneously	**241**	[No immediate change in patient's condition.]
242	Tolbutamide	**242**	[No immediate change in patient's condition.]
243	Calcium chloride intravenously	**243**	[Given.]
244	Packed RBC slowly intravenously	**244**	[No change.]
245	5% dextrose in water, 74 ml per hour	**245**	[Condition deteriorates.]

246	Hypotonic saline (0.5%) 1000 ml intravenously in next four hours	**246**	[Patient improves. IGNORE INSTRUCTIONS AT END OF THIS SECTION; INSTEAD TURN TO SECTION 18-K, PAGE 277 WHEN YOU HAVE COMPLETED THIS SECTION.]
247	1/6 molar sodium lactate, 1000 ml intravenous in next four hours	**247**	[Patient improves. IGNORE INSTRUCTIONS AT END OF THIS SECTION; INSTEAD TURN TO SECTION 18-K, PAGE 277 WHEN YOU HAVE COMPLETED THIS SECTION.]
248	Potassium 20 mEq for each hour of intravenous fluids	**248**	[Patient improves. IGNORE INSTRUCTIONS AT END OF THIS SECTION; INSTEAD TURN TO SECTION 18-K, PAGE 277 WHEN YOU HAVE COMPLETED THIS SECTION.]
249	Add potassium chloride, 60 mg to each bottle of intravenous fluid	**249**	[Patient improves. IGNORE INSTRUCTIONS AT END OF THIS SECTION; INSTEAD TURN TO SECTION 18-K, PAGE 277 WHEN YOU HAVE COMPLETED THIS SECTION.]
250	Central venous pressure catheter placed	**250**	[Done.]
251	Crystalline insulin 70 units stat intravenously and 50 units subcutaneously	**251**	[Rapid improvement of state of consciousness, vomiting decreases. IGNORE INSTRUCTIONS AT END OF THIS SECTION; INSTEAD TURN TO SECTION 18-K, PAGE 277 WHEN YOU HAVE COMPLETED THIS SECTION.]

252 Crystalline insulin every one to two hours depending on blood sugar determination

252 [Patient continues to improve. IGNORE INSTRUCTIONS AT END OF THIS SECTION; INSTEAD TURN TO SECTION 18-K, PAGE 277 WHEN YOU HAVE COMPLETED THIS SECTION.]

253 Phosphate 14 millimoles for each hour of intravenous therapy

253 [Patient improves. IGNORE INSTRUCTIONS AT END OF THIS SECTION; INSTEAD TURN TO SECTION 18 K, PAGE 277 WHEN YOU HAVE COMPLETED THIS SECTION.]

UNLESS OTHERWISE DIRECTED IN THE RESPONSE COLUMN CONTINUE WITH SECTION 18-H

SECTION 18-H

The patient develops moderate hypotension (90/60 mm Hg), tachycardia (147 per minute), and air hunger with labored respirations; he becomes very lethargic, but can be aroused by your shouting at him.

YOU WOULD NOW RECOMMEND (CHOOSE ONE OR MORE):

254 Lumbar puncture

254 [Pressure normal, fluid clear; glucose 160 mg/100 ml, protein 40 mg/100 ml, cells — none.]

255 Emergency laparotomy

255 [The patient fails to recover from his anesthetic. Two hours later he aspirates (while on nasogastric suction) and sustains a cardiac arrest. DO NOT MAKE ANY MORE CHOICES IN THIS SECTION; TURN NOW TO SECTION 18-P, PAGE 283.]

256 Echoencephalogram

256 [Interpreted as normal.]

257	Catheterized urinalysis	**257**	[Color — deep yellow, specific gravity — 1.036, pH — 5.2 protein — trace, glucose — 4+, acetone — 4+, bile — negative, microscopic — normal. IGNORE INSTRUCTIONS AT END OF THIS SECTION; INSTEAD TURN NOW TO SECTION 18-O, PAGE 280.]
258	Endotracheal tube and respirator assisted ventilation	**258**	[No apparent benefit.]
259	Pulmonary scan	**259**	[No localized defect found.]
260	Hepatic scan	**260**	[No concentration or defect in isotope uptake.]
261	Ultrasound scan of abdomen	**261**	[Large fluid filled mass, left upper quadrant.]
262	Intravenous fluids containing ammonium chloride	**262**	[Patient's condition worsens.]
263	Intravenous antibiotics and methylprednisone in appropriate doses	**263**	[No apparent benefit.]

UNLESS OTHERWISE DIRECTED IN THE RESPONSE COLUMN TURN TO SECTION 18-Q, PAGE 284

SECTION 18-I

The patient develops labored deep breathing, slightly slurred speech and a fever of 100 F; his condition is obviously worse.

YOU WOULD NOW (CHOOSE ONLY ONE):

264	Schedule patient for immediate surgery	**264**	[Postoperatively the patient fails to recover from his anesthetic. Two hours later he aspirates (while on nasogastric suction) and sustains a cardiac arrest. TURN TO SECTION 18-P, PAGE 283.]
265	Order routine laboratory and x-ray examinations	**265**	[Patient's condition continues to deteriorate; the nurse advises you he has become comatose. As you enter his room he vomits again and aspirates, becomes cyanotic, and sustains a cardiac arrest. TURN NOW TO SECTION 18-P, PAGE 283.]
266	Obtain more history from patient and family	**266**	[TURN TO SECTION 18-D, PAGE 259.]
267	Examine the patient	**267**	[TURN TO SECTION 18-E, PAGE 263.]

SECTION 18-J

The patient develops labored breathing, slightly slurred speech, and a fever of 100F; his condition is obviously getting worse.

YOU WOULD NOW (CHOOSE ONLY ONE):

268	Call the operating room and schedule patient for immediate surgery	**268**	[Postoperatively the patient fails to recover from his anesthetic; two hours later he aspirates (while on nasogastric suction) and sustains a cardiac arrest. TURN TO SECTION 18-P, PAGE 283.]
269	Obtain appropriate laboratory and x-ray tests	**269**	[TURN TO SECTION 18-F, PAGE 266.]

270	Continue close observation of patient	**270**	[Patient becomes comatose and aspirates vomitus; becomes cyanotic, and sustains a cardiac arrest. TURN TO SECTION 18-P, PAGE 283.]
271	Start appropriate therapy	**271**	[TURN TO SECTION 18-G, PAGE 270.]

SECTION 18-K

The patient is in better condition. Laboratory values at this time are: hematocrit – 38%; blood urea nitrogen – 14 mg/100 ml; serum electrolytes: Na – 138 mEq/L; K – 3.1 mEq/L; Cl – 92 mEq/L; CO_2 – 30 mEq/L; urine electrolytes: Na – 40 mEq/24 hours, K – 30 mEq/24 hours.

YOU WOULD NOW (CHOOSE ONLY ONE):

272	Order intravenous fluids for next 24 hours: 1000 ml 5% dextrose in water, 500 ml Ringer's lactate, 40 mEq KCl given slowly; leave nasogastric tube in place but clamped	**272**	[Patient becomes oliguric. TURN TO SECTION 18-Q, PAGE 284.]
273	Start liquid diet	**273**	[Patient begins to vomit. TURN TO SECTION 18-Q, PAGE 284.]
274	Order intravenous fluids for next 24 hours: 2500 ml 5% dextrose in water, 1500 ml normal saline, 120 mEq KCl; continue nasogastric suction	**274**	[Patient continues to improve. CONTINUE WITH SECTION 18-L.]
275	Pull nasogastric tube, start fluids cautiously by mouth	**275**	[Patient begins to vomit. TURN TO SECTION 18-Q, PAGE 284.]

276	Order intravenous fluids for next 24 hours: 1500 ml 5% dextrose in water, 1000 ml normal saline; continue nasogastric suction	**276**	[Patient develops extreme lethargy and cardiac palpitations. TURN TO SECTION 18-Q, PAGE 284.]

SECTION 18-L

YOU WOULD NOW (CHOOSE ONLY ONE):

277	Schedule the patient for surgery	**277**	[CONTINUE WITH SECTION 18-M.]
278	Continue management without surgical intervention	**278**	[TURN TO SECTION 18-N, PAGE 279.]

SECTION 18-M

YOU WOULD NOW RECOMMEND (CHOOSE ONLY ONE):

279	Cholecystectomy	**279**	[Laparotomy revealed a normal gall bladder; not excised.]
280	Cholecystostomy	**280**	[Laparotomy revealed a normal gall bladder; not drained.]
281	Exploration of common bile duct	**281**	[Laparotomy revealed a normal common duct; not explored.]
282	Vagotomy, antrectomy, and gastroduodenostomy	**282**	[Done; patient recovers from surgery and is discharged well.]
283	Transverse colostomy	**283**	[Laparotomy revealed unobstructured colon; colostomy not done.]
284	Wide gastrotomy and repair of bleeders	**284**	[No bleeding points found.]

285	Vagotomy and gastrojejunostomy	**285**	[Done. Patient recovers from surgery and is discharged well.]
286	50% gastric resection and gastrojejunostomy	**286**	[Done; the patient progressed well initially but you subsequently learn that he eventually developed a stomal ulcer.]
287	Drainage of pancreatic pseudocyst	**287**	[No pseudocyst is found.]
288	Pancreaticojejunostomy	**288**	[Laparatomy revealed normal pancreas; pancreaticojejunostomy not done.]
289	Appendectomy	**289**	[Normal appendix is removed.]
290	Lysis of obstructing adhesions	**290**	[No adhesions are found.]
291	Repair of hiatus hernia	**291**	[Small hiatus hernia repaired; projectile vomiting occurs postoperatively.]

UNLESS OTHERWISE DIRECTED IN THE RESPONSE COLUMN TURN TO SECTION 18-Q, PAGE 284

SECTION 18-N

After two days, nasogastric suction is discontinued and the patient started on a liquid diet. He seems to tolerate this well for three days, but then has another episode of vomiting. The nasogastric tube is replaced, yielding an immediate aspirate of 1800 ml; suction output varies between 2000 and 3000 ml over the next week.

YOU WOULD NOW (CHOOSE ONLY ONE):

292	Schedule the patient for surgery	**292**	[TURN TO SECTION 18-M, PAGE 278.]
293	Continue management without surgical intervention	**293**	[Patient's vomiting persists. TURN TO SECTION 18-Q PAGE 284.]

SECTION 18-O

YOU WOULD NOW ORDER (SELECT AS MANY AS YOU CONSIDER INDICATED):

294	Nothing by mouth	**294**	[Ordered.]
295	Clear liquid diet	**295**	[Patient vomits.]
296	Bland, low-residue diet	**296**	[Patient vomits.]
297	Force fluids	**297**	[Patient vomits.]
298	Nasogastric suction	**298**	[Tube passed, connected to suction; returns partially digested food.]
299	Long intestinal tube for suction	**299**	[Tube passed into stomach.]
300	Gastric lavage	**300**	[Returns particles of partially digested food.]
301	Tap water enema	**301**	[Given; patient develops hypotension.]
302	Open drainage of gastric tube	**302**	[Placed and connected to open drainage.]
303	Maalox, 30 ml every hour	**303**	[Patient vomits.]
304	Type and crossmatch 1500 cc whole blood	**304**	[Blood sent to lab.]
305	Oxygen by nasal catheter at 6 liters per minute flow	**305**	[Started.]
306	Irrigate nasogastric tube every hour	**306**	[Done.]
307	Oxygen tent with high humidity	**307**	[Patient placed in tent.]
308	Atropine 0.4 mg intravenously	**308**	[Given.]
309	Morphine 5 mg intramuscularly	**309**	[Given; no change.]

310	Meperidine 100 mg intramuscularly every four hours	310	[Given, patient becomes semicomatose.]
311	Neomycin by mouth in therapeutic doses	311	[Patient vomits.]
312	Procaine penicillin G in therapeutic doses	312	[Given, no change in condition.]
313	Ampicillin in therapeutic doses	313	[Given, no change in condition.]
314	Clindamycin and gentamycin in therapeutic doses	314	[Given, no change in condition.]
315	Chloramphenicol and penicillin	315	[Given, no change in condition.]
316	Lanatoside C 0.5 mg by mouth	316	[No change in patient's condition.]
317	Digitoxin 0.4 mg intravenously	317	[Auriculoventricular conduction defect develops.]
318	Hydrocortisone intravenously	318	[Patient continues to vomit; condition deteriorates.]
319	NPH insulin 40 units subcutaneously	319	[No immediate change in patient's condition.]
320	Protamine zinc insulin 80 units subcutaneously	320	[No immediate change in patient's condition.]
321	Tolbutamide	321	[No immediate change in patient's condition.]
322	Calcium chloride intravenously	322	[Given.]
323	Packed RBC administered intravenously, slowly	323	[No change.]
324	5% dextrose in water, 74 ml per hour	324	[Condition deteriorates.]

325	Hypotonic saline (0.5%) 1000 ml intravenous in next four hours	**325**	[Patient improves. IGNORE INSTRUCTIONS AT END OF THIS SECTION; INSTEAD TURN TO SECTION 18-K, PAGE 277 WHEN YOU HAVE COMPLETED THIS SECTION.]
326	1/6 molar sodium lactate, 1000 ml intravenous in next four hours	**326**	[Patient improves. IGNORE INSTRUCTIONS AT END OF THIS SECTION; INSTEAD TURN TO SECTION 18-K, PAGE 277 WHEN YOU HAVE COMPLETED THIS SECTION.]
327	Potassium 20 mEq for each hour of intravenous fluids	**327**	[Patient improves. IGNORE INSTRUCTIONS AT END OF THIS SECTION; INSTEAD TURN TO SECTION 18-K, PAGE 277 WHEN YOU HAVE COMPLETED THIS SECTION.]
328	Add potassium chloride, 60 mEq to each bottle of intravenous fluid	**328**	[Patient improves. IGNORE INSTRUCTIONS AT END OF THIS SECTION; INSTEAD TURN TO SECTION 18-K, PAGE 277 WHEN YOU HAVE COMPLETED THIS SECTION.]
329	Central venous pressure catheter placed	**329**	[Done.]
330	Pulmonary artery wedge pressure catheter placed	**330**	[6 mm Hg.]
331	Crystalline insulin 70 units stat intravenously and 50 units subcutaneously	**331**	[Rapid improvement of state of consciousness, vomiting decreases. IGNORE INSTRUCTIONS AT END OF THIS SECTION; INSTEAD TURN TO SECTION 18-K, PAGE 277 WHEN YOU HAVE COMPLETED THIS SECTION.]

332 Crystalline insulin every one to two hours depending on blood sugar determination

332 [Patient continues to improve. IGNORE INSTRUCTIONS AT END OF THIS SECTION; INSTEAD TURN TO SECTION 18-K, PAGE 277 WHEN YOU HAVE COMPLETED THIS SECTION.]

333 Phosphate 14 millimoles for each hour of intravenous therapy

333 [Patient improves. IGNORE INSTRUCTIONS AT END OF THIS SECTION; INSTEAD TURN TO SECTION 18-K, PAGE 277 WHEN YOU HAVE COMPLETED THIS SECTION.]

UNLESS OTHERWISE DIRECTED IN THE RESPONSE COLUMN CONTINUE WITH SECTION 18-Q

SECTION 18-P

334 Record the cause of death below:

____

____

____

____

____

334 [The patient had undiagnosed diabetes mellitus, he was in diabetic coma and died of an accident common in comatose patients. SEE APPENDIX P FOR ADDITIONAL COMMENT AND RECOMMENDED MANAGEMENT. END OF PROBLEM 18.]

NOW DEVELOP RESPONSE 334 FOR FURTHER INFORMATION AND INSTRUCTIONS

SECTION 18-Q

335 Record your diagnoses below:

____

____

____

____

____

____

____

____

335 [This patient had persistent gastric outlet obstruction due to duodenal ulcer and required surgery to relieve the obstruction; management was complicated by his diabetes and resulted in hyponatremia, dehydration, hypokalemia, and acidosis. SEE APPENDIX P FOR ADDITIONAL COMMENT AND RECOMMENDED MANAGEMENT. END OF PROBLEM 18.]

NOW DEVELOP RESPONSE 335 FOR ADDITIONAL INFORMATION AND INSTRUCTIONS

PROBLEM I

HEADACHE IN A CHILD

As the resident on the pediatric service you see a five-year-old boy with known congenital heart disease, who was brought to the pediatric clinic because of severe diffuse headaches of one week duration. There was no relief with the usual analgesics. The parents also noticed that the child has become very irritable and, more recently, that he seems to be extraordinarily sleepy.

NOW CONTINUE WITH SECTION 19-A

SECTION 19-A

YOU WOULD NOW (CHOOSE ONLY ONE):

1	Order laboratory tests on inpatient or outpatient basis	1	[TURN TO SECTION 19-D, PAGE 288.]
2	Perform physical examination	2	[TURN TO SECTION 19-F, PAGE 291.]
3	Initiate therapy	3	[CONTINUE WITH SECTION 19-B, PAGE 286.]
4	Obtain further history from the patient's mother	4	[TURN TO SECTION 19-C, PAGE 287.]
5	Defer further evaluation until symptoms are less vague	5	[TURN TO SECTION 19-G, PAGE 293.]

SECTION 19-B

I WOULD NOW (SELECT AS MANY AS YOU CONSIDER INDICATED):

6	Order parenteral methicillin and streptomycin	6	[Done.]
7	Order digoxin	7	[Atrioventricular block develops.]
8	Order aspirin 0.5 g every four hours	8	[No relief of headaches; child develops ringing in ears.]
9	Order ampicillin IV, 400 mg/kg/day	9	[No improvement in patient's condition.]
10	Order Demerol, 50 mg every six hours	10	[Child becomes very agitated and condition deteriorates.]
11	Order anticoagulants	11	[Given. Patient's condition continues to deteriorate.]
12	Order procaine penicillin G, 250,000 units by mouth every 12 hours	12	[Given. Patient's condition continues to deteriorate.]
13	Order parenteral penicillin and streptomycin	13	[Done.]
14	Obtain emergency neurosurgical consultation	14	[Neurosurgeon advises craniotomy and drainage. This is done and is followed by dramatic improvement and gradual recovery.]
15	Refer to neurology	15	[Done. Patient lost to follow-up.]
16	Suggest sympathectomy	16	[Surgical consultant sees no indication for this operation.]

UNLESS OTHERWISE DIRECTED IN THE RESPONSE COLUMN TURN TO SECTION 19-G

SECTION 19-C

IN TAKING A FURTHER HISTORY FROM THE PATIENT'S MOTHER YOU ARE PARTICULARLY INTERESTED TO INQUIRE ABOUT (SELECT AS MANY AS YOU CONSIDER ESPECIALLY PERTINENT; YOU CAN RETURN TO THIS SECTION AT ANY TIME TO OBTAIN ANY ADDITIONAL HISTORICAL INFORMATION YOU MAY REQUIRE):

17	Fatigue	**17**	[Increased with normal activity.]
18	Dyspnea	**18**	[Present with moderate exertion.]
19	Cyanosis	**19**	[Moderate, increased with exertion.]
20	Developmental history	**20**	[The patient is the smallest child in his kindergarten class.]
21	Family history	**21**	[Noncontributory.]
22	Squatting behavior	**22**	[Occasionally.]
23	Fever	**23**	[100 to 100.8F by mouth for one week.]
24	Recent infection	**24**	[Upper respiratory tract infection two weeks before admission.]
25	Dizziness	**25**	[Yes, progressive in recent days.]
26	Vomiting	**26**	[Yes, projectile on day of admission.]
27	Previous history of headaches	**27**	[None.]
28	Nose bleeds	**28**	[None.]
29	Diarrhea	**29**	[No, bowel movements normal.]
30	Constipation	**30**	[No, bowel movements normal.]
31	Convulsions	**31**	[None.]
32	Allergic history	**32**	[Eczema as an infant.]

33	Chest pain	**33**	[None.]
34	Social history	**34**	[Middle income family; devoted mother; working father; parents are anxious, cooperative, and helpful.]

YOU WOULD NOW (CHOOSE ONLY ONE):

35	Order laboratory tests	**35**	[CONTINUE WITH SECTION 19-D, PAGE 288.]
36	Perform physical examination	**36**	[TURN TO SECTION 19-F, PAGE 291.]
37	Reassure parents of benign nature of the symptoms and ask them to call if other symptoms develop	**37**	[TURN TO SECTION 19-G, PAGE 293.]
38	Initiate therapy	**38**	[TURN TO SECTION 19-B, PAGE 286.]

SECTION 19-D

YOU WOULD NOW ORDER (SELECT AS MANY AS YOU CONSIDER INDICATED):

39	Chest x-ray	**39**	[SEE FIGURES 37 AND 38, PAGE 417.]
40	Throat culture for bacteria	**40**	[Normal flora.]
41	Timed vital capacity	**41**	[Patient's condition deteriorates and procedure must be terminated.]
42	White blood cell count and differential	**42**	[WBC – 15,500/mm^3, differential: segmented neutrophils – 80%, bands – 10%; lymphocytes – 10%.]

43	Lumbar puncture	**43**	[Cerebrospinal fluid: pressure — 300 mm H_2O; cells — 500 segmented neutrophils/mm^3; no red blood cells; protein — 100 mg/100 ml; sugar — 40 mg/100 ml; Gram stained smear — no organisms seen; culture — no report yet.]
44	Fasting blood sugar	**44**	[80 mg/100 ml.]
45	Blood urea nitrogen	**45**	[17 mg/100 ml.]
46	Urinalysis	**46**	[Specific gravity — 1.010, pH — 5.5, protein — negative, glucose — negative, no cells.]
47	Hematocrit	**47**	[60%.]
48	Sedimentation rate	**48**	[30 mm per hour (Wintrobe).]
49	Blood culture for bacteria	**49**	[No growth.]
50	Urine culture for bacteria	**50**	[No growth.]
51	Skull x-rays	**51**	[SEE FIGURES 59 AND 60, PAGE 422.]
52	Electrocardiogram	**52**	[SEE FIGURE 6, PAGE 409.]
53	Serum calcium	**53**	[5.7 mEq/L.]
54	Serum magnesium	**54**	[2.0 mEq/L.]
55	Serum bilirubin (total)	**55**	[1.0 mg/100 ml.]
56	Arterial oxygen saturation	**56**	[82%.]
57	Circulation time (arm to tongue)	**57**	[Done with difficulty, requiring several tries, 10 seconds.]

UNLESS OTHERWISE DIRECTED IN THE RESPONSE COLUMN CONTINUE WITH SECTION 19-E

SECTION 19-E

YOU WOULD NOW ORDER (SELECT AS MANY AS YOU CONSIDER INDICATED):

58	No further tests	**58**	[DO NOT MAKE ANY MORE CHOICES IN ITEMS 59 TO 66, GO DIRECTLY TO ITEMS 67 TO 70.]
59	Cardiac catheterization	**59**	[Done. Patient deteriorates during procedure.]
60	Angiocardiography	**60**	[Done. Patient deteriorates during procedure.]
61	Arterial puncture for determination of oxygen saturation	**61**	[At rest, arterial oxygen saturation — 82%.]
62	Electroencephalogram	**62**	[Tracing shows focal abnormality, right occipital lobe.]
63	Neurologic consultation	**63**	[The patient's symptoms and signs are consistent with space occupying lesion, right occipital lobe, confirmed by cerebral angiography.]
64	Pulmonary function studies	**64**	[Patient cannot cooperate.]
65	Renal arteriogram	**65**	[Procedure done with great difficulty. Patient deteriorates during procedure. X-rays show normal arteries.]
66	Brain scan	**66**	[Brain scan shows increased uptake in right occipital area.]

YOU WOULD NOW (CHOOSE ONLY ONE):

67	Reassure parents of benign nature of the problem and make return appointment in six months	**67**	[TURN TO SECTION 19-G, PAGE 293.]

68	Obtain psychiatric consult	68	[TURN TO SECTION 19-G, PAGE 293.]
69	Initiate emergency treatment	69	[TURN TO SECTION 19-B, PAGE 286.]
70	Discharge patient from your care	70	[TURN TO SECTION 19-G, PAGE 293.]

SECTION 19-F

IN PERFORMING THE PHYSICAL EXAMINATION YOU WOULD BE PARTICULARLY INTERESTED TO CHECK (SELECT AS MANY AS YOU CONSIDER ESPECIALLY PERTINENT; YOU CAN RETURN TO THIS SECTION AT ANYTIME TO OBTAIN ANY ADDITIONAL INFORMATION YOU MAY REQUIRE ABOUT INITIAL PHYSICAL FINDINGS):

71	Mouth	71	[Lips and buccal mucosa moderately cyanotic.]
72	Extremities	72	[Moderate cyanosis and clubbing of digits; no edema.]
73	Ears and throat	73	[Ears normal, throat somewhat injected.]
74	Blood pressure	74	[110/80 mm Hg – right arm; 130/90 mm Hg – right leg.]
75	Optic fundi	75	[Grade 1 papilledema bilaterally.]
76	Neck	76	[Not remarkable.]
77	Palpation of anterior chest	77	[Prominent heave at the lower sternal border, systolic thrill at second and third interspaces, left sternal border.]
78	Auscultation of heart	78	[Second heart sound normal, well heard at third interspace at left sternal border. Grade IV systolic murmur at second and third interspace, left sternal border.]

79	Auscultation of lungs	79	[Normal.]
80	Neurologic examination	80	[Homonymous hemianopsia on right side; hyperactive deep tendon reflexes greater on right side.]
81	Palpation of the abdomen	81	[Liver, kidneys and spleen not palpable, no masses.]
82	Skin	82	[There is cyanosis of digits and lips, rosy cheeks, perioral pallor. The skin is of normal consistency. No petechiae.]
83	Pulse	83	[All pulses felt. Resting rate: 60/minute, regular, synchronous
84	Auscultation of abdomen	84	[Normal bowel sounds. No bruit.]
85	Genitalia	85	[Normal for age. No hernia or hydrocele.]
86	Temperature	86	[101.5F (oral).]
87	Rectal examination	87	[The child objects to procedure, but it is done with difficulty. Small amount of fresh blood on glove. No masses in rectum.]
88	Percussion of abdomen	88	[Resonant; no abnormal dullness
89	Pulse after exercise	89	[Patient faints.]

YOU WOULD NOW (CHOOSE ONLY ONE):

90	Order laboratory tests	90	[TURN TO SECTION 19-D, PAGE 288.]
91	Initiate therapy	91	[TURN TO SECTION 19-B, PAGE 286.]

92	Reassure parents of benign nature of symptoms and ask them to call if further symptoms develop	**92**	[CONTINUE WITH SECTION 19-G, PAGE 293.]
93	Obtain further history from patient's mother	**93**	[TURN TO SECTION 19-C, PAGE 287.]

SECTION 19-G

94	Record your diagnoses below: ____________________ ____________________ ____________________ ____________________ ____________________ ____________________ ____________________ ____________________	**94**	[The complete diagnosis as recorded on the patient's chart was (i) brain abscess, (ii) cyanotic congenital heart disease, tetralogy of Fallot. SEE APPENDIX H FOR ADDITIONAL COMMENT AND RECOMMENDED MANAGEMENT. END OF PROBLEM 19.]

NOW DEVELOP RESPONSE 94 FOR ADDITIONAL INFORMATION AND INSTRUCTIONS

PROBLEM 20

HEADACHES AND SPOTS

A patient whom you have never seen before comes to your office. She is 18 years old and gives the following history spontaneously: "I feel like I'm falling apart. I have for the last few years, been getting some brown spots on my body and my eyesight is getting poorer. I have frequent, funny headaches, and when I get them I feel like I'm going to die. My father is dead. My mother is only 48 years old. She had to be put away in an asylum and I have to look after my brother who can't work."

NOW CONTINUE WITH SECTION 20-A

SECTION 20-A

YOU WOULD NOW (CHOOSE ONLY ONE EACH TIME YOU ARE DIRECTED TO THIS SECTION):

1	Take a complete history	1	[TURN TO SECTION 20-C, PAGE 296.]
2	Perform a physical examination	2	[TURN TO SECTION 20-D, PAGE 301.]
3	Schedule the patient for a return visit and postpone further study until that visit	3	[CONTINUE WITH SECTION 20-B.]
4	Order laboratory tests or special investigations	4	[TURN TO SECTION 20-F, PAGE 313.]
5	Seek consultation	5	[TURN TO SECTION 20-E, PAGE 307.]

6	Initiate therapy	6	[TURN TO SECTION 20-J, PAGE 331.]
7	Order x-ray studies	7	[TURN TO SECTION 20-G, PAGE 322.]
8	Order biopsy studies	8	[TURN TO SECTION 20-H, PAGE 327.]
9	Counsel the patient	9	[TURN TO SECTION 20-I, PAGE 329.]
10	Offer a prognosis	10	[TURN TO SECTION 20-K, PAGE 336.]
11	Discharge the patient	11	[TURN TO SECTION 20-M, PAGE 338.]

SECTION 20-B

AS A FOLLOW–UP YOU WOULD (CHOOSE ONLY ONE EACH TIME YOU ARE DIRECTED TO THIS SECTION):

12	Ask patient to return in two months with special procedures scheduled in the interim	12	[Patient accepts your advice. TURN TO SECTION 20-F, PAGE 313.]
13	Ask patient to return in two months without any special procedures	13	[Patient accepts your advice, she returns in two months with presenting complaint unchanged. Start problem again with statement of presenting complaint and then CONTINUE WITH SECTION 20-A.]
14	Send the patient away without further appointment	14	[Patient accepts your advice.]
15	Ask patient to return in one year	15	[Patient accepts your advice.]

UNLESS OTHERWISE DIRECTED IN THE RESPONSE COLUMN TURN NOW TO SECTION 20-M, PAGE 338

SECTION 20-C

IN OBTAINING THE HISTORY YOU WOULD BE PARTICULARLY INTERESTED TO ASK THE FOLLOWING (SELECT AS MANY AS YOU CONSIDER ESPECIALLY PERTINENT; YOU CAN RETURN TO THIS SECTION AT ANY TIME TO OBTAIN ANY ADDITIONAL HISTORICAL INFORMATION YOU MAY REQUIRE):

16	What is your name?	**16**	[My name is Katherine.]
17	How old are you?	**17**	[I am 18 years old.]
18	What do you do now?	**18**	[I work and I look after my brother who is retarded.]
19	How did your father die?	**19**	[My father died three years ago in a car accident.]
20	How is your mother?	**20**	[My mother is in an asylum and she's only 48 years old.]
21	What brings you here?	**21**	[I get these terrible headaches my eyesight is failing and I feel like I'm falling apart.]
22	What's wrong with your mother?	**22**	[My mother has lumps all over her and she also has a crooked back.]
23	Can your mother come to see me?	**23**	[She can't come to see you; she is not right in the head. Her doctor gave me a picture to give any doctor I may see. Here it is (SEE FIGURE 27, PAGE 414).]
24	Can your brother come to see me?	**24**	[No it's hard for him to get out of the house, but I also have his picture which I only show to doctors (SEE FIGURE 28, PAGE 414).]
25	How old is your brother?	**25**	[My brother is 23 years old.]

26	Is he in good health?	**26**	[He is not in very good health. He also has lumps, he can't hear well and he is mentally retarded.]
27	What sort of diseases run in your family?	**27**	[Well, like these lumps and skin spots.]
28	Has there ever been high blood pressure in your family?	**28**	[My mother has high blood pressure.]
29	Have you ever had an operation?	**29**	[No.]
30	Have you ever been in the hospital?	**30**	[I was in the hospital once after I fainted at work.]
31	Do you take drugs?	**31**	[None except aspirin and Excedrin.]
32	Have you ever had any diseases of childhood?	**32**	[Yes, I had chickenpox and measles and colds.]
33	What else bothers you besides the headaches and the loss of vision?	**33**	[I have brown spots on my body. I have about 13 of them, they are getting more in number and size.]
34	Tell me more about your headaches	**34**	[My headaches are very severe on the left side. I get sick to my stomach and my head feels like it is being squeezed.]
35	How is your vision?	**35**	[I can't see well in my left eye lately.]
36	Do you ever black out?	**36**	[I do black out once every few months, but I can't remember what happens, I have no warning, I just wake up and then stay sleepy.]
37	Do the drugs help?	**37**	[The aspirin and Excedrin don't help my headache or blackouts much.]

38	Do you have stomach trouble?	**38**	[No stomach trouble.]
39	Is there anything wrong with your skin?	**39**	[Just the brown spots.]
40	Have you had any loss of strength in your hands or arms or legs or feet?	**40**	[No, I have had no loss of strength.]
41	How do you feel generally?	**41**	[I get tired easy and feel down in the dumps.]
42	Tell me a little more about your eyes.	**42**	[My vision in my left eye has been getting worse for about three years, I see black and I almost got hit by a car the other day.]
43	How is your hearing?	**43**	[Good.]
44	Do you have any problems with your nose or sinuses?	**44**	[None.]
45	Have you ever had any thyroid or goiter trouble?	**45**	[Never.]
46	Have you ever noticed any lumps or bumps in your neck or under your arms.	**46**	[No lumps in my neck or under my arms.]
47	Do you cough?	**47**	[Only when I get a cold.]
48	Do you get short of breath?	**48**	[Only when I run. Then I get short of breath and I have a pain in my left or right side.]
49	Have you ever had pneumonia?	**49**	[No.]
50	Have you ever had an x-ray?	**50**	[I had a chest x-ray once and it was normal.]
51	Have you ever had any heart murmurs or pain in the chest?	**51**	[No.]

52	Does your heart beat abnormally?	**52**	[No.]
53	Do your feet swell?	**53**	[No.]
54	How is your appetite?	**54**	[My appetite is normal, I eat everything.]
55	Do you have stomach pains?	**55**	[No.]
56	Do you have diarrhea or constipation?	**56**	[No; my bowels have always remained the same.]
57	Do you have nausea or vomiting?	**57**	[No.]
58	Have you ever been yellow?	**58**	[No.]
59	Do you notice that you have excessive bruising or bleeding from your gums or nose?	**59**	[No, I only bleed in my periods.]
60	How often do you pass urine?	**60**	[I pass normal-looking urine about three times a day.]
61	Do you have any pain or burning when you pass urine?	**61**	[No.]
62	Have you ever wet your pants?	**62**	[I wet my pants when I blackout.]
63	Have you any trouble with your sex organs?	**63**	[I have no trouble with my sex organs.]
64	How often do you have periods?	**64**	[Normally, about every month for about five days.]
65	How many pads do you use?	**65**	[About five pads a day, then less the last few days.]
66	Have you ever had a miscarriage?	**66**	[No.]
67	Do you take any pills for preventing pregnancy?	**67**	[No.]

68	Have you ever had any discharges?	68	[No.]
69	Have you ever been told you are anemic?	69	[No, I haven't tired blood.]
70	Has your weight changed?	70	[My weight hasn't changed for many years.]
71	Does the heat or cold bother you?	71	[Not any more than anybody else.]
72	Do you think you're depressed?	72	[I am depressed, but I've never thought about killing myself. I guess having no money is not easy. I look after my brother all day and work, till midnight. You don't get a chance to go out much, especially on my salary.]

YOU WOULD NOW (CHOOSE ONLY ONE):

73	Schedule the patient for a return visit and postpone further study until that time	73	[TURN TO SECTION 20-B, PAGE 295.]
74	Hospitalize the patient if you have not already done so	74	[CONTINUE WITH 82-86 IN THIS SECTION.]
75	Continue your work-up and management on an outpatient basis	75	[CONTINUE WITH 82-86 IN THIS SECTION.]
76	Continue your work-up and management of the patient in the hospital	76	[CONTINUE WITH 82-86 IN THIS SECTION.]
77	Seek consultation	77	[TURN TO SECTION 20-E, PAGE 307.]
78	Transfer the patient to a colleague	78	[TURN TO SECTION 20-M, PAGE 338.]

79 Counsel the patient — [TURN TO SECTION 20-I, PAGE 329.]

80 Offer a prognosis — [TURN TO SECTION 20-K, PAGE 336.]

81 Discharge the patient — [TURN TO SECTION 20-M, PAGE 338.]

YOU WOULD NOW (CHOOSE ONLY ONE):

82 Perform a physical examination if you have not already done so — [CONTINUE WITH SECTION 20-D.]

83 Order laboratory tests or special investigations if you have not already done so — [TURN TO SECTION 20-F, PAGE 313.]

84 Initiate therapy if you have not already done so — [TURN TO SECTION 20-J, PAGE 331.]

85 Order x-ray studies if you have not already done so — [TURN TO SECTION 20-G, PAGE 322.]

86 Order biopsy studies if you have not already done so — [TURN TO SECTION 20-H, PAGE 327.]

SECTION 20-D

IN PERFORMING THE PHYSICAL EXAMINATION, YOU WOULD BE PARTICULARLY INTERESTED TO CHECK (SELECT AS MANY AS YOU CONSIDER ESPECIALLY PERTINENT; YOU CAN RETURN TO THIS SECTION AT ANY TIME TO OBTAIN ANY ADDITIONAL INFORMATION YOU MAY REQUIRE ABOUT THE INITIAL PHYSICAL FINDINGS):

87 General appearance — [Well-nourished, well-developed white girl; she is somewhat sad and chews gum continuously.]

88 Head — [Symmetrical, no scars, bruits, or tenderness.]

89	Hair distribution	89	[Normal female.]

Eyes, Ears, and Throat

90	Eye inspection	90	[Normal.]
91	Eye movement	91	[Full eye movements.]
92	Pupilary reaction	92	[Equally reactive to light and accommodation.]
93	Funduscopic examination	93	[Right eye, normal; left eye, SEE FIGURE 22, PAGE 413.]
94	Visual fields	94	[There is a large defect in the nasal and central fields of the left eye.]
95	Ears and hearing	95	[Ears are normal to inspection; there is no hearing deficit on audiologic determination.]
96	Otoscopic examination	96	[Canals are clear; the tympanic membranes are clear with normal light reflex; no mastoid tenderness.]
97	Throat	97	[There are two moderately enlarged tonsils showing no other abnormality.]

Neck

98	Neck	98	[Supple without adenopathy; no venous distention or abnormal pulsation.]
99	Thyroid	99	[The thyroid is palpable in the midline; there are no nodules and its consistency is normal.]

100	Breasts	**100**	[Full and round without discharge, tenderness, or palpable masses.]

Chest

101	Chest, inspection	**101**	[Appearance symmetrical, with full symmetrical expansion; no visible pulsations.]
102	Chest, percussion, and ausculation	**102**	[Clear to percussion and ausculation.]
103	Heart, palpation	**103**	[Palpation: the point of maximal impulse is palpable in the fifth intercostal space 1.5 cm lateral to midclavicular line; there is no thrill, heave, lift, or abnormal pulsation.]
104	Heart auscultation	**104**	[Auscultation performed in all appropriate positions — normal sinus rhythm, rate 80 per minute; no extra sounds, murmurs, or rubs.]
105	Blood pressure	**105**	[Right arm: 155/95 mm Hg.]

Abdomen and Rectum

106	Abdomen, inspection	**106**	[Normal contour, no visible dilated veins, scars or other abnormalities.]
107	Abdomen, palpation	**107**	[Normal consistency without guarding, tenderness, or spasm; no masses or fluid wave; no palpable enlargement of liver, spleen, kidneys, gallbladder, or urinary bladder; no evidence of hernia.]

108 Rectal examination

108 [No evidence of hemorrhoids; no masses.]

Vaginal

109 Vaginal examination

109 [No abnormalities seen.]

Vascular System, Muscles, and Skeleton

110 Musculature

110 [Normal development without atrophy or fasciculation; normal tone and strength.]

111 Pulses

111 [Equal and strong.]

112 Gait

112 [There is minimal circumduction of the right leg; associated movements are more prominent on the left.]

113 Back examination

113 [No evidence of tenderness, dislocation or subluxation.]

Skin

114 Skin

114 [The only abnormalities found consist of 14 half-inch to three-inch oblong café-au-lait spots scattered over the thorax and abdomen; SEE FIGURES 25 AND 26, PAGE 414. There is axillary freckling bilaterally, a half-inch nonpigmented nevus near the left clavicle, and a small, firm, unencapsulated, fixed nodule behind the right knee; there are three small fibromas on the medial three toes of the right foot.]

Nodes

115	Lymph nodes	**115**	[No palpable cervical, occipital, axillary, supraclavicular, or epitrochlear nodes. There are small bilateral inguinal nodes, discrete, moderately hard, freely moveable, nontender, non-fluctuant, about 1/2 to 1 cm in diameter.]

Neuropsychiatric Examination

116	Mental status	**116**	[Somewhat depressed, but otherwise normal.]
117	Cranial nerves	**117**	[Cranial nerves are normal, except for left optic nerve which demonstrates a macular and temporal area tumor; there is no facial asymmetry and no evidence of facial nerve involvement.]
118	Facial movement	**118**	[Normal, full facial movement; full head movement; normal bilateral full forehead movement.]
119	Motor coordination	**119**	[There is minimal difficulty with rapid alternating movements on the right.]
120	Sensation	**120**	[Light touch, pin prick, deep pain, temperature, position, and vibratory sensations are all intact.]
121	Reflexes	**121**	[There is a mild asymmetry of deep tendon reflexes with the right biceps, patellar, and Achilles tendon reflex more active.]

122	Babinski reflex	**122**	[Right Babinski produces dorsiflexion of the great toe, with fanning of the other toes; left Babinski produces plantar flexion of all toes.]
123	Hoffman reflex	**123**	[Positive Hoffman responses were elicited bilaterally, as were bilateral palmomental reflexes.]
124	Finger to nose test	**124**	[Normal coordination on finger to nose test.]
125	Heel to knee test	**125**	[Normal coordination on heel to knee test.]

YOU WOULD NOW (CHOOSE ONLY ONE):

126	Schedule the patient for a return visit and postpone further study until that time	**126**	[TURN TO SECTION 20-B, PAGE 295.]
127	Hospitalize the patient if you have not already done so	**127**	[CONTINUE WITH 135-139 IN THIS SECTION.]
128	Continue your work-up and management on an outpatient	**128**	[CONTINUE WITH 135-139 IN THIS SECTION.]
129	Continue your work-up and management of the patient in the hospital	**129**	[CONTINUE WITH 135-139 IN THIS SECTION.]
130	Seek consultation	**130**	[CONTINUE WITH SECTION 20-E.]
131	Transfer the patient to a colleague	**131**	[TURN TO SECTION 20-M, PAGE 338.]
132	Counsel the patient	**132**	[TURN TO SECTION 20-I, PAGE 329.]
133	Offer a prognosis	**133**	[TURN TO SECTION 20-K, PAGE 336.]

134	Discharge the patient	**134**	[TURN TO SECTION 20-M, PAGE 338.]

YOU WOULD NOW (CHOOSE ONLY ONE):

135	Take a complete history if you have not already done so	**135**	[TURN TO SECTION 20-C, PAGE 296.]
136	Order laboratory tests or special investigations if you have not already done so	**136**	[TURN TO SECTION 20-F, PAGE 313.]
137	Initiate therapy if you have not already done so	**137**	[TURN TO SECTION 20-J, PAGE 331.]
138	Order x-ray studies if you have not already done so	**138**	[TURN TO SECTION 20-G, PAGE 322.]
139	Order biopsy studies if you have not already done so	**139**	[TURN TO SECTION 20-H, PAGE 327.]

SECTION 20-E

YOU WOULD NOW REQUEST THE FOLLOWING CONSULTATIONS (SELECT AS MANY AS YOU CONSIDER ESPECIALLY PERTINENT; YOU CAN RETURN TO THIS SECTION FOR ADDITIONAL CONSULTATIONS AT ANY TIME):

140	Allergist	**140**	[The patient's physical examination is essentially as stated on the chart. I do not believe that the patient's headaches or cutaneous problems are in any way related to an allergic problem.]
141	Cardiologist	**141**	[The patient's cardiologic status was evaluated and the physical findings are essentially those stated on the chart. There is no cardiomegaly, no murmur, and the electrocardiogram shows an essentially normal tracing.]

142 Endocrinologist

142 [The patient was evaluated from two points of view, that of thyroid status and the possible presence of a pheochromocytoma. As far as the thyroid status is concerned, there is no enlargement of the gland and it has no nodules, there is no tremor, no diarrhea, the sweating pattern appears to be normal, and there is no evidence of exophthalmos. I do not believe that the patient suffers from thyroid disease, although a PBI (protein-bound iodine) and T_4 blood test may help further to rule out this diagnosis. The borderline normal blood pressure plus the presence of neurofibromatosis would be an indication for urine catecholamine and (VMA) vanilmandelic acid tests in the urine. After these studies have been done, I will be happy to evaluate the patient further.]

143 **Ophthalmologist**

143 [Examination of both eyes in this patient who has progressive loss of vision, is essentially that as stated on the chart. The positive findings include: in the right eye, some anisocoria 2 to 3 mm; the pupil reacts to light and accommodation; in the left eye there is a weak reaction to light and it does not react normally to accommodation. Fundus – the right eye shows a type 2 disc with normal vessels, the left eye (SEE FIGURE 22, PAGE 413), shows a marked temporal disc pallor; there is an elevated mass involving the macula and the temporal portion of the fundus. This finding is consistent with Von Recklinghausen's disease and retinal neuroma in the left eye. There is secondary optic atrophy in the left eye and left exotropia secondary to Von Recklinghausen's disease. Advise follow-up in six months. The patient may develop secondary glaucoma.]

144 Orthopedic surgeon

144 [Examination of the skeletal structure by x-ray and functional activity of the bones, joints and muscular systems was essentially normal. I do not believe that the patient's complaints are muscular or skeletal in origin, would advise repeat x-ray of spine in several months, in order to detect possible scoliosis. There are no radiologic findings of neurofibromas involving the bones; examination of the x-ray belonging to the patient's mother (SEE FIGURE 57, PAGE 422) shows severe kyphoscoliosis with collapse of several of the middorsal vertebrae a finding consistent with the patient's apparent diagnosis of neurofibromatosis.]

145 Psychiatrist

145 [The patient is fairly depressed, although there is no evidence of suicidal tendencies. The depression cannot be differentiated from that found in hyperthyroidism but is probably related to the patient's poor family condition. Drugs are not suggested but supportive psychotherapy may be of help to this patient. In view of the good rapport the patient has with you, it is suggested that you continue to provide supportive care for her. Perhaps social service may be of value in helping to alleviate the family situation.]

146 Urologist

146 [The patient is evaluated from the point of view of a possible pheochromocytoma. I do not believe that retroperitoneal air studies are indicated at this time. Radiologic examination of the kidneys is as reported in the intravenous pyelogram; there is no evidence of a suprarenal mass at this time. I would suggest urinary VMA and catecholamine studies.]

147 Plastic surgeon

147 [The patient is evaluated from the point of view of the café-au-lait spots. I do not believe that plastic surgery would be beneficial to this patient at this time; would be happy to reevaluate if neurofibromas develop some time in the future. Thank you for this consultation.]

148 Neurologic consultation

148 [Neurologic examination is essentially as has been described in the chart and is suggestive of a left hemispheral structural lesion. The patient should have a left carotid arteriogram to evaluate this lesion. Computerized axial tomography (or EMI scan) of the head with infusion would be helpful.]

YOU WOULD NOW (CHOOSE ONLY ONE EACH TIME YOU ARE DIRECTED TO THIS SECTION):

149 Schedule the patient for a return visit and postpone further study until that time

149 [TURN TO SECTION 20-L, PAGE 337.]

150 Hospitalize the patient if you have not already done so

150 [CONTINUE WITH 157-162 IN THIS SECTION.]

151	Continue your work-up and management on an outpatient basis	151	[CONTINUE WITH 157-162 IN THIS SECTION.]
152	Continue your work-up and management of the patient in the hospital.	152	[CONTINUE WITH 157-162 IN THIS SECTION.]
153	Transfer the patient to a colleague	153	[TURN TO SECTION 20-M, PAGE 338.]
154	Counsel the patient	154	[TURN TO SECTION 20-I, PAGE 329.]
155	Offer a prognosis	155	[TURN TO SECTION 20-K, PAGE 336.]
156	Discharge the patient	156	[TURN TO SECTION 20-M, PAGE 338.]

YOU WOULD NOW (CHOOSE ONLY ONE):

157	Take a complete history if you have not already done so	157	[TURN TO SECTION 20-C, PAGE 296.]
158	Perform a physical examination if you have not already done so	158	[TURN TO SECTION 20-D, PAGE 301.]
159	Order laboratory tests or special investigations if you have not already done so	159	[CONTINUE WITH SECTION 20-F.]
160	Initiate therapy if you have not already done so	160	[TURN TO SECTION 20-J, PAGE 331.]
161	Order x-ray studies if you have not already done so	161	[TURN TO SECTION 20-G, PAGE 322.]
162	Order biopsy studies if you have not already done so	162	[TURN TO SECTION 20-H, PAGE 327.]

SECTION 20-F

YOU WOULD NOW ORDER THE FOLLOWING DETERMINATIONS (SELECT AS MANY AS YOU CONSIDER INDICATED):

Blood

163	Red blood cell count	**163**	[5.2 X 10^6/mm^3.]
164	White blood cell count	**164**	[6300/mm^3.]
165	Hemoglobin	**165**	[15 g/100 ml.]
166	Hematocrit	**166**	[45%.]
167	Differential	**167**	[Neutrophils – 60%, lymphocytes – 26%, monocytes – 6%, eosinophils – 3%, basophils – 5%.]
168	Red blood cell smear	**168**	[Normal chromicity, no evidence of anisocytosis, no evidence of poikilocytosis.]
169	Mean corpuscular volume	**169**	[87 μm^3.]
170	Mean corpuscular hemoglobin	**170**	[29 pg.]
171	Mean corpuscular hemoglobin concentration	**171**	[34%.]
172	Platelets	**172**	[300,000/mm^3.]
173	Reticulocytes	**173**	[1.2%.]
174	Sickle cell preparation	**174**	[Negative.]
175	Coombs test	**175**	[Negative.]
176	Erythrocyte sedimentation rate	**176**	[8 mm/hour (Wintrobe).]

Urinalysis

177	Appearance	177	[Amber yellow.]
178	pH	178	[6.5.]
179	Diacetic acid	179	[Negative.]
180	Bile pigment	180	[Negative.]
181	Urobilinogen	181	[Negative.]
182	Reducing sugar	182	[Negative.]
183	Protein	183	[0.1 g/24 hours.]
184	Specific gravity	184	[1.019.]
185	Acetone	185	[Negative.]
186	Bacteria	186	[Negative.]
187	Crystals	187	[Negative.]
188	Epithelial cells	188	[0-3/hpf.]
189	Leukocytes	189	[0-3/hpf.]
190	Casts in urine	190	[Negative.]
191	Erythrocytes	191	[0-3/hpf.]
192	Bilirubin in urine	192	[None.]
193	Steroids (24 hours)	193	[17-OH steroids: 6 mg; 17 ketosteroids: 13 mg.]
194	Urine culture, sensitivity and colony count	194	[No growth.]
195	Urine porphobilinogen	195	[Qual: negative; quan: less than 2 mg/24 hours.]

196	Porphyrins	**196**	[Coproporphyrins 130 μg/24 hours, uroporphyrins 2 μg/24 hours.]
197	Bence Jones protein	**197**	[Negative.]
198	Urobilinogen	**198**	[Qual: negative; quan: 3 mg/24 hours.]

Blood Chemistry

199	Sugar	**199**	[85 mg/100 ml random sample.]
200	Urea nitrogen	**200**	[13 mg/100 ml.]
201	Chloride	**201**	[103 mEq/L.]
202	Carbon dioxide combining power	**202**	[27 mEq/L.]
203	Sodium	**203**	[142 mEq/L.]
204	Potassium	**204**	[4.9 mEq/L.]
205	pH	**205**	[7.39.]
206	Creatinine	**206**	[1.5 mg/100 ml.]
207	Uric acid	**207**	[4 mg/100 ml.]
208	Cholesterol total	**208**	[198 mg/100 ml.]
209	Cholesterol-esterified (serum)	**209**	[67% of total.]
210	Amylase	**210**	[95 units/100 ml (Somogyi).]
211	Lipase	**211**	[.86 ml (Cherry-Crandall).]
212	Acid phosphatase	**212**	[0.5 units (King-Armstrong).]
213	Inorganic phosphorus	**213**	[1.0 mEq/L.]

214	Calcium	**214**	[5.1 mEq/L.]
215	Creatine phosphokinase	**215**	[25 IU/ml.]
216	Alkaline phosphatase serum	**216**	[11.5 units (King-Armstrong).]
217	Serum glutamic oxalacetic transaminase	**217**	[18 IU/L.]
218	Serum glutamic pyruvic transaminase	**218**	[24 IU/L.]
219	Lactic dehydrogenase	**219**	[187 units/ml (Wroblewski).]
220	Bromsulphalein clearance	**220**	[5% retention at the end of 45 minutes.]
221	Thymol turbidity	**221**	[2 units/ml.]
222	Cephalin flocculation	**222**	[24 hours – Negative; 48 hours – Negative.]
223	Serum protein	**223**	[7.9 g/100 ml.]
224	Serum albumin	**224**	[4.9 g/100 ml.]
225	Serum globulin	**225**	[3.0 g/100 ml.]
226	Bilirubin-direct	**226**	[0.1 mg/100 ml.]
227	Bilirubin-total	**227**	[0.85 mg/100 ml.]
228	Protein electrophoresis	**228**	[Albumin: 62%, $Alpha_1$ globulin – 7% $Alpha_2$ – 7%, Beta – 11%, Gamma – 13%.]
229	C-Reactive protein	**229**	[Negative.]

Coagulation Studies

230	Partial thromboplastin time	**230**	[67 seconds.]

231	Prothrombin control	**231**	[13 seconds.]
232	Prothrombin time	**232**	[12 seconds; control 13 seconds.]
233	Prothrombin, percent activity	**233**	[95% (approx.).]
234	Fibrinogen	**234**	[0.3 g/100 ml.]
235	Bleeding time (Ivy)	**235**	[Five minutes.]
236	Clotting time (Lee-White)	**236**	[11 minutes.]
237	Rumple-Leeds Test	**237**	[10 petechiae per 2.5 cm.]

Special Hematologic and Biochemcial Studies

238	Lupus erythematosus cell preparation	**238**	[Negative.]
239	Antinuclear antibody	**239**	[Negative.]
240	Serum iron	**240**	[90 μg/100 ml.]
241	Serum iron-binding capacity	**241**	[350 μg/100 ml.]
242	Rheumatoid factor	**242**	[Negative.]
243	Carotenoids	**243**	[235 μg/100 ml.]
244	Vitamin A	**244**	[65 μg/100 ml.]
245	Folic acid (serum)	**245**	[17 ng/ml.]
246	Vitamin B_{12}	**246**	[450 pg/ml.]
247	Radioactive iodine (^{131}I) uptake	**247**	[35%.]
248	Protein-bound iodine	**248**	[6 μg/100 ml.]
249	Plasma norepinephrine	**249**	[.04 μg/L.]
250	Plasma epinephrine	**250**	[None detected.]

251 Blood corticoids – 8 A.M. 251 [15 μg/100 ml.]

252 Glucose tolerance test 252 [

	Blood (mg/ml)	Urine
Fasting	96/100.	Negative
1/2 hr.	140/100.	Negative
2 hrs.	120/100.	Negative
3 hrs.	80/100.	Negative

253 Blood bromide 253 [Negative.]

254 Blood barbituates 254 [None.]

255 Blood ethanol 255 [.1 parts/100 ml.]

256 Blood salicylates 256 [Positive.]

257 Tri-iodothyronine uptake (Resin) 257 [28%.]

258 Thyroxine (Pattee-Murphy) 258 [9 μg/100 ml.]

Serologic Studies

259 Antithyroglobulin 259 [Negative.]

260 STS 260 [Reactive; one dilution.]

261 Mono Spot Test 261 [Negative.]

262 Fluorescent Treponema Antibody Absorption Test 262 [Nonreactive.]

263 Spinal fluid (Colloidal Gold Test) 263 [0001121100.]

Special Studies on Urine

264 Creatinine clearance 264 [110 ml/minute.]

265 Urine creatinine 265 [1.3 g/24 hours.]

266 Phenolsulfonphthalein test

267 Sodium

268 Chloride

269 Calcium

270 Phosphorus

271 Potassium

272 Urine quantitative protein

273 Quantitative glucose

274 Urobilinogen

275 Urine creatinine

276 Metanephrine

277 Catecholamines

278 Vanilmandelic acid

279 Epinephrine

280 Norepinephrine

281 Stool examination

266 [28% excreted in 15 minutes, 70% in two hours.]

267 [180 mEq/24 hours.]

268 [210 mEq/24 hours.]

269 [0.4 mEq/24 hours.]

270 [0.9 g/24 hours.]

271 [60.0 mEq/24 hours.]

272 [0.1 g/24 hours.]

273 [0.3 g/24 hours.]

274 [2.5 mg/24 hours.]

275 [1.3 g/24 hours.]

276 [0.6 mg/24 hours.]

277 [18 μg/100 ml or 103 μg/24 hours.]

278 [4.6 mg/24 hours.]

279 [13 μg/24 hours.]

280 [73 μg/24 hours.]

281 [Stool is soft, brown and formed; blood in stool — negative; pus macroscopic — negative; mucus — negative; occult blood — negative; urobilinogen in stool — 130 mg/24 hours; bile in stool — negative; calcium in stool — 651 mEq/24 hours; ova and parasites — negative.]

282	Gastric analysis	**282**	[Negative for blood and bile; volume and acidity normal.]
283	Spinal tap	**283**	[Opening pressure – 100 mm water; appearance – clear and colorless; protein – 30 mg/100 ml; glucose – 60 mg/100 ml; chloride – 120 mEq/L; culture – negative; cytology – negative; cell count – no cells seen; Pandy – negative.]
284	Cytology for sputum, urine, bronchial washings, gastric washings, breast secretion, pleural fluid, peritoneal fluid	**284**	[Normal cytology, no atypical cells seen.]
285	Electrocardiogram	**285**	[SEE FIGURE 1, PAGE 404.]
286	Electroencephalogram	**286**	[EEG dominant frequency of 9 to 10 cycles per second with activity seen best posteriorly. There is no significant hemispheral asymmetry noted. No epileptogenic activity was seen.]

YOU WOULD NOW (CHOOSE ONLY ONE):

287	Schedule the patient for a return visit and postpone further study until that time	**287**	[TURN TO SECTION 20-L, PAGE 337.]
288	Hospitalize the patient if you have not already done so	**288**	[CONTINUE WITH 296-300 IN THIS SECTION.]
289	Continue your work-up and management on an outpatient basis	**289**	[CONTINUE WITH 296-300 IN THIS SECTION.]
290	Continue your work-up and management of the patient in the hospital	**290**	[CONTINUE WITH 296-300 IN THIS SECTION.]

291 Seek consultation

291 [TURN TO SECTION 20-E, PAGE 307.]

292 Transfer the patient to a colleague

292 [TURN TO SECTION 20-M, PAGE 338.]

293 Counsel the patient

293 [TURN TO SECTION 20-I, PAGE 329.]

294 Offer a prognosis

294 [TURN TO SECTION 20-K, PAGE 336.]

295 Discharge the patient

295 [TURN TO SECTION 20-M, PAGE 338.]

YOU WOULD NOW (CHOOSE ONLY ONE):

296 Take a complete history if you have not already done so

296 [TURN TO SECTION 20-C, PAGE 296.]

297 Perform a physical examination if you have not already done so

297 [TURN TO SECTION 20-D, PAGE 301.]

298 Initiate therapy if you have not already done so

298 [TURN TO SECTION 20-J, PAGE 331.]

299 Order x-ray studies if you have not already done so

299 [CONTINUE WITH SECTION 20-G.]

300 Order biopsy studies if you have not already done so

300 [TURN TO SECTION 20-H, PAGE 327.]

SECTION 20-G

YOU WOULD NOW ORDER THE FOLLOWING RADIOLOGIC EXAMINATIONS (SELECT AS MANY AS YOU CONSIDER INDICATED):

301	Skull	**301**	[Skull films show normal bone contour, density, suture and vessel patterns. The pineal is calcified and in normal position. Sella is normal in size and its floor and clinoid processes are intact. The petrous ridges are intact and the internal auditory canals are normal.]
302	X-ray of cervical spine and neck	**302**	[Films of the neck show normal alignment of the vertebrae, good disc spaces, clear facet lines, and no evidence of arthritic change. The airway and soft tissue shadows are normal. There is no asymmetry of the lower cervical transverse processes or evidence of cervical rib formation. Soft tissues show no calcification.]
303	Radiologic examination of mother's spine	**303**	[SEE FIGURE 57, PAGE 422. IF YOU WISH AN INTERPRETATION OF THIS FIGURE, DEVELOP RESPONSE NUMBER 144 AND THEN CONTINUE WITH THIS SECTION.
304	PA and lateral chest film of the patient	**304**	[The chest film shows well-expanded lung fields without evidence of congestion or consolidation. Diaphragms are smooth, costophrenic angles are clear and the cardiovascular shadow is normal for the age. Bones appear intact and of good density.]

305 Kidneys

305 [Intravenous pyelogram shows normal size, shape and position of the kidneys. Dye appearance time is good in both sides. Calyx, infundibular, and pelvic contours are normal. Ureters shows normal position and increasing density of dye shadow with time. Other soft tissue areas and the bones show no significant localized findings.]

306 Flat plate of the abdomen

306 [The abdomen shows normal distribution of gas in the intestinal tract, the kidneys are well visualized, there are no significant findings in the liver or spleen area. The sacroiliac and hip joint areas are normal.]

307 Upper gastrointestinal tract series

307 [Upper GI series reveals normal passage of barium through the esophagus and no deformity or delay in entering stomach. There is no undue residual fluid in the stomach. The mucosal pattern and peristaltic activity is normal. Pylorus is normal and the duodenal cap fills out nicely. Upper small bowel shows normal course and mucosal pattern.]

308 Barium enema

308 [Barium enema fills the colon without deformity or undue spasm. The sigmoid, splenic flexures, hepatic flexures, and cecum are well visualized on special films. No localized findings are noted in the terminal ileum area. Postevacuation film shows good mucosal pattern.]

309	Left carotid arteriogram	**309**	[A left carotid arteriogram reveals a large arteriovenous malformation in the distribution of the middle cerebral artery. There is no evidence of shift of intercranial structures and no evidence of hydrocephalus. The arteriovenous malformation is deep within the substance of the hemisphere. SEE FIGURE 58, PAGE 422.]
310	Right carotid arteriogram	**310**	[Right carotid arteriogram is entirely within normal limits.]
311	Brain scan	**311**	[There is increased uptake deep in the left hemisphere. No superficial uptake is seen on the AP view. Lateral view is entirely within normal limits.]
312	Liver scan	**312**	[Rose bengal scan of the liver reveals the organ to be of normal size and without demonstrable parenchymal defects. Method not reliable for lesions of less than 2 cm in diameter.]
313	Scan of the lung	**313**	[Pulmonary perfusion scan with macro aggregates of albumin reveals normal perfusion in all views.]
314	Skeletal scans	**314**	[Scans of the thoracolumbar spine and pelvis fail to reveal evidence of reactive bone formation.]
315	Cardiac pool and hepatic blood pool	**315**	[The cardiac blood pool is not enlarged, it corresponds closely to the cardiac shadow on the correlation shadow graph; there is no separation between the cardiac and hepatic pools.]

316 Pancreas scan

317 Renal scan

318 Thyroid scan

319 Myelogram

320 Pneumoencephalogram

321 Carotid arteriogram

322 Ventriculogram

YOU WOULD NOW (CHOOSE ONLY ONE):

323 Schedule the patient for a return visit and postpone further study until that time

324 Hospitalize the patient if you have not already done so

325 Continue your work-up and management on an outpatient basis

326 Continue your work-up and management of the patient in the hospital

327 Seek consultation

316 [Head, midportion, and tail of the pancreas are visualized in normal position; no intrinsic defects are demonstrated.]

317 [The kidneys are well visualized and exhibit normal size, shape and position. Tracer distribution is uniform.]

318 [The thyroid gland is normal in size, shape and position. Tracer distribution is uniform.]

319 [Patient refuses this procedure.]

320 [Patient refuses this procedure.]

321 [SEE FIGURE 58, PAGE 422.]

322 [Patient refuses the procedure.]

323 [TURN TO SECTION 20-L, PAGE 337.]

324 [CONTINUE WITH 332-336 IN THIS SECTION.]

325 [CONTINUE WITH 332-336 IN THIS SECTION.]

326 [CONTINUE WITH 332-336 IN THIS SECTION.]

327 [TURN TO SECTION 20-E, PAGE 307.]

328	Transfer the patient to a colleague	**328**	[TURN TO SECTION 20-M, PAGE 338.]
329	Counsel the patient	**329**	[TURN TO SECTION 20-I, PAGE 329.]
330	Offer a prognosis	**330**	[TURN TO SECTION 20-K, PAGE 336.]
331	Discharge the patient	**331**	[TURN TO SECTION 20-M, PAGE 338.]

YOU WOULD NOW (CHOOSE ONLY ONE):

332	Take a complete history if you have not already done so	**332**	[TURN TO SECTION 20-C, PAGE 296.]
333	Perform a physical examination, if you have not already done so	**333**	[TURN TO SECTION 20-D, PAGE 301.]
334	Order laboratory tests or special investigations if you have not already done so	**334**	[TURN TO SECTION 20-F, PAGE 313.]
335	Initiate therapy if you have not already done so	**335**	[TURN TO SECTION 20-J, PAGE 331.]
336	Order biopsy studies if you have not already done so	**336**	TURN TO SECTION 20-H, PAGE 327.]

SECTION 20-H

YOU WOULD NOW ORDER (SELECT AS MANY AS YOU CONSIDER INDICATED):

337	Liver biopsy	**337**	[The liver shows a normal architectural pattern, the portal spaces are well preserved, there is no inflammatory reaction, the liver parenchymal cells appear normal without cloudy swelling.]
338	Brain biopsy	**338**	[Patient refuses this procedure.]
339	Skin biopsy	**339**	[A biopsy taken from one of the hyperpigmented areas demonstrates some increase in the pigmentary deposit in the basal layer of the epidermis; the dermal structures are intact. There is no inflammatory reaction. Biopsy taken from a nodule behind the knee demonstrates an intradermal mass consisting of Schwann cell elements, the intradermal neural mass is nonencapsulated, the cells form masses and swirls.]
340	Skin biopsy from lesion near left clavicle	**340**	[The epidermis appears to be normal. Entirely within the dermis lie strands and nests of cuboid epithelioid cells, with a pale cytoplasm and with large regular nuclei. There is a small amount of pigment within some of the cells. There is no junctional activity.]
341	Rectal mucosal biopsy	**341**	[Patient refuses this procedure.]
342	Renal biopsy	**342**	[Renal biopsy was attempted, during biopsy the patient developed a hypotensive episode.]

YOU WOULD NOW (CHOOSE ONLY ONE):

343	Schedule the patient for a return visit and postpone further study until that time	**343**	[TURN TO SECTION 20-L, PAGE 337.]
344	Hospitalize the patient if you have not already done so	**344**	[CONTINUE WITH 352-356 IN THIS SECTION.]
345	Continue your work-up and management on an outpatient basis	**345**	[CONTINUE WITH 352-356 IN THIS SECTION.]
346	Continue your work-up and management of the patient in the hospital	**346**	[CONTINUE WITH 352-356 IN THIS SECTION.]
347	Seek consultation	**347**	[TURN TO SECTION 20-E, PAGE 307.]
348	Transfer the patient to a colleague	**348**	[TURN TO SECTION 20-M, PAGE 338.]
349	Counsel the patient	**349**	[CONTINUE WITH SECTION 20-I.]
350	Offer a prognosis	**350**	[TURN TO SECTION 20-K, PAGE 336.]
351	Discharge the patient	**351**	[TURN TO SECTION 20-M, PAGE 338.]

YOU WOULD NOW (CHOOSE ONLY ONE):

352	Take a complete history if you have not already done so	**352**	[TURN TO SECTION 20-C, PAGE 296.]
353	Perform a physical examination if you have not already done so	**353**	[TURN TO SECTION 20-D, PAGE 301.]
354	Order laboratory tests or special investigations if you have not already done so	**354**	[TURN TO SECTION 20-F, PAGE 313.]

355	Initiate therapy if you have not already done so	**355**	[TURN TO SECTION 20-J, PAGE 331.]
356	Order x-ray studies if you have not already done so	**356**	[TURN TO SECTION 20-G, PAGE 332.]

SECTION 20-I

OU WOULD NOW (SELECT AS MANY AS YOU CONSIDER INDICATED):

357	Advise the patient not to marry	**357**	[Patient becomes more depressed.]
358	Advise the patient not to have children	**358**	[Patient becomes more depressed.]
359	Advise the patient that she may marry but she should have a genetic inquiry into prospective mate	**359**	[Patient asks whom to see for advice.]
360	Advise the patient to see a psychiatrist	**360**	[Patient requests a referral. IF YOU WISH TO SEE THE PSYCHIATRIST'S REPORT, DEVELOP RESPONSE NUMBER 145, PAGE 310 AND THEN CONTINUE WITH THIS SECTION.
361	Refer patient to social service	**361**	[Done.]
362	Refer patient to occupational therapy	**362**	[Done.]
363	Explain the risk of genetic transfer of patient's disability by advising her that each child has a 50% chance of inheriting the disease	**363**	[Done.]

364	Explain the risk of genetic transfer of patient's disability by advising her that each child has a 25% chance of inheriting the disease	**364**	[Done.]

YOU WOULD NOW (CHOOSE ONLY ONE):

365	Schedule the patient for a return visit and postpone further study until that time	**365**	[TURN TO SECTION 20-L, PAGE 337.]
366	Hospitalize the patient if you have not already done so	**366**	[CONTINUE WITH 373-378 IN THIS SECTION.]
367	Continue your work-up and management on an outpatient basis	**367**	[CONTINUE WITH 373-378 IN THIS SECTION.]
368	Continue your work-up and management of the patient in the hospital	**368**	[CONTINUE WITH 373-378 IN THIS SECTION.]
369	Seek consultation	**369**	[TURN TO SECTION 20-E, PAGE 307.]
370	Transfer the patient to a colleague	**370**	[TURN TO SECTION 20-M, PAGE 338.]
371	Offer a prognosis	**371**	[TURN TO SECTION 20-K, PAGE 336.]
372	Discharge the patient	**372**	[TURN TO SECTION 20-M, PAGE 338.]

YOU WOULD NOW (CHOOSE ONLY ONE):

373	Take a complete history if you have not already done so	**373**	[TURN TO SECTION 20-C, PAGE 296.]
374	Perform a physical examination if you have not already done so	**374**	[TURN TO SECTION 20-D, PAGE 301.]

375 Order laboratory tests or special investigations if you have not already done so 375

376 Initiate therapy if you have not already done so 376

377 Order x-ray studies if you have not already done so 377

378 Order biopsy studies if you have not already done so 378

SECTION 20-J

YOU WOULD NOW ORDER (SELECT AS MANY AS YOU CONSIDER INDICATED):

379 Phenobarbital 15 mg three times a day 379

380 Phenobarbital 30 mg three times a day 380

381 Dilantin 100 mg three times a day 381

382 Dilantin 100 mg three times a day plus phenobarbital 30 mg three times a day 382

383 Dilantin 1 g three times a day 383

384 Phenobarbital discontinued 384

385 Dilantin discontinued 385

386	Benadryl 50 mg four times a day	386	[Given, patient became extremely lethargic.]
387	Benadryl discontinued	387	[Done.]
388	Chlorpromazine 25 mg four times a day	388	[Given, patient has three seizures within the next seven days.]
389	Chlorpromazine discontinued	389	[Done.]
390	Dextroamphetamine 5 mg three times a day	390	[Given, patient notices no change in seizure pattern, but feels more nervous and complains of pounding heart beats.]
391	Dextroamphetamine discontinued	391	[Done.]
392	Milontin 100 mg four times a day	392	[No apparent change in seizure pattern, patient complains of gait difficulties.]
393	Milontin discontinued	393	[Done.]
394	Peganone 125 mg four times a day	394	[No change in seizure pattern.]
395	Phenurone 1 mg four times a day	395	[Patient becomes seizure free, but notes a yellowish tinge to her skin.]
396	Phenurone discontinued	396	[Done.]
397	Tegretol 100 mg three times a day	397	[Given, no change in seizure pattern.]
398	Tegretol discontinued	398	[Done.]
399	Cafergot	399	[Given, this appears to ameliorate the individual headaches.]
400	Cafergot discontinued	400	[Done.]

401	Oral contraceptives	**401**	[Given, patient's headaches become much more severe and she feels she is having more difficulty with her right arm and leg.]
402	Oral contraceptives discontinued	**402**	[Done.]
403	Insulin 40 units	**403**	[Given, patient had three seizures late in the morning following the first dose of insulin.]
404	Insulin discontinued	**404**	[Done.]
405	Monoamine oxidase inhibitors	**405**	[Given, patient complained of increased generalized throbbing headaches.]
406	Monoamine oxidase inhibitors discontinued	**406**	[Done.]
407	Aspirin 10 grains every four hours	**407**	[Given, patient complains of some ringing in the ears.]
408	Aspirin discontinued	**408**	[Done.]
409	Digitalis	**409**	[Given, patient develops bradycardia.]
410	Digitalis discontinued	**410**	[Done.]
411	Hydrochlorothiazide 50 mg every two days	**411**	[Given, patient develops phototoxic eruption.]
412	Hydrochlorothiazide discontinued	**412**	[Done.]
413	Plaquenil 100 mg every day	**413**	[Given, patient develops blurring of vision.]
414	Plaquenil discontinued	**414**	[Done.]

415	Reserpine	**415**	[Given; patient develops orthostatic hypotension.]
416	Reserpine discontinued	**416**	[Done.]
417	Methoxalen	**417**	[Given; patient's sensitivity to sunlight increases.]
418	Methoxalen discontinued	**418**	[Done.]
419	Librium 20 mg three times a day	**419**	[Given; patient becomes drowsy.]
420	Librium discontinued	**420**	[Done.]
421	Phentolamine 5 mg three times a day	**421**	[Pharmacist asks you whether you want it for intravenous, intramuscular, or oral administration.]
422	Phentolamine discontinued	**422**	[Done.]
423	Coal tar ointment 3%	**423**	[Given.]
424	Coal tar ointment discontinued	**424**	[Done.]
425	Steroid ointment (1% hydrocortisone)	**425**	[Given.]
426	Benzophenone cream	**426**	[Given; patient develops some hypopigmentation around the café-au-lait spots.]
427	Benzophenone cream discontinued	**427**	[Done.]
428	Pilocarpine eyedrops	**428**	[Given.]
429	Pilocarpine eyedrops discontinued	**429**	[Done.]
430	Atropine eyedrops	**430**	[Given.]

431	Atropine eyedrops discontinued	431
432	Chloromycetin capsules	432
433	Chloromycetin capsules discontinued	433
434	Chloromycetin eye ointment	434
435	Chloromycetin eye ointment discontinued	435
436	Steroid eye ointment or drops	436
437	Steroid eye treatment discontinued	437

YOU WOULD ALSO RECOMMEND (SELECT AS MANY AS YOU CONSIDER INDICATED):

438	Psychotherapy	438
439	Plastic repair of skin	439
440	Adrenal surgery	440
441	Renal surgery	441
442	Thoracic surgery	442

443	Craniotomy and implantation of shunt	**443**	[The neurosurgeon advises that the procedure is not indicated, patient has no evidence of raised intracranial pressure.]
444	Exploratory craniotomy	**444**	[Neurosurgeon advises that although patient has a definite A-V malformation, its location in the dominant hemisphere is such as to contraindicate surgery at this time. Patient should return monthly for the first six months and after that as necessary for control of seizures.]

UNLESS OTHERWISE DIRECTED IN THE RESPONSE COLUMN CONTINUE WITH SECTION 20-K

SECTION 20-K

WITH REGARD TO HER SKIN CONDITION, YOUR PROGNOSIS IS THAT THE CONDITION WILL (SELECT AS MANY AS YOU CONSIDER INDICATED):

445	Improve	**445**	[Patient accepts your advice.]
446	Stay about the same	**446**	[Patient accepts your advice.]
447	Become worse with more brown spots	**447**	[Patient seems unhappy but accepts your advice.]
448	Become worse with the development of other lesions	**448**	[Patient becomes somewhat anxious and asks when she must return.]

WITH RESPECT TO THE CENTRAL NERVOUS SYSTEM DISORDER YOUR PROGNOSIS IS THAT (SELECT AS MANY AS YOU CONSIDER INDICATED):

449	There was no lesion and no change will occur	**449**	[Patient accepts your prognosis.]
450	Psychiatric condition will be worsened	**450**	[Patient becomes more depressed

451	Psychiatric treatment will help	**451**	[Patient requests referral to a psychiatrist.]
452	Drugs will help	**452**	[Patient accepts your advice.]
453	Surgery may become necessary	**453**	[Patient asks when she may return.]

UNLESS OTHERWISE DIRECTED IN THE RESPONSE COLUMN CONTINUE WITH SECTION 20-L

SECTION 20-L

AS A FOLLOW-UP YOU WOULD NOW (CHOOSE ONLY ONE):

454	Ask patient to return in two months with special procedures scheduled in the interim	**454**	[Patient accepts your advice; CONTINUE WITH SECTION 20-M.]
455	Ask patient to return in two months without any special procedures scheduled in the interim	**455**	[Patient accepts your advice; CONTINUE WITH SECTION 20-M.]
456	Send the patient away without further appointment	**456**	[Patient accepts your advice; CONTINUE WITH SECTION 20-M.]
457	Ask patient to return in one year	**457**	[Patient accepts your advice; CONTINUE WITH SECTION 20-M.]
458	Offer genetic counseling, if you have not already done so	**458**	[TURN TO SECTION 20-N, PAGE 338.]

SECTION 20-M

459 Record your diagnostic impressions below:

____
____
____
____
____
____

459 [The diagnosis as recorded on this patient's chart was (I) neurofibromatosis, (II) cerebral arteriovenous malformation. SEE APPENDIX B FOR ADDITIONAL COMMENT AND RECOMMENDED MANAGEMENT. END OF PROBLEM 20.]

NOW DEVELOP RESPONSE 459 OPPOSITE FOR ADDITIONAL INFORMATION AND INSTRUCTIONS

SECTION 20-N

YOU WOULD NOW (SELECT AS MANY AS YOU CONSIDER INDICATED):

460 Advise the patient not to marry — **460** [Patient becomes more depressed

461 Advise the patient not to have children — **461** [Patient becomes more depressed

462 Advise the patient that she may marry but she should have a genetic inquiry into prospective mate — **462** [Patient asks whom to see for advice.]

463 Advise the patient to see a psychiatrist — **463** [Patient requests a referral. IF YOU WISH TO SEE THE PSYCHIATRIST'S REPORT, DEVELOP RESPONSE NUMBER 145, PAGE 310 AND THEN CONTINUE WITH THIS SECTION.]

464 Refer patient to social service — **464** [Done.]

465 Refer patient to occupational therapy — **465** [Done.]

466 Explain the risk of genetic transfer of patient's disability by advising her that each child has a 50% chance of inheriting the disease

466 [Done.]

467 Explain the risk of genetic transfer of patient's disability by advising her that each child has a 25% chance of inheriting the disease

467 [Done.]

AS A FOLLOW-UP YOU WOULD NOW (CHOOSE ONLY ONE):

468 Ask patient to return in two months with special procedures scheduled in the interim

468 [Patient accepts your advise; CONTINUE WITH SECTION 20-M, PAGE 338.]

469 Ask patient to return in two months without any special procedures scheduled in the interim

469 [Patient accepts your advise; CONTINUE WITH SECTION 20-M, PAGE 338.]

470 Send the patient away without further appointment

470 [Patient accepts your advice; CONTINUE WITH SECTION 20-M, PAGE 338.]

471 Ask patient to return in one year

471 [Patient accepts your advice; CONTINUE WITH SECTION 20-M, PAGE 338.]

APPENDICES

APPENDIX A

COMMENT

The signs and symptoms – sudden onset of severe upper abdominal pains accompanied by a silent exquisitely tender abdomen – presented by this patient are classic for perforated duodenal ulcer. The flat film of the abdomen, showing free air in the peritoneal cavity confirms the diagnosis of a ruptured viscus beyond any doubt, and makes operation mandatory.

This problem stresses the importance of obtaining a complete medical history, including a review of the patient's drug therapy, even while beginning management of an emergency situation. Correct management in this instance depends on ascertaining a history of drug allergy and drug usage. A helpful mnemonic to remember in history taking in all acutely ill patients is to take an *AMPLE* history, in addition to the usual anamnesis.

A – Allergies, previous reactions
M – Any medications presently or recently taken, especially steroids, salicylates, cardiac drugs, diuretics, and anticoagulants. Remember that drugs for "rheumatism" and "arthritis" frequently contain steroids.
P – Previous illnesses, hospitalizations, operations
L – Last meal (time, nature, amount of food ingested, anorexia)
E – Events immediately preceding onset of illness

This patient is allergic to penicillin, has been taking steroids for arthritis, and furthermore has been on phenformin for diabetes. Failure to support the patient with steroids during the operative and postoperative periods may result in marked hypotension, fever, and irrational behavior, which responds only to intravenous hydrocortisone. Administration of penicillin may lead to an anaphylactic reaction. Other therapeutic pitfalls to be avoided are wrong drugs, wrong dosage, and wrong route of administration.

Options for nonoperative management are provided but this soon fails. The treatment indicated is clearly surgical.

APPENDIX A

RECOMMENDED MANAGEMENT

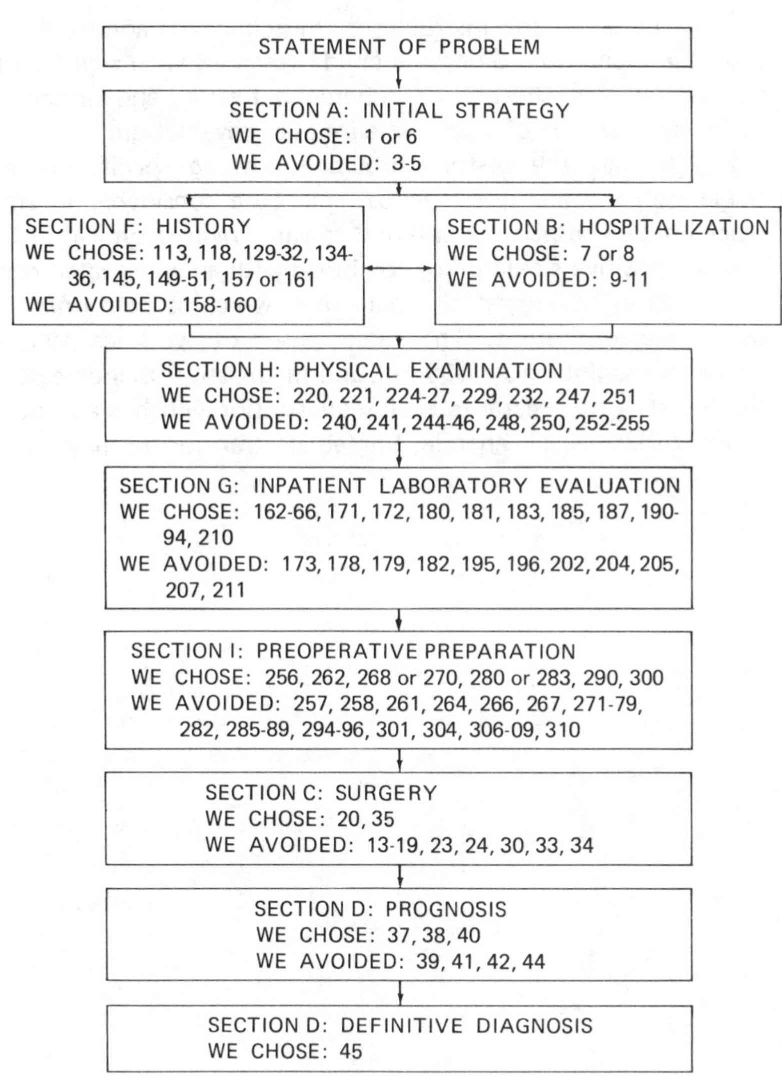

STATEMENT OF PROBLEM
SECTION A: INITIAL STRATEGY
WE CHOSE: 1 or 6
WE AVOIDED: 3-5
SECTION F: HISTORY
WE CHOSE: 113, 118, 129-32, 134-36, 145, 149-51, 157 or 161
WE AVOIDED: 158-160
SECTION B: HOSPITALIZATION
WE CHOSE: 7 or 8
WE AVOIDED: 9-11
SECTION H: PHYSICAL EXAMINATION
WE CHOSE: 220, 221, 224-27, 229, 232, 247, 251
WE AVOIDED: 240, 241, 244-46, 248, 250, 252-255
SECTION G: INPATIENT LABORATORY EVALUATION
WE CHOSE: 162-66, 171, 172, 180, 181, 183, 185, 187, 190-94, 210
WE AVOIDED: 173, 178, 179, 182, 195, 196, 202, 204, 205, 207, 211
SECTION I: PREOPERATIVE PREPARATION
WE CHOSE: 256, 262, 268 or 270, 280 or 283, 290, 300
WE AVOIDED: 257, 258, 261, 264, 266, 267, 271-79, 282, 285-89, 294-96, 301, 304, 306-09, 310
SECTION C: SURGERY
WE CHOSE: 20, 35
WE AVOIDED: 13-19, 23, 24, 30, 33, 34
SECTION D: PROGNOSIS
WE CHOSE: 37, 38, 40
WE AVOIDED: 39, 41, 42, 44
SECTION D: DEFINITIVE DIAGNOSIS
WE CHOSE: 45

APPENDIX B

COMMENT

As noted in the instructions, the child was admitted to the hospital for evaluation. Since the child presented with significant disease, it was felt that chest films, tuberculin testing, and urinalysis should be included as part of a complete inpatient evaluation.

Although the history provided nothing specifically suggesting sickle cell anemia, this diagnosis must be considered in any anemic black child. The peripheral blood smear shown is typical of SS disease and the positive sickle prep, combined with an an elevated reticulocyte count, strongly suggest the diagnosis, which is confirmed by hemoglobin electrophoresis. The rapid onset of weakness and lethargy, the low hemoglobin (3 g/100 ml), and the massive splenomegaly indicate the presence of visceral red cell sequestration which is a serious complication of sickle cell anemia. Immediate transfusion may be lifesaving.

APPENDIX B

RECOMMENDED MANAGEMENT

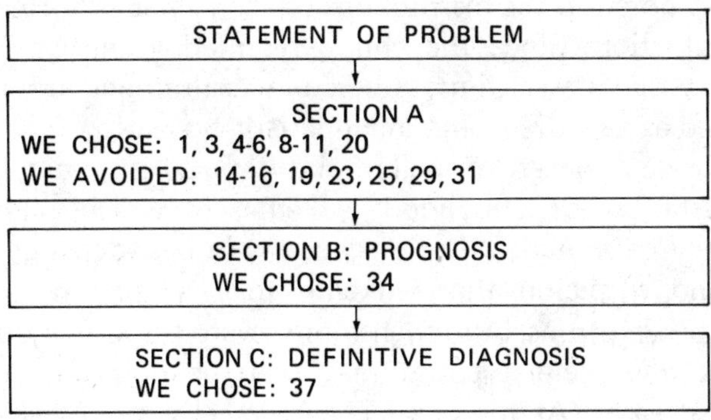

APPENDIX C

COMMENT

As noted in the instructions the child was admitted to the hospital for evaluation. Since the child presented with significant disease, it was felt that chest films, tuberculin testing, and urinalysis should be included as part of a complete inpatient evaluation.

Gradual onset of pallor and fatigue is a common presenting manifestation of childhood leukemia in which physical abnormalities may be minimal. The diagnosis is in part dependent on an awareness and suspicion that leukemia may be present in children with minimal symptoms. Although more severe thrombocytopenia is usually present, the platelet count may even be normal if the condition is detected early. At the onset leukemic cells are not always seen in the peripheral blood. The essential diagnostic test is the bone marrow examination which reveals significant replacement of normal marrow cells by blast (stem cells, lymphoblasts) forms.

An increased level of serum uric acid results from the breakdown of leukemic cells and consequent increased load of purines excreted as uric acid. Measurement of uric acid levels and use of adjunctive therapy to prevent uric acid nephropathy, a potentially life-threatening complication, is one essential act early in the treatment of leukemia.

APPENDIX C

RECOMMENDED MANAGEMENT

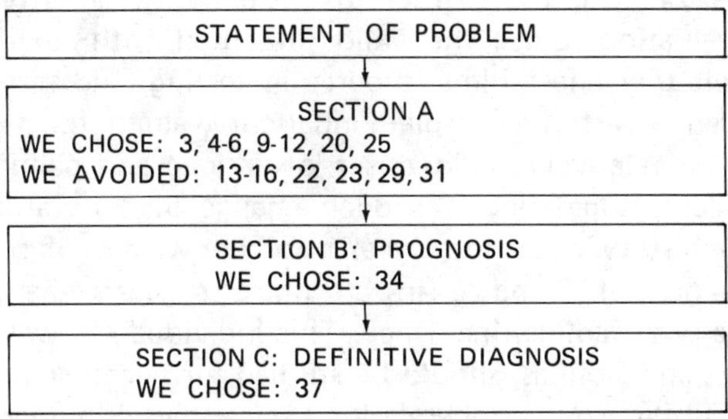

APPENDIX D

COMMENT

As noted in the instructions the child was admitted to the hospital for evaluation. Since the child presented with significant disease, it was felt that chest films, tuberculin testing, and urinalysis should be included as part of a complete inpatient evaluation.

The relatively rapid onset of fatigue and pallor in this child is significant, suggesting a sudden change in his status. Although the family history does not reveal prior knowledge of spherocytosis, the occurrence of jaundice in an uncle suggests the possibility of a disease with familial incidence. This individual, as well as the patient's parents and siblings, should be studied further since the disease may be quite subtle. The peripheral blood smear reveals numerous spherocytes, and the increased osmotic fragility of the red cells further confirms the diagnosis of the disorder. The previously mentioned rapid onset of symptoms and the finding of a low reticulocyte count suggest the occurrence of an aplastic crisis which is confirmed by bone marrow examination revealing erythroid hypoplasia. This is a frequent presenting complication of hereditary spherocytosis in which the hemolytic process has been compensated by increased red cell production. If such a patient is transfused before the diagnosis is recognized, the proper diagnosis may be delayed due to a dilution of spherocytes in the peripheral blood by normal donor red cells.

Splenectomy is the treatment of choice and should optimally be performed at 4 to 5 years of age in order to avoid the increased incidence of cholelithias. In older children and adults, splenectomy should be performed at the time of diagnosis unless the patient is in the aplastic phase, in which case splenectomy should be postponed until the aplastic crisis has been adequately treated by medical means. Splenectomy should be avoided in children under two years of age because of the increased risk of serious infection following such a procedure in this age group. Because of the autosomal dominant pattern of inheritance of this disease, blood counts, reticulocyte counts, and osmotic fragility tests should be performed on the parents and siblings of affected patients.

APPENDIX D

RECOMMENDED MANAGEMENT

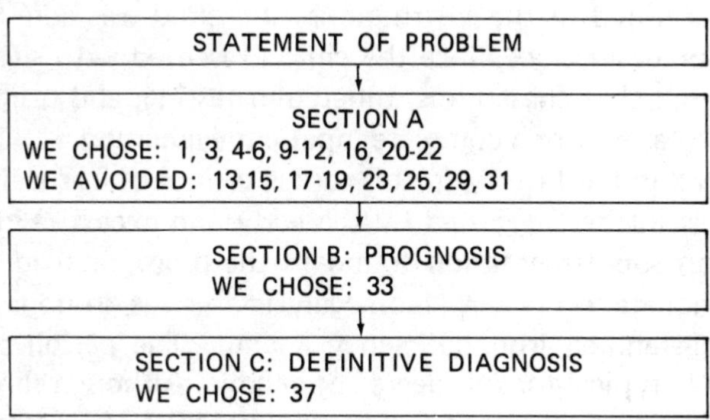

APPENDIX E

COMMENT

As noted in the instructions, the child was admitted to the hospital for evaluation. Since the child presented with significant disease, it was felt that chest films, tuberculin testing, and urinalysis should be included as part of a complete inpatient evaluation.

The initial history in this case is typical of iron deficiency anemia, which is further suggested by the early and excessive milk intake without iron supplementation found in the more detailed dietary history. The findings of slight splenomegaly in this age group is not uncommon in long-standing iron deficiency anemia. The peripheral blood smear shown is typical for this degree of anemia. Although thrombocytopenia is not the rule, it is found in approximately 10% of cases of severe iron deficiency anemia. The finding of a positive sickle cell test, which is a necessary part of the evaluation of a black child with anemia, must be further investigated by hemoglobin electrophoresis, which in this case documents the presence of a sickle cell trait. Although sickle cell trait could have been suspected because of the low reticulocyte count and the absence of morphologic abnormalities of sickle cell disease in the peripheral smear, it should be confirmed by hemoglobin electrophoresis.

The presence of gastrointestinal blood loss indicated by a positive stool guaiac test can be documented in a significant number of children with iron deficiency anemia. In some cases this may be due to a direct toxic effect of cow's milk protein on the intestinal mucosa. In addition, frank protein-losing enteropathy may occur leading to hypoalbuminemia and edema.

APPENDIX E

RECOMMENDED MANAGEMENT

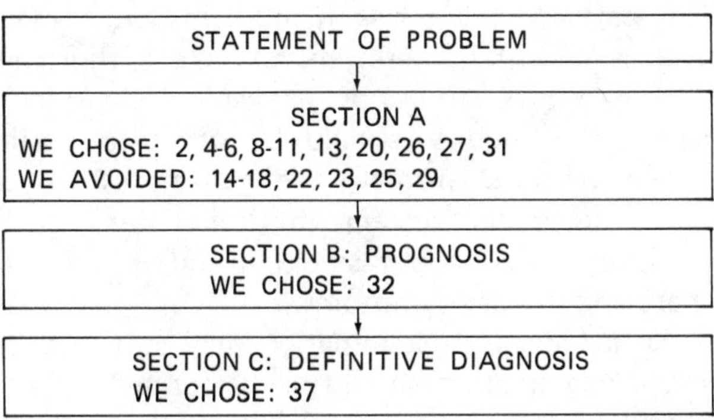

APPENDIX F

COMMENT

This patient has a series of problems which may occur in his age group. It is essential, therefore, to take a thorough history before initiating laboratory studies or medication. Considering the presenting complaints, the inquiry should be occupied particularly with the family and personal history, the gastrointestinal system, the liver and the cardiovascular system. In view of his age, the patient should be specifically asked about smoking and drinking habits and about pulmonary and urinary symptoms.

A partial physical examination may suffice as an initial step but a complete examination should be performed either as an outpatient or in hospital. In the physical examination, special attention should be given to the cardiovascular and pulmonary systems, the gastrointestinal system, and the lower urinary tract. Sigmoidoscopic examination at this juncture is not desirable given the history of angina, congestive failure, and electrocardiographic evidence of myocardial insufficiency. Hospitalization will be required and should take place when the examiner has concluded that surgical management is necessary.

Laboratory studies may be focused on essentials if the early management has been adequate: stools should be studied for fat content, the upper gastrointestinal tract and bile tract should be examined radiologically, and an electrocardiogram and chest x-ray should be done. Excessive or unessential radiologic and hematologic investigations, as well as exotic studies undertaken to rule out metabolic or endocrine disease, should be avoided.

Immediate management of the congestive failure includes digitalization, low-salt diet, diuretics, and antihypertensive therapy; a low-fat diet and cessation of smoking would also benefit the patient. Definitive treatment includes, in addition to long-term management of the congestive cardiac failure, cholecystectomy and exploration of the common bile duct, as well as visual and tactile examination of the pancreas. More radical surgery is not indicated. Purely medical management of the gastrointestinal complaints is not adequate.

APPENDIX F

RECOMMENDED MANAGEMENT

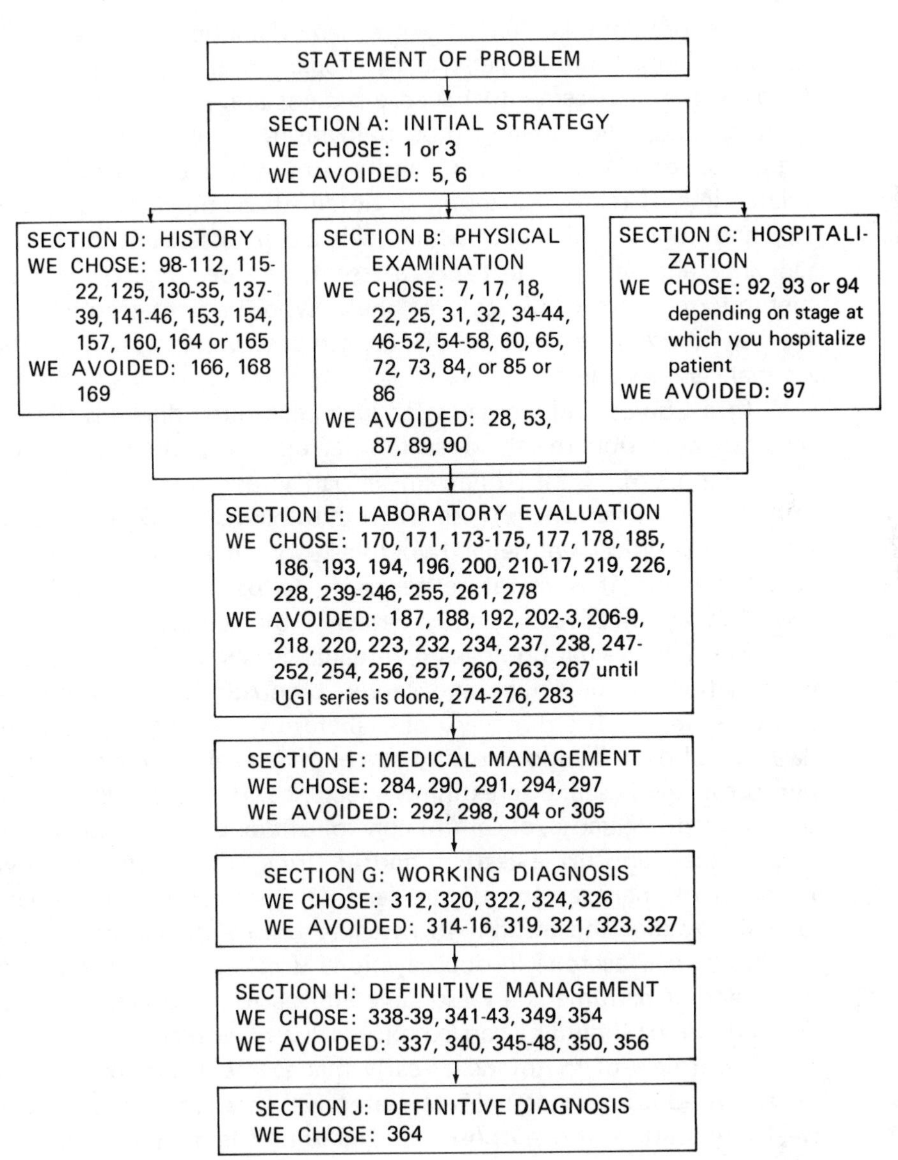

STATEMENT OF PROBLEM
SECTION A: INITIAL STRATEGY
WE CHOSE: 1 or 3
WE AVOIDED: 5, 6
SECTION D: HISTORY
WE CHOSE: 98-112, 115-22, 125, 130-35, 137-39, 141-46, 153, 154, 157, 160, 164 or 165
WE AVOIDED: 166, 168 169
SECTION B: PHYSICAL EXAMINATION
WE CHOSE: 7, 17, 18, 22, 25, 31, 32, 34-44, 46-52, 54-58, 60, 65, 72, 73, 84, or 85 or 86
WE AVOIDED: 28, 53, 87, 89, 90
SECTION C: HOSPITALIZATION
WE CHOSE: 92, 93 or 94 depending on stage at which you hospitalize patient
WE AVOIDED: 97
SECTION E: LABORATORY EVALUATION
WE CHOSE: 170, 171, 173-175, 177, 178, 185, 186, 193, 194, 196, 200, 210-17, 219, 226, 228, 239-246, 255, 261, 278
WE AVOIDED: 187, 188, 192, 202-3, 206-9, 218, 220, 223, 232, 234, 237, 238, 247-252, 254, 256, 257, 260, 263, 267 until UGI series is done, 274-276, 283
SECTION F: MEDICAL MANAGEMENT
WE CHOSE: 284, 290, 291, 294, 297
WE AVOIDED: 292, 298, 304 or 305
SECTION G: WORKING DIAGNOSIS
WE CHOSE: 312, 320, 322, 324, 326
WE AVOIDED: 314-16, 319, 321, 323, 327
SECTION H: DEFINITIVE MANAGEMENT
WE CHOSE: 338-39, 341-43, 349, 354
WE AVOIDED: 337, 340, 345-48, 350, 356
SECTION J: DEFINITIVE DIAGNOSIS
WE CHOSE: 364

APPENDIX G

COMMENT

The problem is that of a pregnant diabetic with the incidental finding of an abnormal cervical cytologic smear. The important principles in the management of such a patient are: (1) meticulous control of the metabolic disease (hospitalization, frequent prenatal visits, regulation of diet and insulin, and so on); (2) selection of the appropriate time of rehospitalization to obtain those biochemical, biophysical, and sonographic tests which will aid in assessing potential fetal jeopardy and fetal maturity, data essential to deciding the timing and method of delivery; (3) care of the newborn infant (respiratory distress syndrome), as well as (4) conservative management of the abnormal cervical smear.

In a 28-year-old woman with well-controlled diabetes there is no medical indication for therapeutic interruption of the pregnancy. Nor does a report of a Class III Pap smear justify radical measures. However, in a significant percent of cases such cytology is the *first* indication of either an atypical epithelial hyperplasia or an in situ intra-epithelial carcinoma and it is therefore necessary to perform a cone biopsy if less than an invasive cancer is detected by cervical punch biopsies.

Routine evaluation in early pregnancy should include speculum examination of the vagina and cervix, blood and urine examinations, and chest x-ray. The discovery of diabetes may lead to a two to three-day initial hospitalization, ideally at a high-risk center, for the following purposes: a) baseline creatinine clearance determination, b) renal thresholds for glucose, c) careful control of diabetes, d) instructions for insulin, diet, and urine testing, and e) urine culture and sensitivities. If inpatient management is not feasible, then outpatient control of diabetes by diet and insulin with weekly follow-up and close attention to glucose and acetone in double-voided urine specimens taken before meals and at bedtime is a reasonable alternative. Frequent blood sugar determinations should be carried out — usually weekly.

Regardless of the mode of early management, this patient should be admitted to a maternal-fetal intensive care unit at or about 34 weeks' gestation for purposes outlined in the first paragraph. The working protocol at this time should include: decreased activity (bed rest as much as possible), careful control of diabetes, creatinine clearance, urine culture, daily 24-hour urinary estriol determinations, and weekly oxytocin challenge test (to assess the respiratory "placental" reserve under the stress of simulated labor), weekly amniocentesis for lecithin-sphingomyelin ratio and creatinine concentration and weekly ultrasonic fetal biparietal diameter determinations (a guide to fetal age and/or maturity and, in some instances, an early warning of possible fetal growth retardation secondary to intrauterine undernutrition).

If the known gestational age is confirmed by fetal maturity studies (B-Scan cephalotometry at least 9.0 cm, L/S ratio greater than 2, and amniotic fluid creatinine greater than 2 mg%) the pregnancy is terminated at 38 to 39 weeks' gestation. In determining the method of delivery, it is important to assess the adequacy of the pelvis (x-ray pelvimetry) and the ripeness of the cervix. Since the estimated fetal weight in this case was between 2800 and 3200 grams and examination indicated an adequate pelvis as well as a cervix amenable to induction, the ideal management was induction of labor with oxytocin administered via infusion pump together with amniotomy. Continuous monitoring of the fetal heart rate and uterine contraction pattern to detect early signs of possible fetal hypoxia are essential throughout labor and delivery. If signs of fetal distress (hypoxia) are persistent and progressive and if corrective measures fail to alleviate these ominous signs within a 20- to 30-minute period, cesarean section is indicated. (See Recommended Management for the details of combined electronic and biochemical surveillance of the high-risk fetus.)

If a large fetus is suspected, primary cesarean section should be carried out to avoid difficult labor. If the dates are uncertain in such a patient under continuous inpatient surveillance, she should be followed until the onset of spontaneous labor or until signs of fetal jeopardy (such as a significant fall in 24-hour estriol determinations and a positive oxytocin challenge test, which serves to confirm the low estriol excretion rates) dictate premature delivery if fetal maturity is probable (as judged by L/S ratio).

The procedures outlined in this discussion have reduced perinatal loss from stillbirth and prematurity among pregnant diabetics.

At birth the infant should be placed in an intensive care unit. If there is no evidence of respiratory distress, early feedings should be considered. The chest should be examined radiologically, vital signs obtained frequently and baseline serum electrolytes, glucose, calcium, pH and blood gases established.

The treatment of a three-hour-old acidotic infant (with hyaline membrane disease and hypoglycemia) includes intravenous glucose and sodium bicarbonate and an enriched O_2 environment. If, despite a high-oxygen environment (greater than 60%), arterial oxygenation cannot be maintained over 50 mm Hg, CPAP (continuous positive airway pressure) breathing should be instituted. Other intravenous treatment is to be avoided unless cardiac failure ensues. Jaundice present at three days in this infant required a conservative approach since the serum bilirubin did not rise precipitously above 18 mg per 100 ml and there were no clinical signs of central nervous system involvement.

Purulent conjunctivitis until proven otherwise should be considered a bacterial disease (staphylococcal, streptococcal, Gram-negative organisms) and appropriate cultures should be taken. Gonococcal conjunctivitis has been adequately prevented by the previous administration of silver nitrate which itself rarely causes any severe conjunctival reaction.

Management of High-Risk Pregnancies

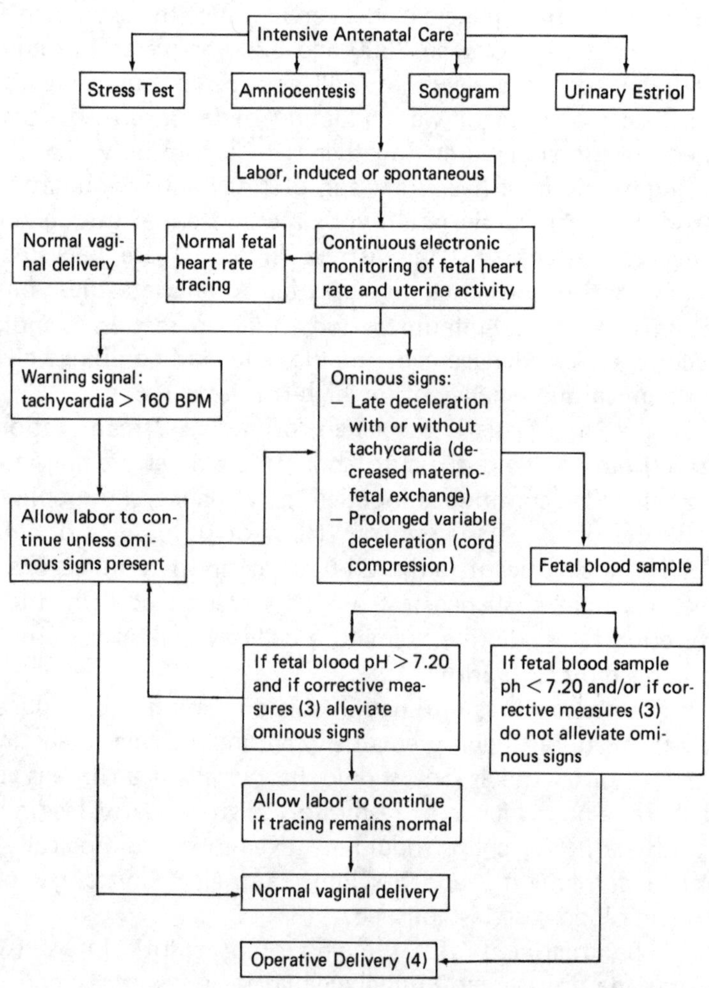

1. Diabetes, chronic hypertension, preeclampsia, premature onset of labor, third trimester bleeding.
2. Ausculated fetal heart rate > 160 or < 120 per minute or meconium staining of amniotic fluid.
3. Change maternal position to alleviate maternal hypotension and/or cord compression. Decrease or stop intravenous oxytocin infusion to alleviate uterine hyperactivity.
4. Anticipate birth of depressed newborn and have available obstetric or pediatric personnel skilled in direct resuscitative techniques.

APPENDIX G

RECOMMENDED MANAGEMENT

STATEMENT OF PROBLEM

↓

SECTION A: INITIAL VISIT
WE CHOSE: 2, 4, 5, 7, 9, 10, 14
WE AVOIDED: 1, 3, 6

↓

SECTION B: INITIAL LABORATORY EVALUATION
WE CHOSE: 16, 18, 19, 23, 24, 26, 28, 40
WE AVOIDED: 22, 25, 29, 32-35, 38, 39, 41, 42

↓

SECTION C: HOSPITALIZATION
WE CHOSE: 43, 46, 51 or 53, 58, 60
WE AVOIDED: 44, 47-50, 55, 56, 59, 61

↓

SECTION D: DECISION REGARDING VAGINAL SMEAR
WE CHOSE: 63 or 66, 67
WE AVOIDED: 64, 65

↓

SECTION E: DECISION REGARDING PREGNANCY
WE CHOSE: 70
WE AVOIDED: 68, 69, 71-75

↓

SECTION F: REGULAR OFFICE VISITS
WE CHOSE: 78, 79, 82, 83, 85, 86
WE AVOIDED: 77, 87, 88, 91, 92

↓

SECTION G: HOSPITALIZATION
WE CHOSE: 93, 95, 96, 98, 99, 106, 108
WE AVOIDED: 94, 97, 105, 107

↓

SECTION H: CONTINUE HOSPITALIZATION
WE CHOSE: 109, 116-20, 129
WE AVOIDED: 112, 114, 121-23, 125, 216-228

↓

SECTION I: INFANT AT BIRTH
WE CHOSE: 131, 133, 134, 137-139, 141, 142, 147, 152
WE AVOIDED: 130, 132, 135, 144, 146, 148, 151

↓

SECTION J: INFANT AT 3 HOURS
WE CHOSE: 155, 157, 160-162, 164, 166
WE AVOIDED: 154, 156, 158, 159, 163, 165

↓

SECTION K: INFANT AT 36 HOURS
WE CHOSE: 167-169, 171, 173, 175-177
WE AVOIDED: 170, 172, 174, 178, 179

↓

SECTION L: INFANT AT 14 DAYS
WE CHOSE: 181 or 182 or 183
WE AVOIDED: 184, 185

↓

SECTION R: DEFINITIVE DIAGNOSIS
WE CHOSE: 191

APPENDIX H

COMMENT

This problem is designed to emphasize the need to consider persistent headache in a child with cyanotic congenital heart disease as an indicator of brain abscess until proved otherwise. Furthermore, one should consider brain abscess as a life-threatening situation which requires emergency treatment and a need for action leading to prompt surgical repair. The older view that brain abscess *requires* the demonstration of an infection elsewhere, such as bacterial endocarditis, middle ear or sinus infection, has been superceded by the understanding that the cyanotic child may develop intravascular sludging in a small cerebral artery, with subsequent occlusion of a vessel and encephalomalacia leading to abscess formation.

The order in which the laboratory, radiologic, and other studies should be done is dictated by the difficulties imposed on the patient. It is preferable to start with an electroencephalogram and/or brain scan, followed by cerebral arteriogram, if necessary. Once the data have been gathered, burr holes are made and an air study may be added. Finally, if needed, craniotomy may be performed. Our neurologic consultants all agreed that a lumbar puncture was not necessary or desirable in this patient. Other laboratory procedures which are time consuming, such as pulmonary function studies, angiocardiography, or those which make the patient uncomfortable and add little to the solution of the urgent problem at hand should be avoided.

Methicillin and Streptomycin were the drugs of choice in this patient.

The electrocardiogram was supportive of the underlying diagnosis here — that of tetralogy of Fallot. The tracing suggested evidence of right ventricular overload and right atrial enlargement.

APPENDIX H

RECOMMENDED MANAGEMENT

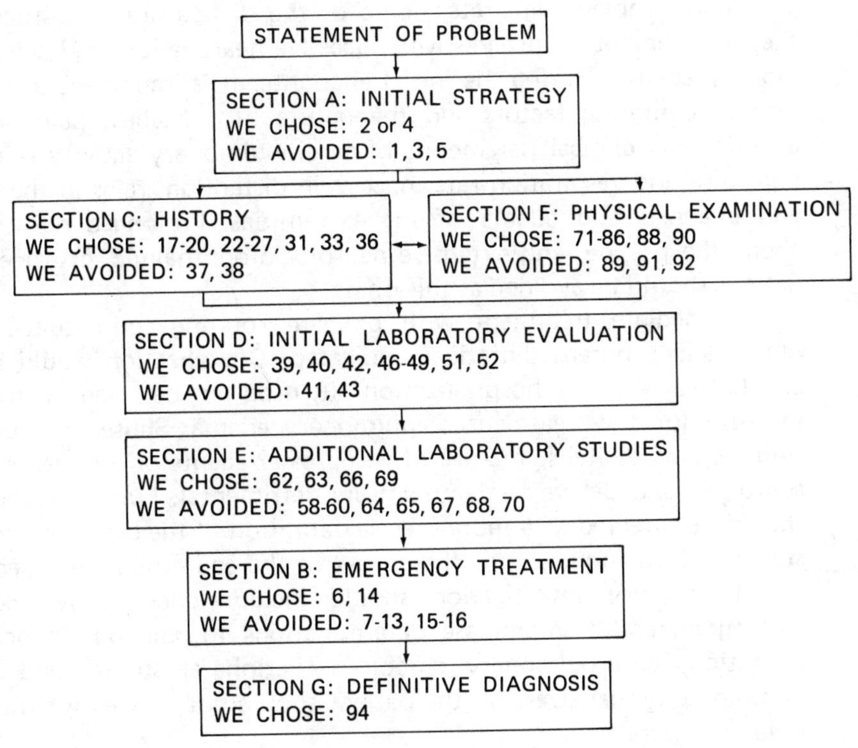
STATEMENT OF PROBLEM
SECTION A: INITIAL STRATEGY
WE CHOSE: 2 or 4
WE AVOIDED: 1, 3, 5
SECTION C: HISTORY
WE CHOSE: 17-20, 22-27, 31, 33, 36
WE AVOIDED: 37, 38
SECTION F: PHYSICAL EXAMINATION
WE CHOSE: 71-86, 88, 90
WE AVOIDED: 89, 91, 92
SECTION D: INITIAL LABORATORY EVALUATION
WE CHOSE: 39, 40, 42, 46-49, 51, 52
WE AVOIDED: 41, 43
SECTION E: ADDITIONAL LABORATORY STUDIES
WE CHOSE: 62, 63, 66, 69
WE AVOIDED: 58-60, 64, 65, 67, 68, 70
SECTION B: EMERGENCY TREATMENT
WE CHOSE: 6, 14
WE AVOIDED: 7-13, 15-16
SECTION G: DEFINITIVE DIAGNOSIS
WE CHOSE: 94

APPENDIX I

COMMENT

This problem illustrates some of the difficulties encountered in the management of progressive congestive heart failure and acute pulmonary edema. During the initial encounter it is important to inquire into precipitating factors and the nature of the chest pain, and to examine the clinical parameters of cardiopulmonary activity – including pulse and respiration rate, neck vein distention, rales in the chest, and cyanosis and edema of the extremities. Prolonged questioning about the psyche, and extensive neurologic ophthalmic, or ear examinations should be avoided at this point.

Immediate treatment with oxygen, rotating tourniquets, morphine, and a potent diuretic is indicated. Digitalization would be instituted early in the hospitalization but need not be given as an acute measure for the treatment of pulmonary edema. Subsequent discontinuation of digitalis, the use of vasopresser agents or intravenous salt solutions, and delays of treatment are detrimental. Further evaluation should be directed at a more precise definition of the cardiopulmonary status and an inquiry into the causes of the acute pulmonary edema.

Laboratory investigation should include chest x-ray, electrocardiogram and transaminase determinations to rule out myocardial infarction, and pulmonary embolism. Peripheral studies and those imposing physical stress on the patient should not be attempted at this time.

Long-term management should include sodium restriction, digitalization, and the judicious use of diuretics if necessary. If heart failure recurs, the precipitating causes both extrinsic (patient doesn't follow therapy) and intrinsic (electrolyte imbalance, digitalis intoxication), should be considered. Treatment of recurrent heart failure demands study of electrolytes, fluid restriction, and replacement of potassium and chloride loss. The potent diuretics may induce severe electrolyte deficiencies which may in turn render diuretic therapy less effective and increase the risk and likelihood of digitalis toxicity. Increased administration of fluid and digitalis may be detrimental unless electrolyte balance has been restored through the use of potasium chloride supplements and in some cases even the addition of sodium chloride. Although the more potent diuretics may be helpful in maintaining a diuresis, they may lead to severe potassium loss which must be recognized and treated appropriately.

APPENDIX I

RECOMMENDED MANAGEMENT

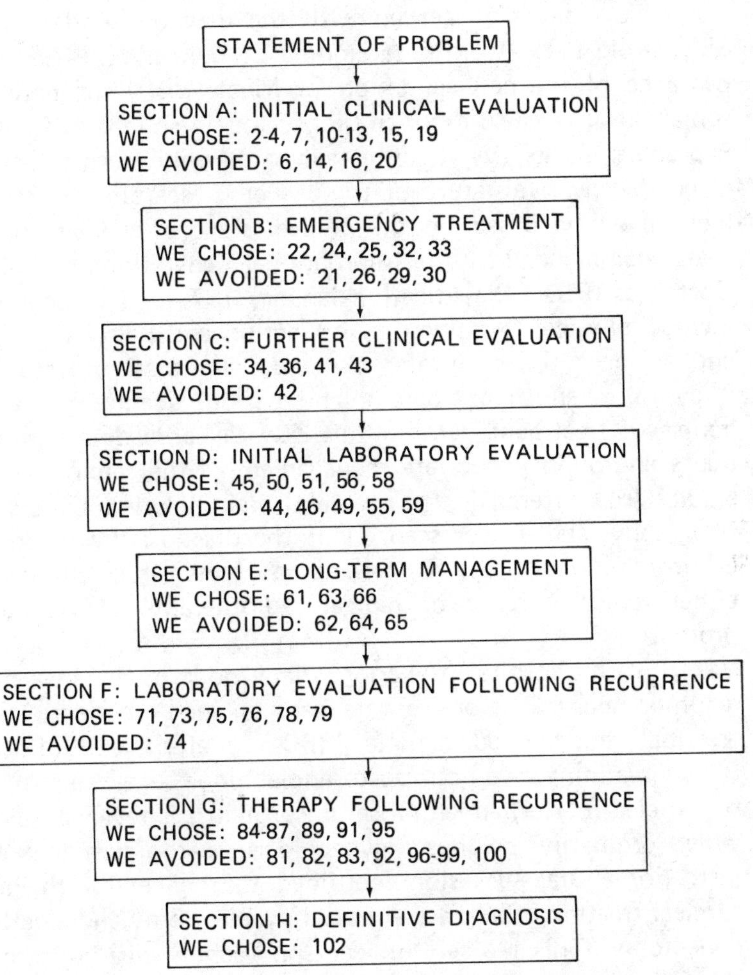

STATEMENT OF PROBLEM
SECTION A: INITIAL CLINICAL EVALUATION
WE CHOSE: 2-4, 7, 10-13, 15, 19
WE AVOIDED: 6, 14, 16, 20
SECTION B: EMERGENCY TREATMENT
WE CHOSE: 22, 24, 25, 32, 33
WE AVOIDED: 21, 26, 29, 30
SECTION C: FURTHER CLINICAL EVALUATION
WE CHOSE: 34, 36, 41, 43
WE AVOIDED: 42
SECTION D: INITIAL LABORATORY EVALUATION
WE CHOSE: 45, 50, 51, 56, 58
WE AVOIDED: 44, 46, 49, 55, 59
SECTION E: LONG-TERM MANAGEMENT
WE CHOSE: 61, 63, 66
WE AVOIDED: 62, 64, 65
SECTION F: LABORATORY EVALUATION FOLLOWING RECURRENCE
WE CHOSE: 71, 73, 75, 76, 78, 79
WE AVOIDED: 74
SECTION G: THERAPY FOLLOWING RECURRENCE
WE CHOSE: 84-87, 89, 91, 95
WE AVOIDED: 81, 82, 83, 92, 96-99, 100
SECTION H: DEFINITIVE DIAGNOSIS
WE CHOSE: 102

APPENDIX J

COMMENT

This case is concerned with the diagnosis and treatment of a 38-year-old Para IV with carcinoma of the cervix. Because of the appearance of the cervical lesion (a friable mass) the patient must be subjected at once to a punch biopsy for, in spite of a frankly positive Pap smear (Class IV), treatment is based only on histologic diagnosis. Once the invasive nature of the cancer is ascertained, definitive treatment must be based on the clinical stage of the disorder following that recommended by the International Federation of Gynecology and Obstetrics (FIGO Classification-January 1971).* The recommendations include physical examination, inspection and palpation of the cervix and adjacent tissues (preferably under anesthesia), cystoscopy, chest x-ray, intravenous pyelogram, and barium enema. To proceed to a course of treatment without this essential core data base risks inadequate and/or inappropriate management of the carcinoma. Additional studies (not offered in the problem) may include a bone survey, lymphography, and a liver scan. Once the diagnosis has been established as (International Stage IB) carcinoma of the cervix, proper treatment, either radical surgery or radical radiotherapy, should be instituted promptly.

In many hospitals the appropriate mode of therapy is decided by a tumor board. The entire data base on such a patient, including the essential general medical data (CBC, urinalysis, culture as indicated, BUN, creatinine, two-hour postprandial blood sugar, electrocardiogram, serum electrolytes, and total serum proteins) is reviewed by the board which ordinarily includes a gynecologist, pathologist, and radiotherapist. For a Stage I lesion (confined to the cervix) the appropriate surgical treatment includes a radical hysterectomy and a pelvic lymphadenectomy. This radical surgical approach is clearly indicated when the following criteria are met: (1) the patient is in good general health and not too obese; (2) the lesion is in an early stage of development, and (3) a surgeon who is experienced in radical pelvic operations is available. The operative approach is preferable to radiotherapy when such conditions as the following obtain: previous total removal of the uterus, pelvic inflammatory disease, adnexal masses, large uterine

* *International Journal of Gynaecology and Obstetrics* 9:172, 1971.

myomata or pregnancy. In early lesions, such as the one described here, preservation of functional ovarian tissue is possible.

In the majority of hospitals throughout the United States, radiotherapy is the most common method of treating invasive carcinoma of the cervix. Not only is this method appropriate for lesions in an early stage of invasiveness (such as was found in this patient), but it is indispensable in the more advanced stages of invasive cervical carcinoma (Stage II-IV). Radiation therapy of cervical carcinoma is usually delivered by an external and internal source of x-rays. Megavoltage teletherapy is usually employed to deliver cancericidal doses to the primary lesions as well as to the contiguous areas of the pelvis and to the pelvic lymph nodes. Complimentary therapy, delivered to the primary lesion typically consists of intrauterine and intravaginal sources containing radioisotopes such as radium or cesium. The recommended plan calls for total radiation doses to points A of 8000 rads and to points B of 6000 rads, delivered during a period of five or six weeks.

Surgical treatment is necessary for successful eradication of radio-resistant lesions and for recurrences after optimal radiation has been achieved. Pelvic recurrences following radical hysterectomy for cervical cancer may be treated by pelvic radiation therapy.

In some instances palliation may be achieved for recurrences of cervical carcinoma which have extended beyond the true pelvis; for example, by spot radiation to areas of vertebral metastases. As a final measure, cordotomy may be utilized for pain relief.

No chemotherapeutic agents are presently known to be effective against cervical carcinoma.

In summary, treatment of invasive carcinoma of the uterine cervix requires a well-integrated team approach involving gynecologists, pathologists, radiotherapists, urologists, internists, sometimes psychiatrists, and other appropriate nursing and paramedical personnel highly skilled in this specialized area. Continuous care from diagnosis and initial treatment through careful follow-up should lead to early recognition of any complications of treatment, persistence, or recurrence, so that corrective or secondary treatment may be initiated at the earliest possible time.

APPENDIX J

RECOMMENDED MANAGEMENT

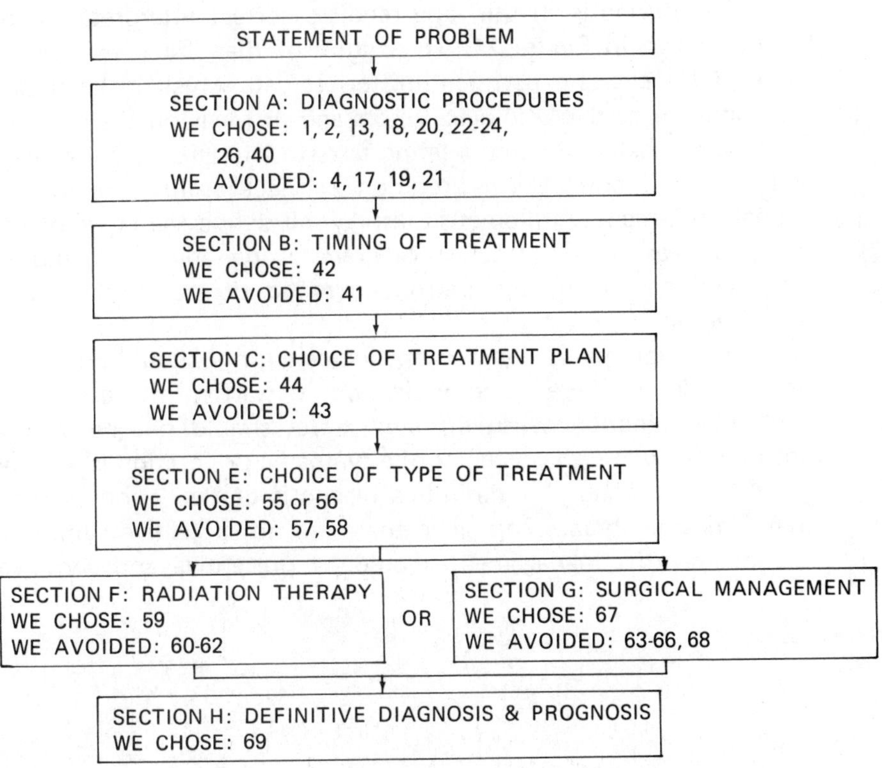

STATEMENT OF PROBLEM
SECTION A: DIAGNOSTIC PROCEDURES
WE CHOSE: 1, 2, 13, 18, 20, 22-24,
26, 40
WE AVOIDED: 4, 17, 19, 21
SECTION B: TIMING OF TREATMENT
WE CHOSE: 42
WE AVOIDED: 41
SECTION C: CHOICE OF TREATMENT PLAN
WE CHOSE: 44
WE AVOIDED: 43
SECTION E: CHOICE OF TYPE OF TREATMENT
WE CHOSE: 55 or 56
WE AVOIDED: 57, 58
SECTION F: RADIATION THERAPY
WE CHOSE: 59
WE AVOIDED: 60-62
OR
SECTION G: SURGICAL MANAGEMENT
WE CHOSE: 67
WE AVOIDED: 63-66, 68
SECTION H: DEFINITIVE DIAGNOSIS & PROGNOSIS
WE CHOSE: 69

APPENDIX K

COMMENT

The diagnosis in this case requires correct interpretation of the lesion shown in Figure *21*. The nature of that lesion can be further defined by eliciting pertinent historical data which make it possible to eliminate certain etiologic factors and to focus on the hearing loss. In making that evaluation hearing tests to lateralize any loss are helpful and their correct interpretation provides useful data for a functional assessment. Audiometric testing will define the range of hearing loss; whereas uncomfortable rotational testing, spinal tap, and expensive laminograms of the petrous pyramid do not provide valuable information.

Myringotomy is likewise not indicated; nor should a cold caloric test be done. There is no indication to warrant the assessment of vestibular function sensitivity and water should not be introduced into an ear where the patency of a tympanic perforation is not known.

After arriving at a definitive diagnosis of the lesion of the right tympanic membrane, and since there are no subjective symptoms or complaints, the management should be preventive and conservative.

APPENDIX K

RECOMMENDED MANAGEMENT

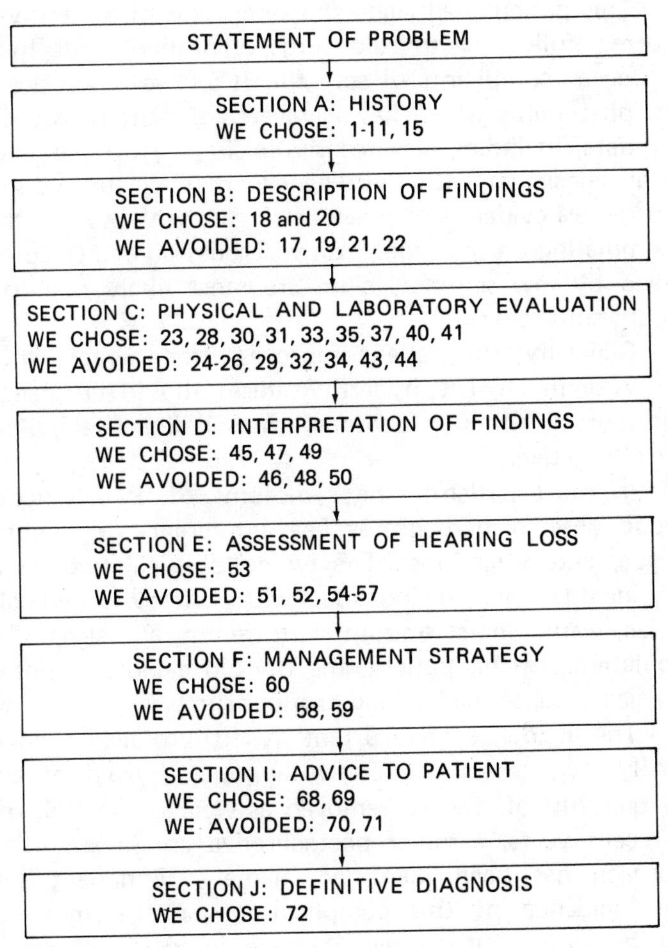

STATEMENT OF PROBLEM
SECTION A: HISTORY
WE CHOSE: 1-11, 15
SECTION B: DESCRIPTION OF FINDINGS
WE CHOSE: 18 and 20
WE AVOIDED: 17, 19, 21, 22
SECTION C: PHYSICAL AND LABORATORY EVALUATION
WE CHOSE: 23, 28, 30, 31, 33, 35, 37, 40, 41
WE AVOIDED: 24-26, 29, 32, 34, 43, 44
SECTION D: INTERPRETATION OF FINDINGS
WE CHOSE: 45, 47, 49
WE AVOIDED: 46, 48, 50
SECTION E: ASSESSMENT OF HEARING LOSS
WE CHOSE: 53
WE AVOIDED: 51, 52, 54-57
SECTION F: MANAGEMENT STRATEGY
WE CHOSE: 60
WE AVOIDED: 58, 59
SECTION I: ADVICE TO PATIENT
WE CHOSE: 68, 69
WE AVOIDED: 70, 71
SECTION J: DEFINITIVE DIAGNOSIS
WE CHOSE: 72

APPENDIX L

COMMENT

This patient had signs and symptoms of hyperthyroidism, which recurred following thyroid surgery, probably for hyperthyroidism. Her recent complaints of sore throat and fever are probably due to a viral pharyngitis which has aggravated the thyrotoxicosis. The laboratory data, including elevated serum T_4, T_3 uptake, and I^{131} uptake, are all consistent with the diagnosis of hyperthyroidism. The thyroid scan reveals evidence of previous surgery with most of the radioisotope accumulating on one side. Positive Trousseau and Chvotek signs accompanied by low serum calcium are most likely due to postoperative hypoparathyroidism.

Clinically, the patient improves after therapy with oral calcium and Vitamin D. The hyperthyroidism should be managed with propylthiouracil although treatment with radioactive iodine is an acceptable alternative.

In most patients, the symptoms of thyrotoxicosis begin with gradual onset of nervousness, heat intolerance, irritability, palpatation, fatigue, and weight loss. The typical physical findings are many and may include a nervous individual with goiter; widened palpebral fissure; lid lag; warm, moist smooth skin; tremor; and signs of hyperdynamic circulation. In this patient, the thyroid gland was not symmetrically enlarged because she had had previous surgery.

The incidence of recurrent hyperthyroidism following surgery is usually low, as is postoperative hypoparathyroidism, and varies with the quantity of thyroid removed as well as the skill of the surgeon. In recent years, a major postoperative complication of the surgical approach has been identified, namely permanent hypothyroidism. The incidence of this complication varies from 4 percent to 30 percent with a progressive increase in incidence with time, similar to that produced by radioactive iodine, although not quite as high.

APPENDIX L

RECOMMENDED MANAGEMENT

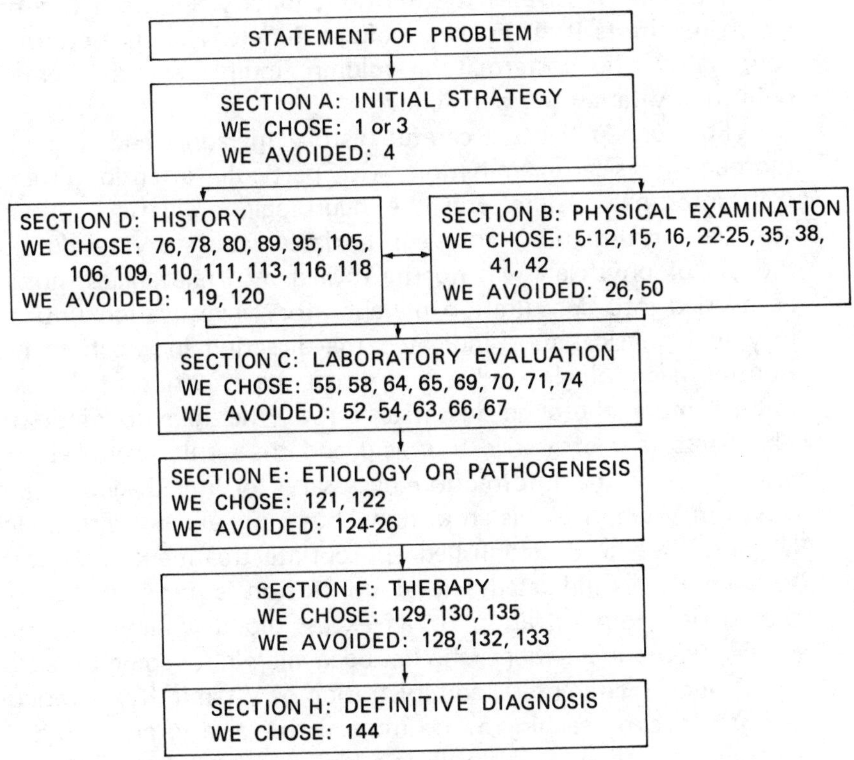

STATEMENT OF PROBLEM
SECTION A: INITIAL STRATEGY
WE CHOSE: 1 or 3
WE AVOIDED: 4
SECTION D: HISTORY
WE CHOSE: 76, 78, 80, 89, 95, 105, 106, 109, 110, 111, 113, 116, 118
WE AVOIDED: 119, 120
SECTION B: PHYSICAL EXAMINATION
WE CHOSE: 5-12, 15, 16, 22-25, 35, 38, 41, 42
WE AVOIDED: 26, 50
SECTION C: LABORATORY EVALUATION
WE CHOSE: 55, 58, 64, 65, 69, 70, 71, 74
WE AVOIDED: 52, 54, 63, 66, 67
SECTION E: ETIOLOGY OR PATHOGENESIS
WE CHOSE: 121, 122
WE AVOIDED: 124-26
SECTION F: THERAPY
WE CHOSE: 129, 130, 135
WE AVOIDED: 128, 132, 133
SECTION H: DEFINITIVE DIAGNOSIS
WE CHOSE: 144

APPENDIX M

COMMENT

This case illustrates the multidisciplinary approach to a problem which manifests itself as a neurologic deficit. The characteristic polyneuropathy, the posterolateral column findings and the dementia all point to a Vitamin B_{12} deficiency.

For such patients a careful history (personal and family) and a thorough physical examination, with particular attention given to the gastrointestinal system and the neurologic evaluation, provide the essential information for appropriate laboratory evaluation. The thoughtful physician will not be misled by irrelevancies, nor will he be hurried into consultation or laboratory investigation until the history and physical have indicated the direction in which to proceed. Routine hematologic studies will direct the attention of the examiner toward more thorough investigation of the hematopoietic system. The assessment of gastric free acid and the results from the Schilling test complete the information necessary for the diagnosis. Bioassay of serum Vitamin B_{12} is an optional but more expensive test. Once the diagnosis has been established appropriate treatment with parenteral Vitamin B_{12} is indicated. Blood transfusion is *not* indicated because the sudden administration of an excess blood volume may result in cardiac failure in a patient who has been anemic for some time.

Following parenteral administration of Vitamin B_{12}, a reticulocyte response occurs reaching a maximum within five to eight days. Such a response is frequently helpful as a last diagnostic test or "therapeutic trial." Subjective improvement, including a sense of well-being, gain in appetite, and disappearance of sore tongue, may occur within several days of the first B_{12} injection. The neurologic symptoms do not change as quickly, but are usually reversible except where death of nerve cells has occured. Since the incidence of carcinoma of the stomach is much higher among patients with a B_{12} deficiency than in the general population, this dreaded complication should be kept in mind during follow-up visits.

APPENDIX M

RECOMMENDED MANAGEMENT

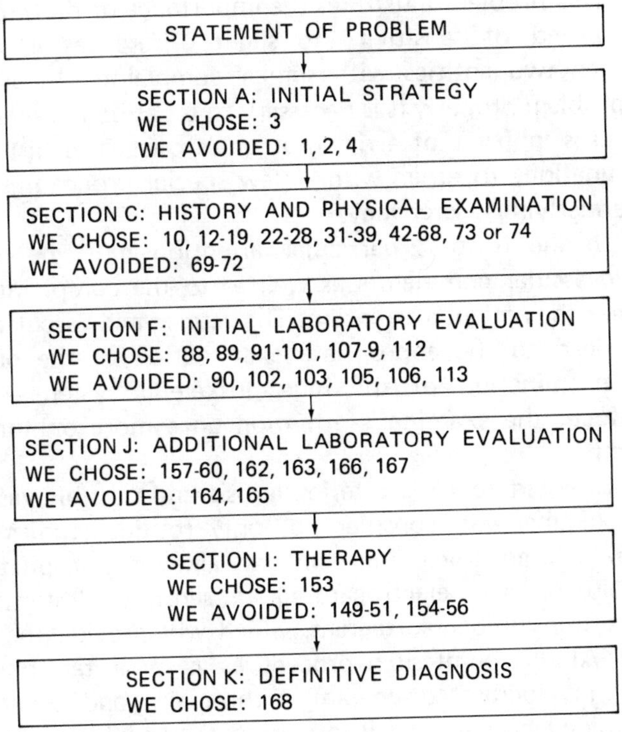

STATEMENT OF PROBLEM

SECTION A: INITIAL STRATEGY
WE CHOSE: 3
WE AVOIDED: 1, 2, 4

SECTION C: HISTORY AND PHYSICAL EXAMINATION
WE CHOSE: 10, 12-19, 22-28, 31-39, 42-68, 73 or 74
WE AVOIDED: 69-72

SECTION F: INITIAL LABORATORY EVALUATION
WE CHOSE: 88, 89, 91-101, 107-9, 112
WE AVOIDED: 90, 102, 103, 105, 106, 113

SECTION J: ADDITIONAL LABORATORY EVALUATION
WE CHOSE: 157-60, 162, 163, 166, 167
WE AVOIDED: 164, 165

SECTION I: THERAPY
WE CHOSE: 153
WE AVOIDED: 149-51, 154-56

SECTION K: DEFINITIVE DIAGNOSIS
WE CHOSE: 168

APPENDIX N

COMMENT

This problem illustrates the importance of thoroughness in investigation and of sensitivity to slight differences in symptomatology between two entities with similar complaints. In order to approach the problem properly it is necessary to set aside the referring physician's diagnosis in favor of arriving at one's own. The history and physical examination, together with a few special procedures, will illuminate the underlying discrepancy.

In the history, particular attention must be paid to previous cardiovascular complaints as well as to the complaints that currently occupy the patient's attention. The cardiac and vascular complaints will then lead to the appropriate examination of the peripheral pulses. The examination of the musculoskeletal system – free of pain – will focus the examiner's attention once more on the peripheral vasculature.

Oriented towards arteriosclerosis and possible vascular occlusion, the examiner will consider not only routine studies relative to the spinal column (including acid and alkaline phosphatase levels), but will also order an electrocardiogram, serum cholesterol determination, and a translumbar aortagram, which will provide the definitive diagnosis. At this point such procedures as spinal tap, pneumoencephalogram, myelogram, discogram, arthrogram, and bronchogram should be avoided because the information they yield is not worth the risk they entail. Consultations with appropriate specialists (orthopedist, cardiologist, and particularly the vascular surgeon) are necessary for therapeutic resolution of the problem. The other consultations are peripheral to the central problem.

APPENDIX N

RECOMMENDED MANAGEMENT

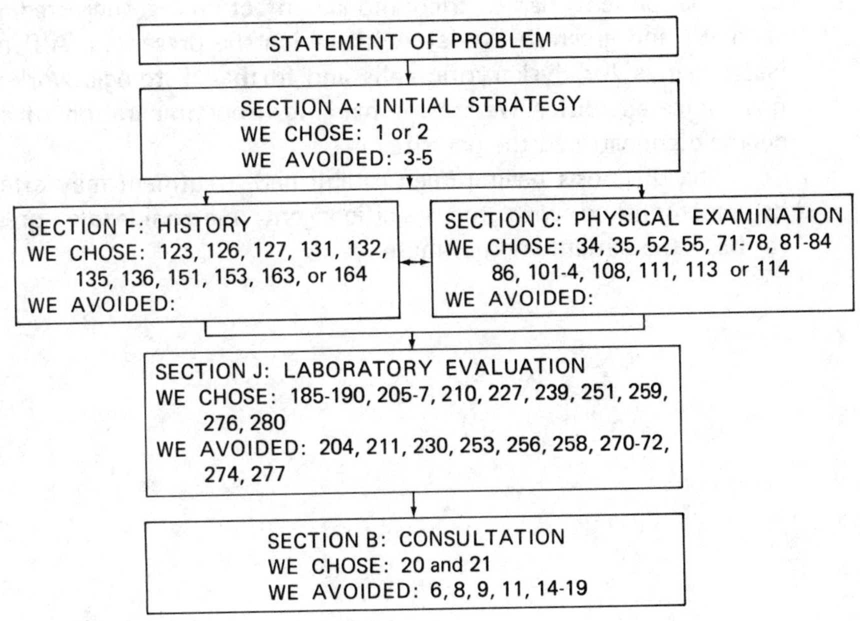

STATEMENT OF PROBLEM
SECTION A: INITIAL STRATEGY
WE CHOSE: 1 or 2
WE AVOIDED: 3-5
SECTION F: HISTORY
WE CHOSE: 123, 126, 127, 131, 132, 135, 136, 151, 153, 163, or 164
WE AVOIDED:
SECTION C: PHYSICAL EXAMINATION
WE CHOSE: 34, 35, 52, 55, 71-78, 81-84 86, 101-4, 108, 111, 113 or 114
WE AVOIDED:
SECTION J: LABORATORY EVALUATION
WE CHOSE: 185-190, 205-7, 210, 227, 239, 251, 259, 276, 280
WE AVOIDED: 204, 211, 230, 253, 256, 258, 270-72, 274, 277
SECTION B: CONSULTATION
WE CHOSE: 20 and 21
WE AVOIDED: 6, 8, 9, 11, 14-19

APPENDIX O

COMMENT

The patient has a trichomonas infection as suggested by the cervicitis and greenish exudate with which she presented. A Pap smear was negative for dyskaryotic cells and further histologic work-up was not indicated, but a wet smear hanging drop preparation of the discharge demonstrated the parasite.

The diagnosis having been established, treatment may effectively be accomplished with the specific agent, metronidazole, prescribed for both the patient and her mate.

APPENDIX O

RECOMMENDED MANAGEMENT

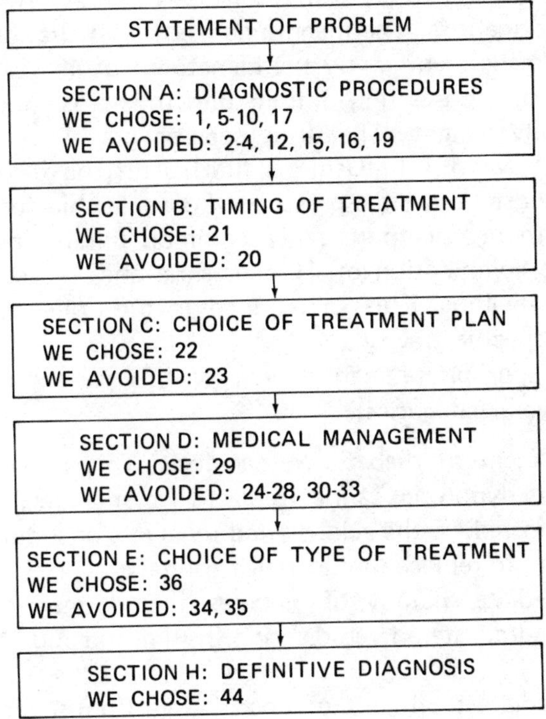

STATEMENT OF PROBLEM
SECTION A: DIAGNOSTIC PROCEDURES
WE CHOSE: 1, 5-10, 17
WE AVOIDED: 2-4, 12, 15, 16, 19
SECTION B: TIMING OF TREATMENT
WE CHOSE: 21
WE AVOIDED: 20
SECTION C: CHOICE OF TREATMENT PLAN
WE CHOSE: 22
WE AVOIDED: 23
SECTION D: MEDICAL MANAGEMENT
WE CHOSE: 29
WE AVOIDED: 24-28, 30-33
SECTION E: CHOICE OF TYPE OF TREATMENT
WE CHOSE: 36
WE AVOIDED: 34, 35
SECTION H: DEFINITIVE DIAGNOSIS
WE CHOSE: 44

APPENDIX P

COMMENT

Though the patient ultimately required surgery to relieve the persistent gastric obstruction due to duodenal ulcer, it is first necessary to recognize and to control his diabetes and to correct his fluid-electrolyte abnormalities. The magnitude of the dehydration (hemoconcentration) is made manifest by the hematocrit of 48% and the hemoglobin of 16.8 g, representing a fluid deficit expressed as 6 to 8% of the total body weight. The urine specific gravity of 1.036 (osmolality would be over 1200 mOsm per liter) signifying maximal concentration further substantiates the presence of considerable dehydration. Furthermore, although acetonuria is a common finding in states of dehydration, the combination of 4+ glucosuria and 4+ acetonuria speaks for diabetes mellitus. This solute load in the urine may further explain the high specific gravity.

The appropriate management of this patient may be considered under several categories:

A. Treatment of diabetic ketoacidosis. This should include administration of hypotonic saline (replaces water and salt), lactate or bicarbonate (to reduce the acidosis and renal loss of sodium and potassium), potassium, to replace that lost electrolyte, and phosphate.
B. Immediate therapy of diabetes. Include intravenous and subcutaneously administered rapid-acting insulin and monitor blood or urine glucose.
C. Immediate treatment of obstruction. Continue nasogastric suction until it can be ascertained whether the obstruction has been relieved and continue maintenance of electrolyte balance by intravenous infusions.
D. Surgical treatment of obstruction. To be instituted either when fluid-electrolyte disequilibrium and diabetes have been corrected or, if copious bile returns through the Levine tube and the gastric decompensation can be corrected following enteric hyperalimentation, in 10 days to two weeks. Vagotomy and pyloroplasty may be performed, but best results would be anticipated with vagotomy, antrectomy (50% gastric resection), and gastroduodenostomy (Billroth I operation).

The patient may be expected to recover from surgery and his electrocardiogram should no longer show hypokalemic changes. He should subsequently be treated with lente insulin to provide long-term management of the diabetes.

APPENDIX P

RECOMMENDED MANAGEMENT

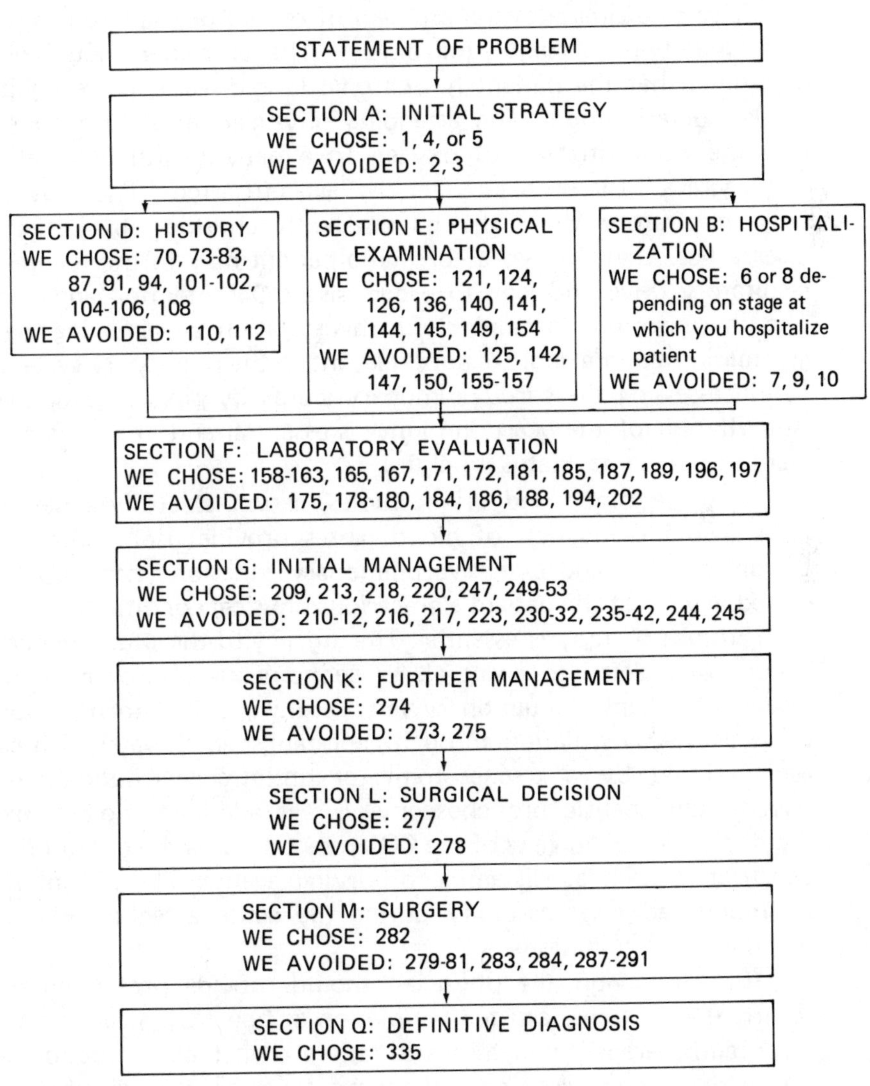

STATEMENT OF PROBLEM
SECTION A: INITIAL STRATEGY
WE CHOSE: 1, 4, or 5
WE AVOIDED: 2, 3
SECTION D: HISTORY
WE CHOSE: 70, 73-83, 87, 91, 94, 101-102, 104-106, 108
WE AVOIDED: 110, 112
SECTION E: PHYSICAL EXAMINATION
WE CHOSE: 121, 124, 126, 136, 140, 141, 144, 145, 149, 154
WE AVOIDED: 125, 142, 147, 150, 155-157
SECTION B: HOSPITALIZATION
WE CHOSE: 6 or 8 depending on stage at which you hospitalize patient
WE AVOIDED: 7, 9, 10
SECTION F: LABORATORY EVALUATION
WE CHOSE: 158-163, 165, 167, 171, 172, 181, 185, 187, 189, 196, 197
WE AVOIDED: 175, 178-180, 184, 186, 188, 194, 202
SECTION G: INITIAL MANAGEMENT
WE CHOSE: 209, 213, 218, 220, 247, 249-53
WE AVOIDED: 210-12, 216, 217, 223, 230-32, 235-42, 244, 245
SECTION K: FURTHER MANAGEMENT
WE CHOSE: 274
WE AVOIDED: 273, 275
SECTION L: SURGICAL DECISION
WE CHOSE: 277
WE AVOIDED: 278
SECTION M: SURGERY
WE CHOSE: 282
WE AVOIDED: 279-81, 283, 284, 287-291
SECTION Q: DEFINITIVE DIAGNOSIS
WE CHOSE: 335

APPENDIX Q

COMMENT

This case simulates the problem of respiratory failure in a patient with underlying chronic lung disease. The examiner should quickly determine that the patient has chronic lung disease and recognize his sudden deterioration. The attending physician must also appreciate that the administration of oxygen to a patient with CO_2 retention may aggravate the problem. The low levels of arterial P_{O_2} may be the only respiratory drive the patient with chronic obstructive lung disease has. Giving oxygen to such a patient may further depress this respiratory drive and lead to progressive CO_2 retention and acidosis. The physician must act quickly in this situation by removing the oxygen mask, taking a short history relevant to the pulmonary system, and rapidly assessing the cardiopulmonary status by physical examination. Auscultation of the heart and lungs is essential and in this case assessment of the mental status is helpful.

Routine blood and urine studies, serum electrolyte determinations, and investigation of blood gasses provide useful information. Barium swallow and extensive pulmonary function tests are not warranted in view of the patient's precarious physical condition.

Prompt therapy is essential. The urgency of the situation demands action. Any delay to await either spontaneous improvement or the results of extensive pulmonary tests is unwise. Treatment should include assisted ventilation through an established airway which can be accomplished by a tracheostomy or endotracheal intubation and possibly therapeutic bronchoscopy. Direct administration of oxygen is contraindicated in view of the CO_2 retention as is the use of bronchoconstrictors such as histamine or drying agents. The patient should be monitored very carefully during the acute episode by frequent blood-gas determinations.

For follow-up the physician should provide protection against recurrent infections, assisted ventilation at home by means of a respirator, and therapeutic measures to relieve bronchial obstruction. Monitoring of blood-gasses and pulmonary function periodically may be desirable.

APPENDIX Q

RECOMMENDED MANAGEMENT

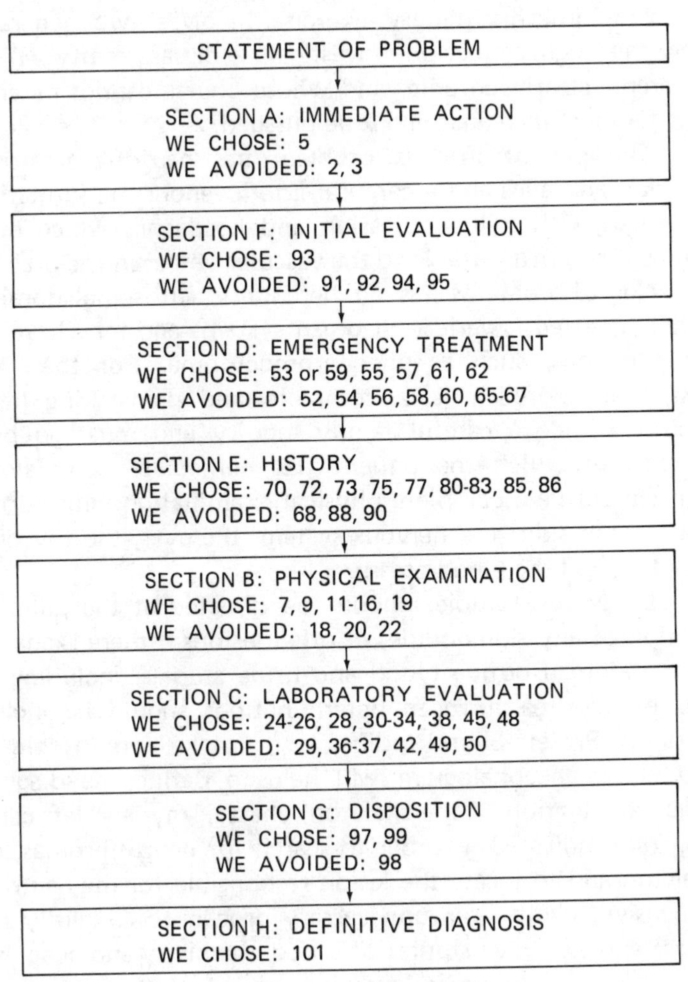

STATEMENT OF PROBLEM
SECTION A: IMMEDIATE ACTION
WE CHOSE: 5
WE AVOIDED: 2, 3
SECTION F: INITIAL EVALUATION
WE CHOSE: 93
WE AVOIDED: 91, 92, 94, 95
SECTION D: EMERGENCY TREATMENT
WE CHOSE: 53 or 59, 55, 57, 61, 62
WE AVOIDED: 52, 54, 56, 58, 60, 65-67
SECTION E: HISTORY
WE CHOSE: 70, 72, 73, 75, 77, 80-83, 85, 86
WE AVOIDED: 68, 88, 90
SECTION B: PHYSICAL EXAMINATION
WE CHOSE: 7, 9, 11-16, 19
WE AVOIDED: 18, 20, 22
SECTION C: LABORATORY EVALUATION
WE CHOSE: 24-26, 28, 30-34, 38, 45, 48
WE AVOIDED: 29, 36-37, 42, 49, 50
SECTION G: DISPOSITION
WE CHOSE: 97, 99
WE AVOIDED: 98
SECTION H: DEFINITIVE DIAGNOSIS
WE CHOSE: 101

APPENDIX R

COMMENT

This interdisciplinary exercise involves two general questions: How thoroughly must one investigate a disease entity which is quickly apparent, clearly chronic, and whose course cannot be changed? And how far must its management be pursued?

The patient in this problem has neurofibromatosis involving the skin and eyes and a cerebral arteriovenous malformation. She also presented with mild depression and headaches which may not have been entirely attributable to the vascular defect in the brain.

Neurofibromatosis is an hereditary autosomal dominant disease that may affect a variety of organ systems and may have recognizable complications, such as pheochromocytoma. For these reasons, the best first approach is a complete and painstaking history which should include a careful family inquiry and must go beyond those systems of which the patient has immediate complaint. The next step should be a complete physical examination with particular attention to the skin, the nervous system, the eyes, the thyroid gland, the skeleton, and the blood pressure.

Laboratory studies should be directed at the pathologic identification of any skin nodules or other lesions if there is any doubt about their nature. Routine blood and urine studies, including blood sugar and blood urea nitrogen determinations should be included in the work-up. Protein-bound iodine, I^{131} uptake and thyroid scan, VMA, and electroencephalogram will help to define the diagnosis. Radiologic examination of the skeleton, chest x-ray, and left cartoid arteriogram are indicated in order to search for neurofibromas involving the skeleton and to locate the lesion responsible for the neurologic deficit. Expensive, painful, or unnecessary procedures (including red cell indices) and excessive studies of blood chemistry and coagulation should be avoided. Radiologic examination of the gastrointerstinal tract, contrast studies of the central nervous system (other than those mentioned), ventriculography, biopsy of the liver, brain, and rectal mucosa will add no useful information and may be dangerous. Consultation needs will vary with the training of the primary physician contacted. Certain of the suggested possibilities are probably unnecessary.

Because the vascular defect was not accessible to surgical intervention, proper therapeutic management includes a conservative approach to management of the seizures. Excessive drug therapy (including mood elevators, ointments, contraceptive pills, and eye drops) is to be avoided; these may aggravate the seizures or cause other undesirable side effects without helping the patient. It is important to counsel the patient as to the prognosis and genetic hazards and to see the patient for follow-up. Should the vascular defect bleed, surgical intervention would become mandatory.

APPENDIX R

RECOMMENDED MANAGEMENT

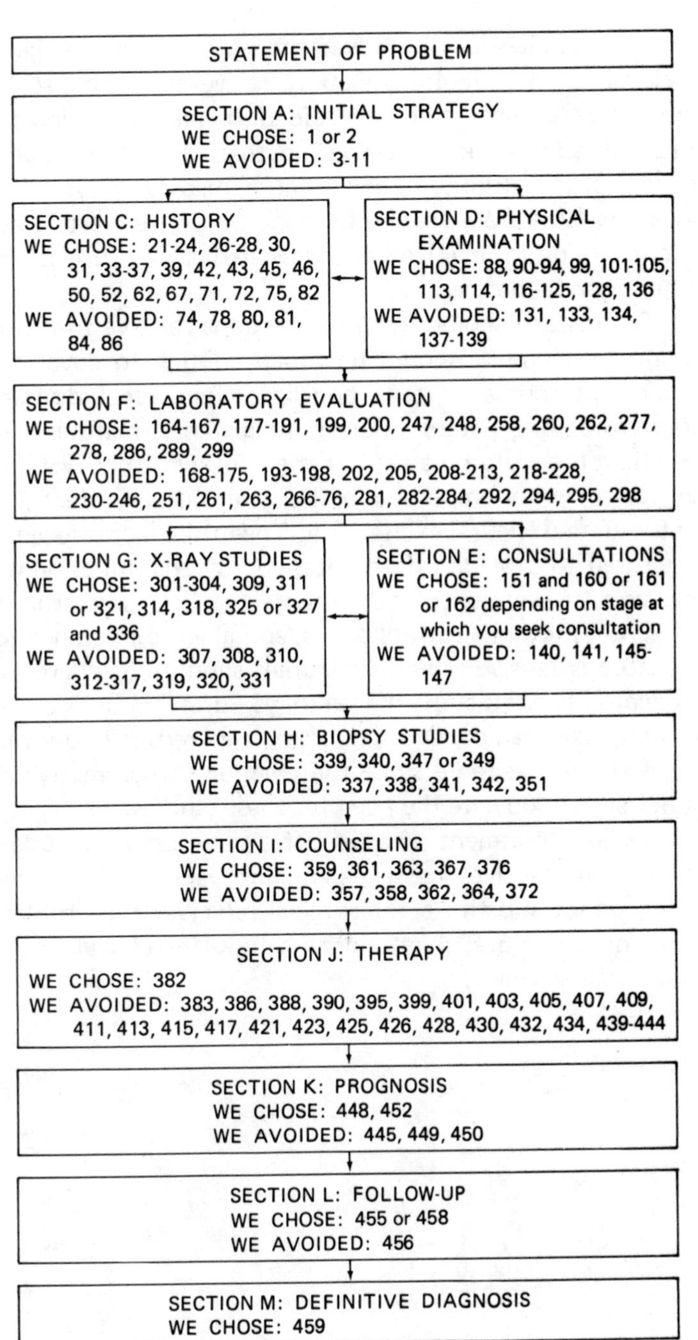

STATEMENT OF PROBLEM
SECTION A: INITIAL STRATEGY
WE CHOSE: 1 or 2
WE AVOIDED: 3-11
SECTION C: HISTORY
WE CHOSE: 21-24, 26-28, 30, 31, 33-37, 39, 42, 43, 45, 46, 50, 52, 62, 67, 71, 72, 75, 82
WE AVOIDED: 74, 78, 80, 81, 84, 86
SECTION D: PHYSICAL EXAMINATION
WE CHOSE: 88, 90-94, 99, 101-105, 113, 114, 116-125, 128, 136
WE AVOIDED: 131, 133, 134, 137-139
SECTION F: LABORATORY EVALUATION
WE CHOSE: 164-167, 177-191, 199, 200, 247, 248, 258, 260, 262, 277, 278, 286, 289, 299
WE AVOIDED: 168-175, 193-198, 202, 205, 208-213, 218-228, 230-246, 251, 261, 263, 266-76, 281, 282-284, 292, 294, 295, 298
SECTION G: X-RAY STUDIES
WE CHOSE: 301-304, 309, 311 or 321, 314, 318, 325 or 327 and 336
WE AVOIDED: 307, 308, 310, 312-317, 319, 320, 331
SECTION E: CONSULTATIONS
WE CHOSE: 151 and 160 or 161 or 162 depending on stage at which you seek consultation
WE AVOIDED: 140, 141, 145-147
SECTION H: BIOPSY STUDIES
WE CHOSE: 339, 340, 347 or 349
WE AVOIDED: 337, 338, 341, 342, 351
SECTION I: COUNSELING
WE CHOSE: 359, 361, 363, 367, 376
WE AVOIDED: 357, 358, 362, 364, 372
SECTION J: THERAPY
WE CHOSE: 382
WE AVOIDED: 383, 386, 388, 390, 395, 399, 401, 403, 405, 407, 409, 411, 413, 415, 417, 421, 423, 425, 426, 428, 430, 432, 434, 439-444
SECTION K: PROGNOSIS
WE CHOSE: 448, 452
WE AVOIDED: 445, 449, 450
SECTION L: FOLLOW-UP
WE CHOSE: 455 or 458
WE AVOIDED: 456
SECTION M: DEFINITIVE DIAGNOSIS
WE CHOSE: 459

APPENDIX S

COMMENT

This problem can be solved by asking for a urologic consultation at several stages in its investigation. However, the indiscriminate use of consultative services can be avoided if the examining physician will undertake appropriate investigation to narrow the scope of the problem. It is therefore desirable that a history, physical examination, and a few laboratory studies be done before requesting a consultation so that the organ involved and the medical or surgical nature of the problem can be defined.

The history should include questions relative to the genitourinary system; this inquiry should be broad enough to cover the possibility of congenital renal disease and infectious renal disease, as well as parathyroid or dietary-induced renal abnormalities. The physical examination should be aimed at the cardiovascular system, the abdominal cavity (with emphasis on the genitourinary tract), the skeleton, and the state of neural excitability. The initial laboratory studies should be selected to provide information about renal function while avoiding unnecessary complexity and expense (eg, iron and iron-binding capacity, serum protein electrophoresis, and glucose tolerance tests).

More extensive radiologic studies should be ordered to determine the anatomic status of the kidneys, ureters, and urinary bladder. Renal biopsy, radioactive renogram, and red cell survival are neither indicated nor desirable since the cystourethrogram (which should be done first) will obviate the need for these studies.

Medical treatment of a palliative nature may include calcium gluconate, hypotensive agents, penicillin, and bicarbonate. But these agents cannot substitute for surgical repair of the problem. Definitive treatment, therefore, may consist simply in referral to a urologist for surgical management.

APPENDIX S

RECOMMENDED MANAGEMENT

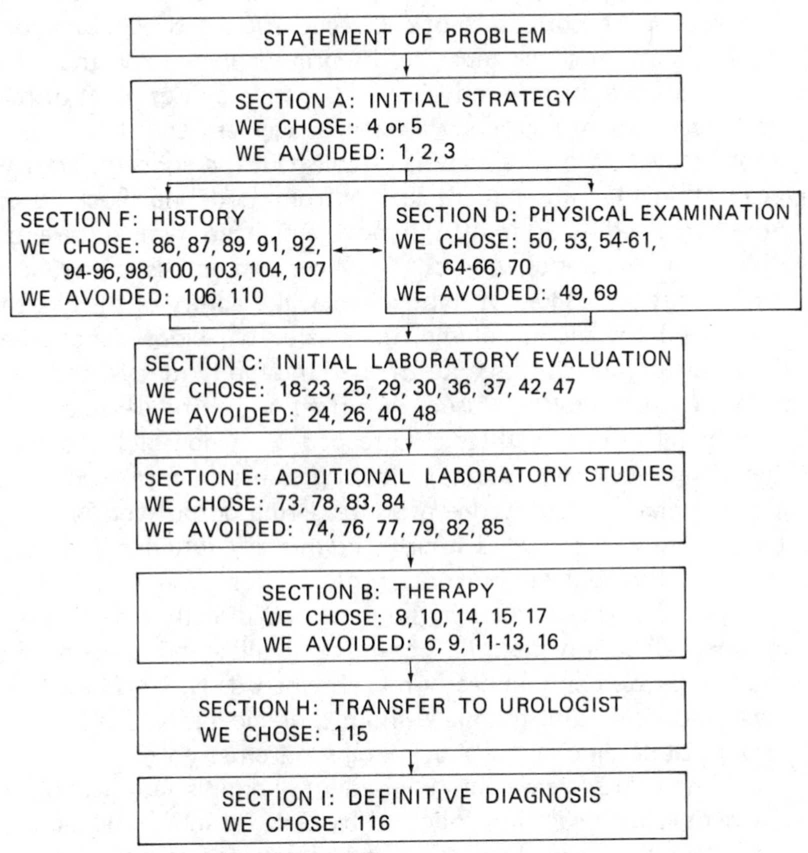

STATEMENT OF PROBLEM
SECTION A: INITIAL STRATEGY
WE CHOSE: 4 or 5
WE AVOIDED: 1, 2, 3
SECTION F: HISTORY
WE CHOSE: 86, 87, 89, 91, 92, 94-96, 98, 100, 103, 104, 107
WE AVOIDED: 106, 110
SECTION D: PHYSICAL EXAMINATION
WE CHOSE: 50, 53, 54-61, 64-66, 70
WE AVOIDED: 49, 69
SECTION C: INITIAL LABORATORY EVALUATION
WE CHOSE: 18-23, 25, 29, 30, 36, 37, 42, 47
WE AVOIDED: 24, 26, 40, 48
SECTION E: ADDITIONAL LABORATORY STUDIES
WE CHOSE: 73, 78, 83, 84
WE AVOIDED: 74, 76, 77, 79, 82, 85
SECTION B: THERAPY
WE CHOSE: 8, 10, 14, 15, 17
WE AVOIDED: 6, 9, 11-13, 16
SECTION H: TRANSFER TO UROLOGIST
WE CHOSE: 115
SECTION I: DEFINITIVE DIAGNOSIS
WE CHOSE: 116

APPENDIX T

COMMENT

This exercise poses the problem faced by the physician who encounters a patient with multiple injuries and who appears to be in shock. For its correct solution, recognition and classification of the clinical state of shock must be the prime concern and the other problems relating to history, physical and complete assessment of the injury, and treatment of pain must await management and stabilization of the shock state. Once an airway is established, the concerns start with the realization that this patient suffers from moderate shock: Blood pressure decreased by 20 to 40%; hypovolemia, cool temperature, pale skin, thirst, and mental cloudiness. The next step entails gathering information about the degree of hypovolemia, the ability of the heart to move (circulate) the blood volume, the degree of acidosis and other metabolic disturbances, the state of the lungs and kidneys, and other vital signs. A vast amount of such information can be gathered by placing indwelling arterial catheters (attached to a console) and monitoring heart rate, respiratory rate, blood pressure, central venous pressure or pulmonary artery wedge pressure. Urine output and intravenous intake should be recorded hourly. Pulmonary function may be studied every two to four hours to offer information about arterial P_{O_2}, P_{CO_2}, and pH. Cardiac output may be measured directly by the dye dilution or thermodilution method. Serum osmolality and proteins should be studied as well and a chest x-ray obtained daily. This patient suffered from multiple blunt trauma without thoracic injury, but had a very real chance of developing the shock lung syndrome.

Immediate treatment required the administration of intravenous Ringer's lactate solution followed by dextran and whole blood, as soon as it becomes available. Typing and crossmatch should have been done on arrival. Vasopressors should not have been given to this patient since fluid replacement was of prime importance and would have increased peripheral resistance at the expense of tissue perfusion. Vasodilators were not offered here since their use in the patient with moderate hypovolemia would not normally be considered until after volume replacement had been vigorously tried and found to be ineffective. The ultimate decision about further or more intensive approaches to the shock state is made on clinical grounds: return of normal cerebration, urine output, skin color, and stabilization of blood pressure, heart and respiratory rates. Since this patient responded to a conservative approach, more radical measures were not indicated.

Despite the pain associated with fractures, Demerol or morphine has an unfortunate effect both on cerebral centers (eg, respiratory, vasomotor) and on peripheral tissue oxygen extraction, and should not be used until the patient is stable. Once circulatory stability has been achieved, morphine or Demerol should be given to relieve pain. Because of the compound fracture, a wide-spectrum antibiotic was prescribed. The patient had been in good health prior to the accident and there was no evidence of heart failure so that neither steroids nor digitalis were indicated.

Once circulatory stability has been achieved and CNS and other internal injury excluded, the lacerations, leg and hip injuries may be diagnosed and treated by the methods indicated in Section D.

BIBLIOGRAPHY

1. Schumer W, Nyhus LM: Treatment of Shock: Principles and Practice. Philadelphia, Lea and Febiger, 1974
2. Shires GT, Carrico CJ, Canizaro PD: Shock. Philadelphia, Saunders, 1973

APPENDIX T

RECOMMENDED MANAGEMENT

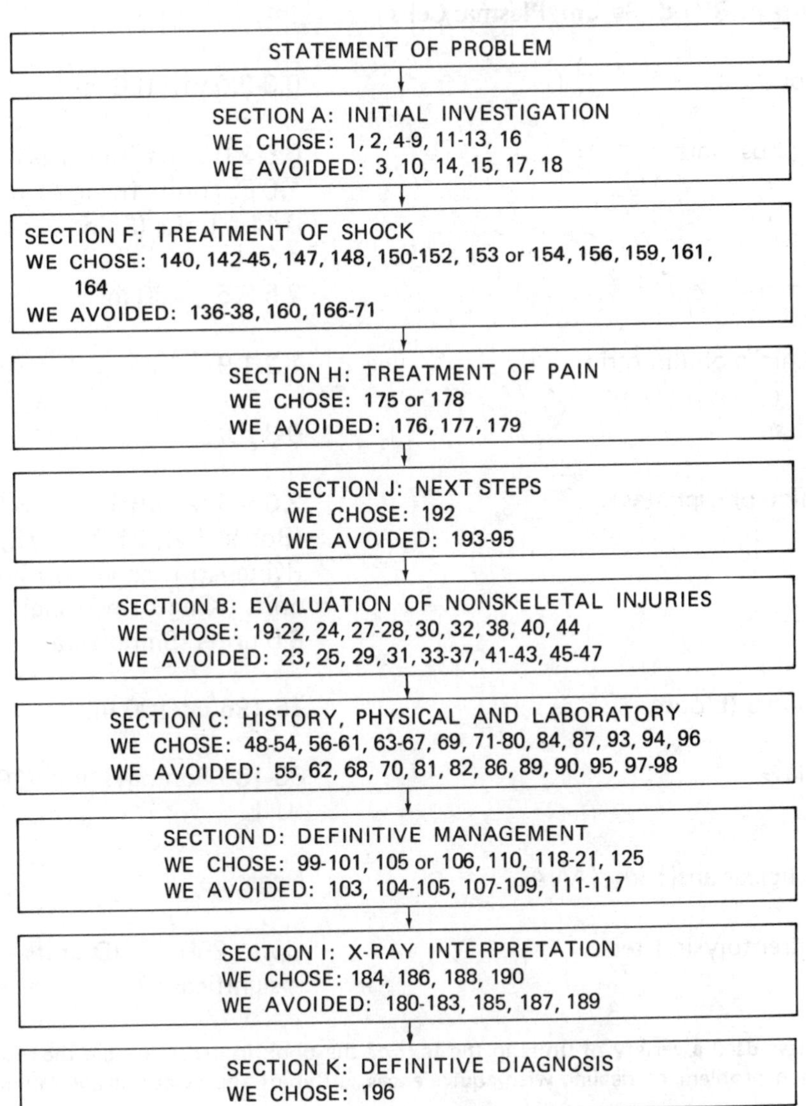

STATEMENT OF PROBLEM

SECTION A: INITIAL INVESTIGATION
WE CHOSE: 1, 2, 4-9, 11-13, 16
WE AVOIDED: 3, 10, 14, 15, 17, 18

SECTION F: TREATMENT OF SHOCK
WE CHOSE: 140, 142-45, 147, 148, 150-152, 153 or 154, 156, 159, 161, 164
WE AVOIDED: 136-38, 160, 166-71

SECTION H: TREATMENT OF PAIN
WE CHOSE: 175 or 178
WE AVOIDED: 176, 177, 179

SECTION J: NEXT STEPS
WE CHOSE: 192
WE AVOIDED: 193-95

SECTION B: EVALUATION OF NONSKELETAL INJURIES
WE CHOSE: 19-22, 24, 27-28, 30, 32, 38, 40, 44
WE AVOIDED: 23, 25, 29, 31, 33-37, 41-43, 45-47

SECTION C: HISTORY, PHYSICAL AND LABORATORY
WE CHOSE: 48-54, 56-61, 63-67, 69, 71-80, 84, 87, 93, 94, 96
WE AVOIDED: 55, 62, 68, 70, 81, 82, 86, 89, 90, 95, 97-98

SECTION D: DEFINITIVE MANAGEMENT
WE CHOSE: 99-101, 105 or 106, 110, 118-21, 125
WE AVOIDED: 103, 104-105, 107-109, 111-117

SECTION I: X-RAY INTERPRETATION
WE CHOSE: 184, 186, 188, 190
WE AVOIDED: 180-183, 185, 187, 189

SECTION K: DEFINITIVE DIAGNOSIS
WE CHOSE: 196

APPENDIX U

NORMAL VALUES*

Constituents of Blood: Serum; Plasma; Cells

Acetone	0.3-2.0 mg/100 ml
Acid phosphatase	0.5-2.0 units (Bodansky); 0.2-1.8 IU; 1.0-5.0 units (King-Armstrong); 0-11.0 units (Shinowara)
Albumin	3.5-5.5 g/100 ml
Albumin/globulin ratio	1.2-1.9
Aldolase	0-8 IU/L
Alkaline phosphatase	2.0-4.5 (Adults), 3.0-13.0 (Children), (Bodansky); 21-91 IU/L; 10-20 units (King-Armstrong), (Children); 5.0-13.0 units (King-Armstrong), (Adults); 2.2-8.6 units (Shinowara)
Ammonia (blood)	75-196 μg/100 ml
Amylase	60-180 Somogyi units/100 ml; 0.8-3.2 IU/L
Antinuclear antibody (ANA)	Negative
Antistreptolysin titer	Up to 250 TODD units – A rise in titer is significant

*We have used a variety of units in the text of the book in order to help the reader adapt to the common problem of dealing with equivalences, different abbreviations and laboratory individual differences.

Antithyroglobulin	0
Barbiturates	0
Basal metabolic rate	–15% to +15% of mean standard
Bicarbonate (Astrup)	24-30 mEq/L
Bilirubin – direct	0.1-0.3 mg/100 ml
Bilirubin – total	0.3-1.0 mg/100 ml
Bleeding time (IVY)	1-9 minutes
Blood urea nitrogen (BUN)	10-20 mg/100 ml Newborn – 16 mg/100 ml
Bromide	0
Bromsulphalein clearance (BSP)	5% or less retention after 45 minutes
Calcium	4.5-5.5 mEq/L; 9-11 mg/100 ml Newborn – 8.4 mg/100 ml
Carbon dioxide (combining power)	21-30 mEq/L; 50-70 vol. %; cord blood 20.6 mEq/L
Carotenoids	50-300 μg/100 ml
Catecholamines – Epinephrine	.05-.07 μg/L
Norepinephrine	0.30-0.36 μg/L
Cephalin flocculation (obsolete)	0-1/24 hour
Chlorides	98-106 mEq/L Cord blood 98-110 mEq/L
Cholesterol – esterified total	100-180/100 ml 180-240 mg/100 ml
Chorionic gonadotrophins	0 IU/ml. In pregnancy 40-90 days approximately 50 IU/ml

Clot retraction (quantitative) (Didisheim)	75%
Clotting time (Lee-White)	9-15 minutes (majority); 2-19 minutes (range)
Cortisol	2-20 μg/100 ml at 8:00 A.M.
Corticosteroids (Plasma)	13 ± 6 μg/ml at 8:00 A.M.
Complete Blood Count (CBC)	
Hemoglobin	Adults: 14-16 g/100 ml Children: 12-14 g/100 ml Newborn: 17-20 g/100 ml
Hematocrit	Men—45%; Women—40% Children—38%; Newborn—47-58%
Red blood cells	$5 \pm 1 \times 10^6$/mm^3
White blood cells (total)	7000/mm^3 : (At birth), 14-18000/mm^3
White blood cells (differential)	Polynuclear 25-60% (segmental) 0-20% (band) Lymphocytes 20-50% Mononuclear 2.4-11% Eosinophils 3-5% Basophils 0.6-1.8%
Reticulocytes	0-2%
Platelets	300,000/mm^3, ± 50,000
Smear	No abnormal cells seen
Coomb's test	Negative
C-reactive protein (CRP)	Negative
Creatine	0.2-0.8 mg/100 ml

Creatine phosphokinase	Female: 5-25 U/ml Male: 5-35 U/ml
Creatinine	1-1/5 mg/100 ml
Creatinine clearance	(Corrected to 1.73 m^3 body surface area) 91-130 ml/minute
Culture for bacteria	No growth
Differential white blood count (see CBC)	
Erythrocyte sedimentation rate (ESR) (Wintrobe)	Male: 0-9 mm/one hour Female: 0-20 mm/one hour
Ethanol	0
Fibrinogen (plasma)	160-415 mg/100 ml
Fluorescent treponemal antibody absorption test (FTA)	Nonreactive
Folic acid	6-15 ng/ml
Globulins	2.0-30 g/100 ml
Glucose (Blood) Fasting	60-90 mg/100 ml
– Random	80-160 mg/100 ml
– Renal Threshold	180 mg/100 ml
– Two hour postprandial	80-120 mg/100 ml
– Newborn	40-97 mg/100 ml
Glucose-6-phosphate-dehydrogenase (plasma)	0-5-2.4 IU
Glucose tolerance test (oral)	Not more than 160 mg/100 ml "true glucose" after one-half hour. Return to normal (less than 120 mg/100 ml) by two hours. Glucose not present in any urine specimen.
Glutamic oxalacetic transaminase (SGOT)	6-18 IU/L

Glutamic pyruvic transaminase (SGPT)	3-26 IU/L
Hematocrit (see CBC)	
Hemoglobin (see CBC)	
Hemoglobin electrophoresis	Hemoglobin AA, 85% or more; Hemoglobin A_2 1.5-3%; Fetal hemoglobin <2%
Hemogram (see CBC)	
Heterophile antibody determination for infectious mononucleosis	Usually reported as "positive" or "negative." Significant titers (for infectious mononucleosis) are usually in the range of 1:320
I^{131}, uptake/24 hours	15-45%; mean 35%
Iron	107 ± 31 μg/100 ml
Iron-binding capacity (unsaturated) Saturation:	305 ± 32 μg/100 ml 20-45%
Lactic dehydrogenase (LDH)	120-419 units/ml (Wroblewski)
Latex fixation titer	(See Rheumatoid factor – latex)
Lead	<20 μg/100 ml
Lipase	1.5 ml N/20 NaOH (Cherry-Crandall)
Liver function studies	(See SGOT, SGPT, BSP)
Lupus erythematosus cell preparation (LE prep)	None found
Magnesium	1.5-2.5 mEq/L; 2-3 mg/100 ml
Mean corpuscular hemoglobin concentration (MCHC)	34 ± 2 g/100 ml
Mean corpuscular hemoglobin (MCH)	29 ± 2 pg
Mean corpuscular volume (MCV)	90 ± 7 μ

Mean Corpuscular Diameter (MCD)	$75 \pm 0.3\ \mu m$
Mono spot test	Negative
Nonprotein nitrogen (NPN)	15-35 mg/100 ml
Osmotic fragility of red cells	Slight hemolysis 0.45-0.39% Complete hemolysis 0.33-0.30%
Oxytocinase	Values vary considerably. It is usually reported as "normal" to "markedly elevated" (normally found elevated in later stages of pregnancy).
Oxygen saturation (arterial blood) (venous blood)	97 vol. % 60-95 vol. % } at sea level
Partial Thromboplastin time	60-70 seconds
P_{CO_2} (arterial blood)	38 mm Hg (± 2.9 SD)
P_{CO_2} (venous blood) At birth	35-45 mm Hg 42.8 mm Hg
pH (blood) At birth	7.38-7.44 7.29
P_{O_2} (arterial blood)	104.2 mm Hg − 0.27 X age in years, seated.
Adult At birth-venous blood (infant breathing)	Usually 75-100 mm Hg 60% O_2 − 45 mm Hg
Phosphorus	1-1.5 mEq/L; 3-4.5 mg/100 ml
Platelet count (see CBC)	
Potassium	3.5-5.0 mEq/L Cord blood − 5.6-12 mEq/L
Protein (total)	5.5-8.0 g/100 ml
Protein bound iodine (PBI)	$4.0\text{-}8.0\ \mu g/100$ ml

Test	Normal value
Protein electrophoresis	Albumin: 3.5-5.5 g/100 ml (50-65%) Globulin: 2.0-3.5 g/100 ml (35-50%) $Alpha_1$: 0.2-0.4 g/100 ml (5.0-7.0%) $Alpha_2$: 0.5-0.9 g/100 ml (7.0-12%) Beta: 0.6-1.1 g/100 ml (10-15%) Gamma: 0.7-1.7 g/100 ml (13-20%)
Prothrombin consumption (% activity)	Over 80% in one hour
Prothrombin control	11-16 seconds } Should be comparable
Prothrombin time	11-16 seconds } Should be comparable
Red cell survival time (Cr^{51})	T 1/2: 28 days
Red cell galactose-1-phosphate uridyl transferase	Normal
Red cell glucose-6-phosphate-dehydrogenase	Usually reported as "normal" = Type B; or "deficient" = Type A
Reticulocyte count (See CBC)	
Rheumatoid factor (latex)	Negative = 1:40 Doubtful = 1:80-1:160 Positive = 1:320
Salicylates	0
Schilling test	Excretion in urine of orally administered Vitamin B_{12} following parenteral injection of B_{12}: 7-40%.
Serological test for syphilis (STS, RPR, VDRL, or Wasserman)	Nonreactive
Sheep cell agglutination	Negative
Sickle cell preparation	Negative
Sodium	136-145 mEq/L Cord blood – 126-166 Emq/L

Tri-iodothyronine (RBC-T_3)	15%
T_3 (Radioimmunoassay)	96-172 ng/100 ml
Thyroxine (Pattee-Murphy test)	4-11 μg/100 ml
Thymol turbidity (obsolete)	0-5 units
Tri-iodothyronine daily for one week followed by I^{131} uptake:	Below 20% in 24 hours.
Tri-iodothyronine uptake (Resin)	25-35% (expressed as a ratio: 0.82-1.17)
Uric acid	3-7 mg/100 ml
Vitamin A	50-100 μg/100 ml
Vitamin B_{12}	200-600 pg/ml
Volume (blood)	Men: 6.0-7.5% of body weight (depends on obesity and muscularity) Normal build, 7.0% Women: 5.5-7.0% Normal build, 6.5%
White blood cell count (see CBC)	
Zinc turbidity (obsolete)	2-12 units

Urine

Acetone	0
Addis count (24 hours)	RBC: 0-130,000 WBC: 0-650,000 CASTS-Hyaline: 0-2000
Amylase	35-260 units/hour (Somogyi)
Appearance	Clear, straw colored
Bacteria	None on clean catch
Bence-Jones protein	0
Bile pigment (bilirubin)	0

Calcium (quantitative)	<7.5 mEq/24 hours; <150 mg/24 hours
Catecholamines	Epinephrine and norepinephrine: 100 μg/24 hour Metanephrine and normetanephrine: 1.3 mg/24 hour Metanephrine: Up to 1.0 mg/24 hour VMA: 0.7-6.8 mg/24 hour
Casts	Up to one hyaline cast
Chlorides	120-240 mEq/24 hours
Chorionic Gonadotrophins	0
Concentration test	After 24 hour fluid restiction, specific gravity 1.025 or more
Creatine (expressed as creatinine)	Males <50 mg/24 hours; Females <100 mg/24 hours
Creatinine (24 hour)	1.0-1.6 g/24 hours
Crystals	Uric acid crystals may be present.
Diacetic acid	0
Electrolytes	Potassium 25-100 mEq/24 hours – varies with intake. Sodium 100-260 mEq/24 hours – varies with intake
Epithelial cells	1-5/HPF
Estriol excretion – 24 hours (oxidase method)	50-300 mg/24 hours
Glucose	0
Lead	30-80 μg/24 hours
pH (titrable acidity 125-150 mEq/24 hours)	pH 4.6-8.0

Phenosulfonphthalein excretion	Excrete > 25% in 15 minutes; >40% in 30 minutes; >55% in two hours
Phosphorus	0.8-2 g/24 hours
Porphobilinogen (Watson-Schwartz Test)	Negative
Porphobilinogen/24 hours	0.38-2.42 mg
Porphyrins – Coproporphyrins (I & III) – Uroporphyrins	100-300 μg/24 hours 1-5 μg/24 hours
Potassium (See Electrolytes)	
Protein	<50 mg/24 hours
17-Hydroxycorticoids	2-10 mg/24 hours
17-Ketosteroids	7-25 mg/24 hours – male 4-15 mg/24 hours – female
Sodium (See Electrolytes)	
Pregnanediol excretion	1-8 mg/24 hours in non-Gravid females. Increases in pregnancy from about 6-40 mg/24 hours. A small decrease may occur at 40 weeks
Pregnanetriol excretion	2.5 mg/24 hours (Adult)
Specific gravity	1.003 to 1.025
Urobilinogen	1-3.5 mg/24 hours
Vanilmandelic acid	0.7-6.8 mg/24 hours

Gastrointestinal Tract

Culture (stool)	Reported as "normal flora"
Diagnex blue test	>1.6 mg excreted/two hours

Test	Normal value
D-xylose absorption test	Five-hour collection 5-8 g (or >20% of ingested dose). Serum xylose should be 25-40 mg/100 ml one hour after oral dose.
Examination (stool)	Well formed, brown, no ova or parasites.
Fat analysis – Chemical – Radioactive	Less than 6.0 g/24 hours or Less than 25% of dry weight
Gastric analysis	Volume/24 hours = 2-3 L Reaction pH 1.6-1.8 Basal acid output: Female 2.0 ± 1.8 mEq/hour Male 3.0 ± 2.0 mEq/hour After histamine: Female 16 ± 5 mEq/hour Male 23 ± 5 mEq/hour
Occult blood (stool)	Guaiac or Benzidine tests: 0 Urobilinogen: 80-150 mg/24 hours Calcium: 15-65 mEq/24 hours
Pancrozymin secretin test	Bicarbonate and protein should be reported as "normal." Interpretation of the results is usually supplied.

Cerebrospinal Fluid

Test	Normal value
Cells	Fewer than 5/mm^3 (mononuclears)
Chloride	120-130 mEq/L
Colloidal gold test	Not more than one in any tube
Glucose	50-75 mg/100 ml
Pressure	70-180 mm H_2O
Protein	15-45 mg/100 ml Albumin – 58% Alpha$_1$ globulin – 5% Alpha$_2$ globulin – 14% Beta globulin – 10% Gamma globulin – 13%

Miscellaneous Studies

Study	Normal value
Amniocentesis: lecithin/sphingomyelin ratio	1:1 (Rises as term approaches)
Amniotic fluid: creatinine spectrophotometric analysis	Normal curve
Circulation time (arm-tongue) Decholin	10-16 seconds
Cold caloric test	Normal symmetrical reactions of nystagmus, past-pointing, and falling
Cold pressor test	Increased response in essential hypertension and pheochromocytoma.
Darkfield examination	No *Treponema pallidum* found
Donovan Bodies', search for	Negative
Frei test	0.66 mm nodule at 48 hours = Positive test
Gellé test	Normal response: change in pressure against the drum alters hearing.
Liver scan	No localized defects seen. No "hot" or "cold" areas found. Uniform uptake.
Nasal smear for eosinophil	1-2 seen/low-power field
Nerve conduction time: sciatic nerve	Normal
Pap smear	No abnormal or dyskaryotic cells seen.
Pulmonary wedge pressure	3-11 mm Hg
Vital capacity	see below
Timed vital capacity	Expiration of 70-80% of forced vital capacity in one second.

Vital capacity:

Age	Men	Women
20-39	3.35-5.90 L	2.45-4.38 L
40-59	2.72-5.30 L	2.09-4.02 L
>60	2.42-4.70 L	1.91-3.66 L

Test	Normal value
Purified protein derivative skin test (PPD)	Less than 1 cm erythema at 72 hours. No induration.
Rinne test	Positive = no obstructive deafness present.
Rumple-Leeds test	Compared to normal control: 10 or fewer petechiae/2.5 cm.
Rotation test	Nystagmus duration 25-40 seconds for each horizontal canal.
Schwabach test	Hearing in test subject is identical to that of the examiner (who has perfect hearing).
Stenger test	No evidence of malingering.
Tine test	Less than 1 cm erythema and no induration at 72 hours.
Vaginal smear for cornification	Number of cornified cells depend on age, place in cycle and pregnancy.
Venous pressure (antecubital)	70-140 mm H_2O
Weber test	Hearing identical in both ears: no suggestion of nerve or conduction deafness.
Wet smear from vagina	
— hanging drop preparation	No trichomonas seen
— Gram's stain of wet smear	Normal flora
— KOH preparation	No hyphae or chlamydospores seen

ILLUSTRATIONS

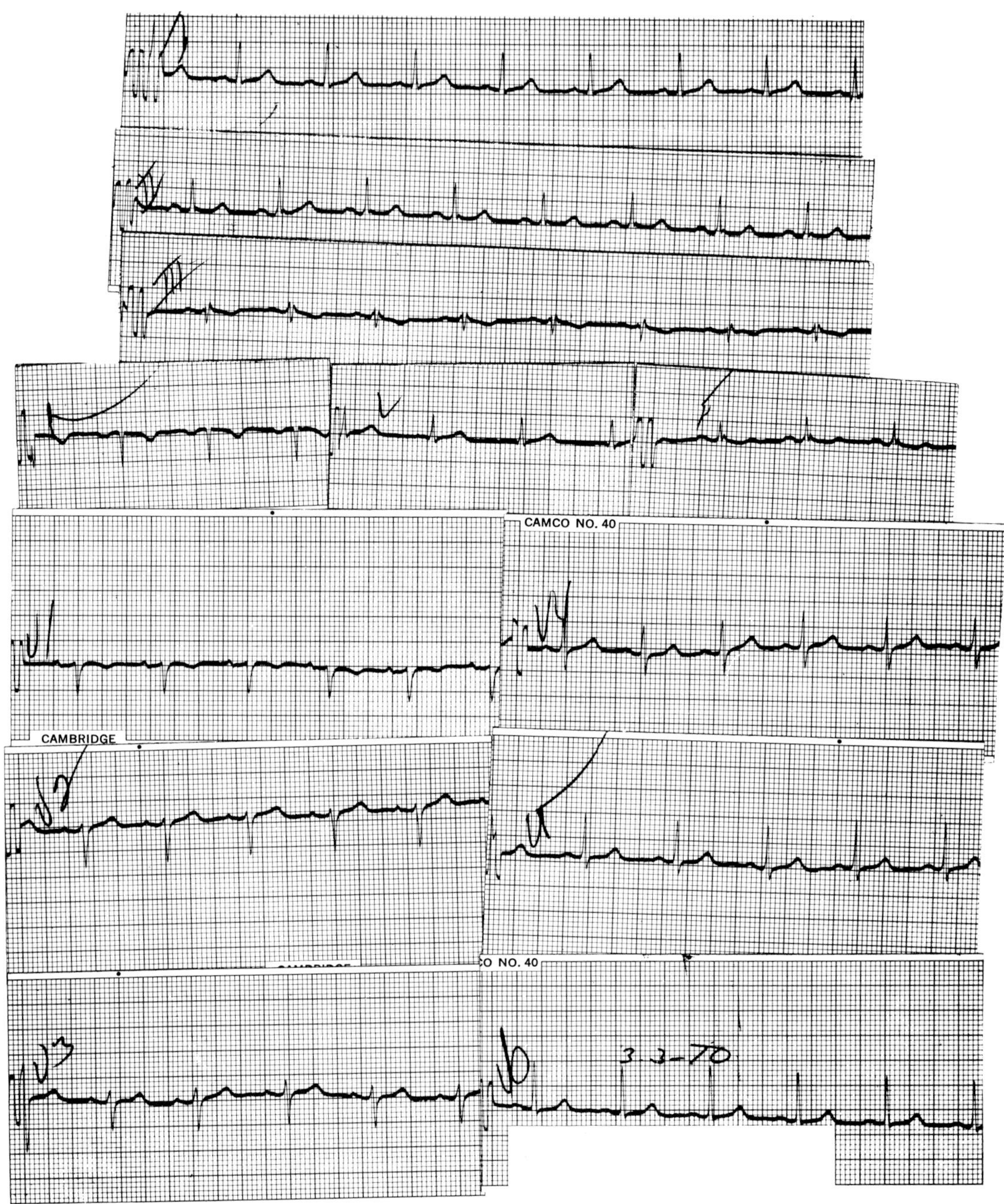

FIGURE 1

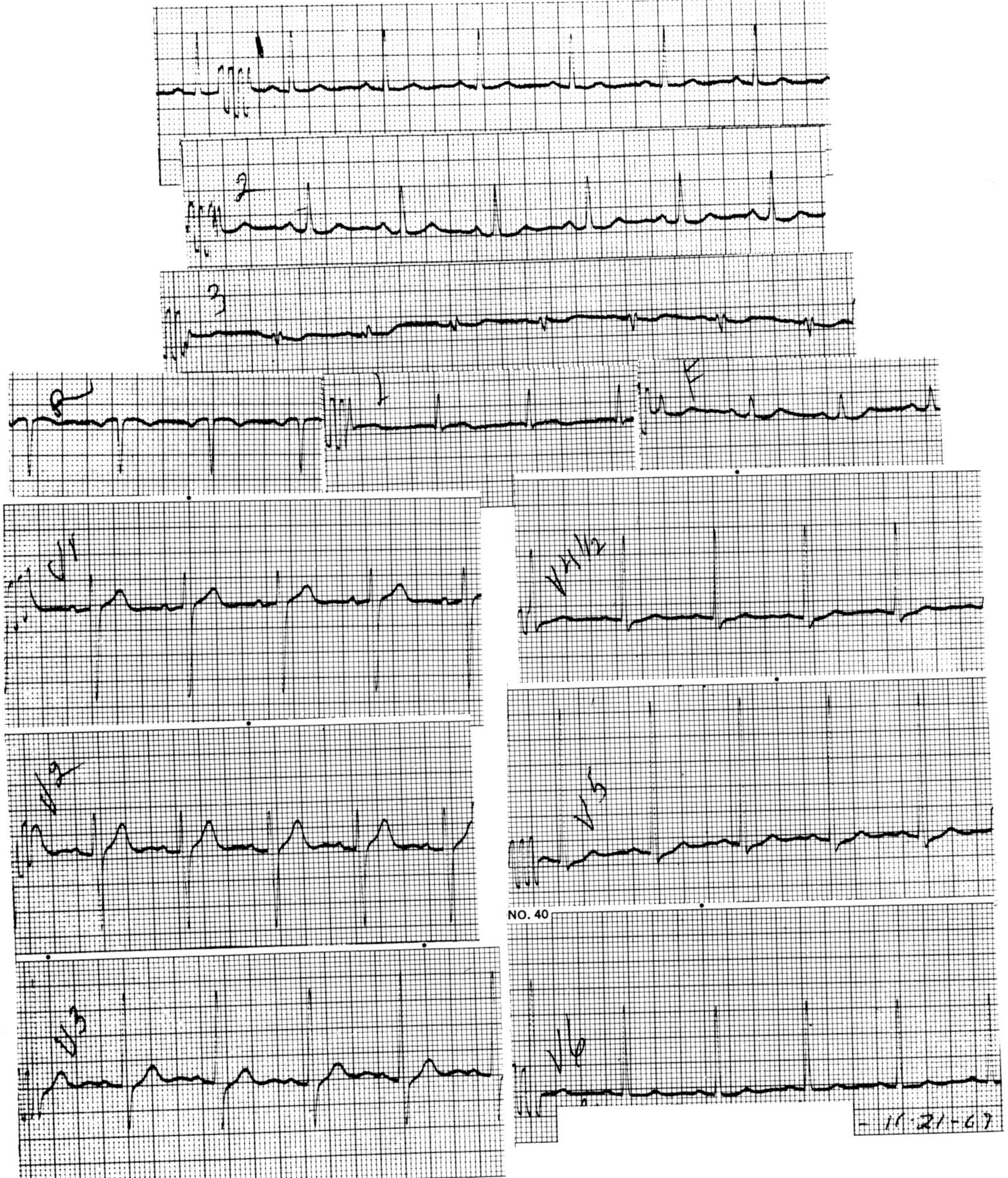

FIGURE 2

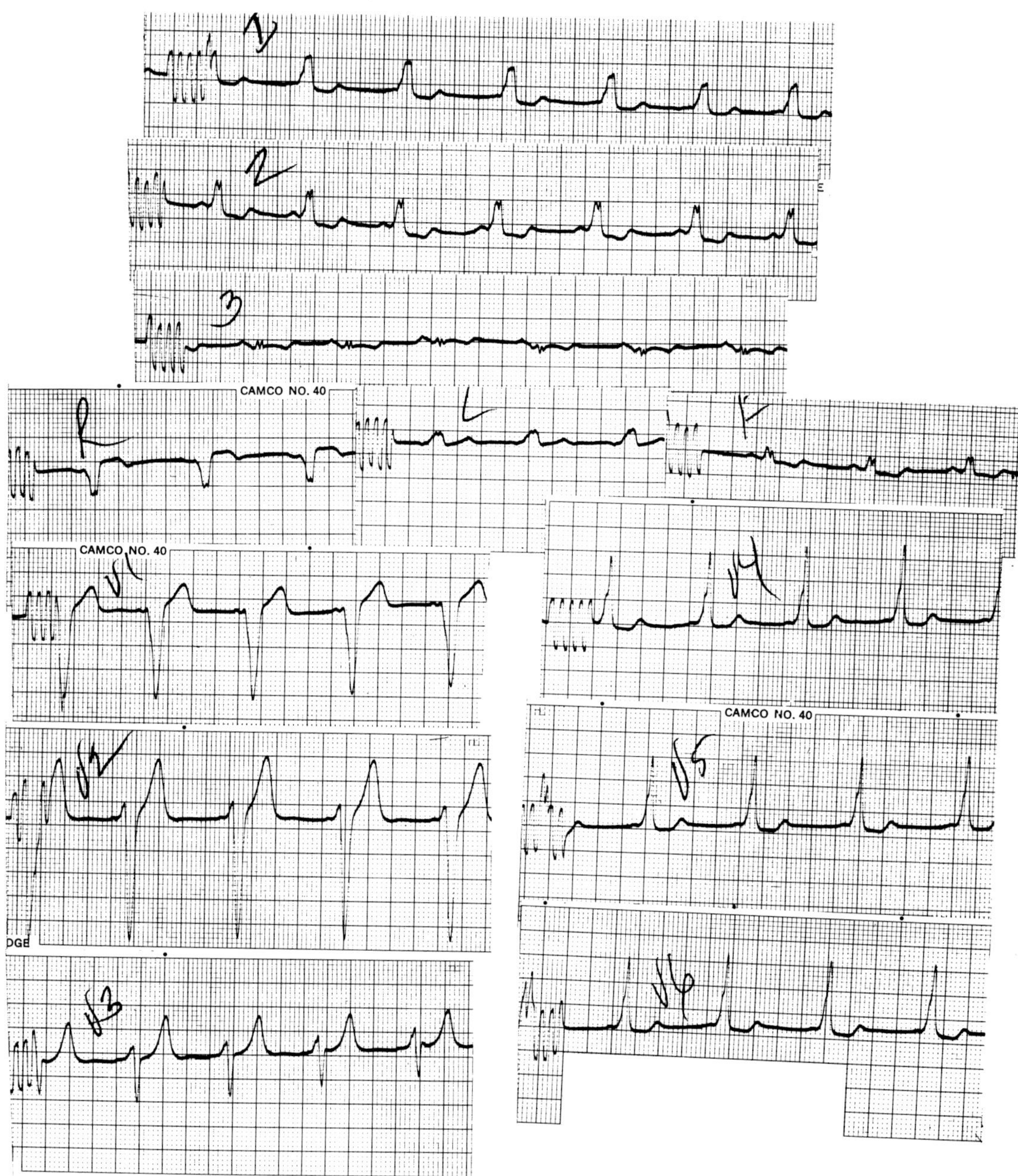

FIGURE 3

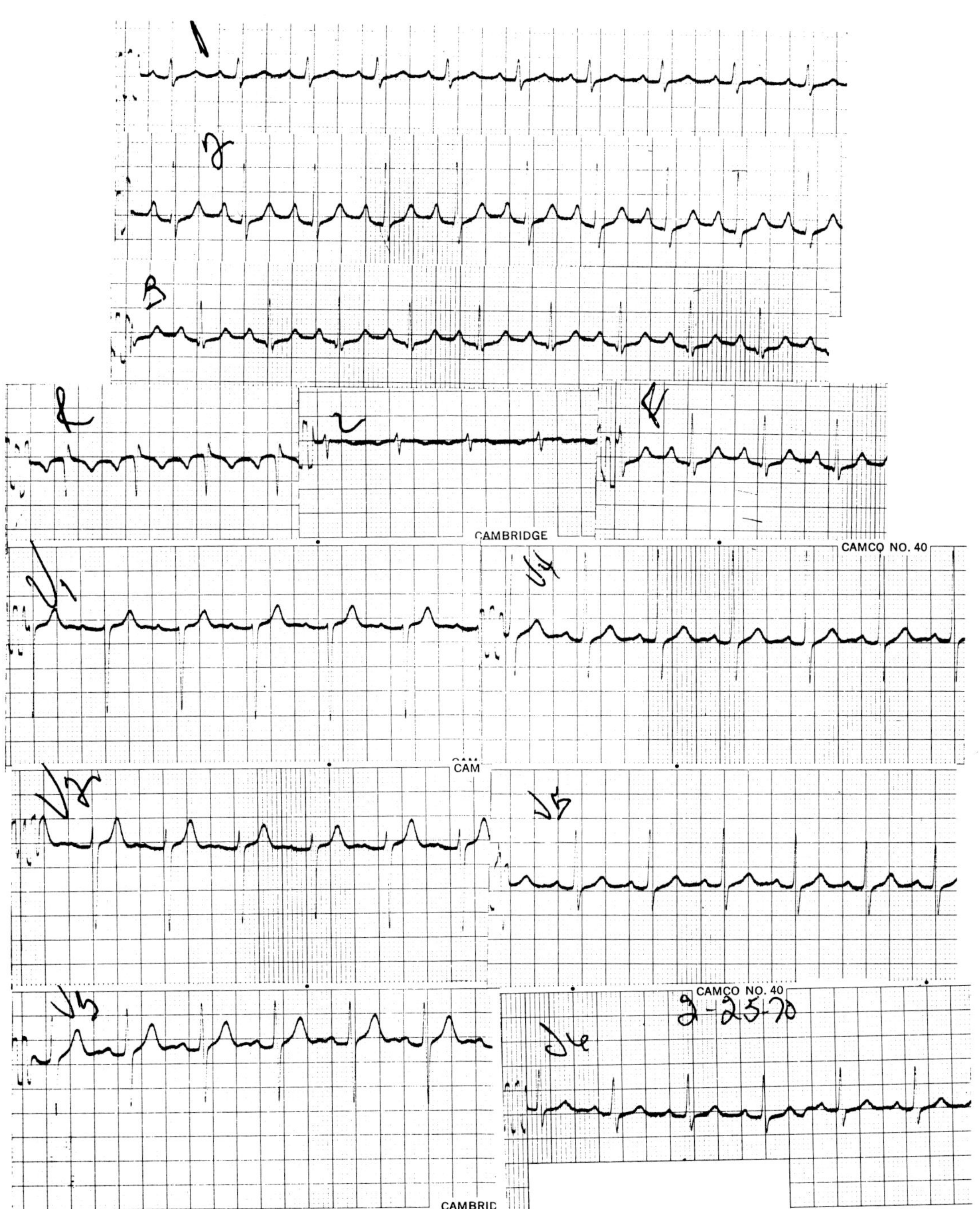

FIGURE 4

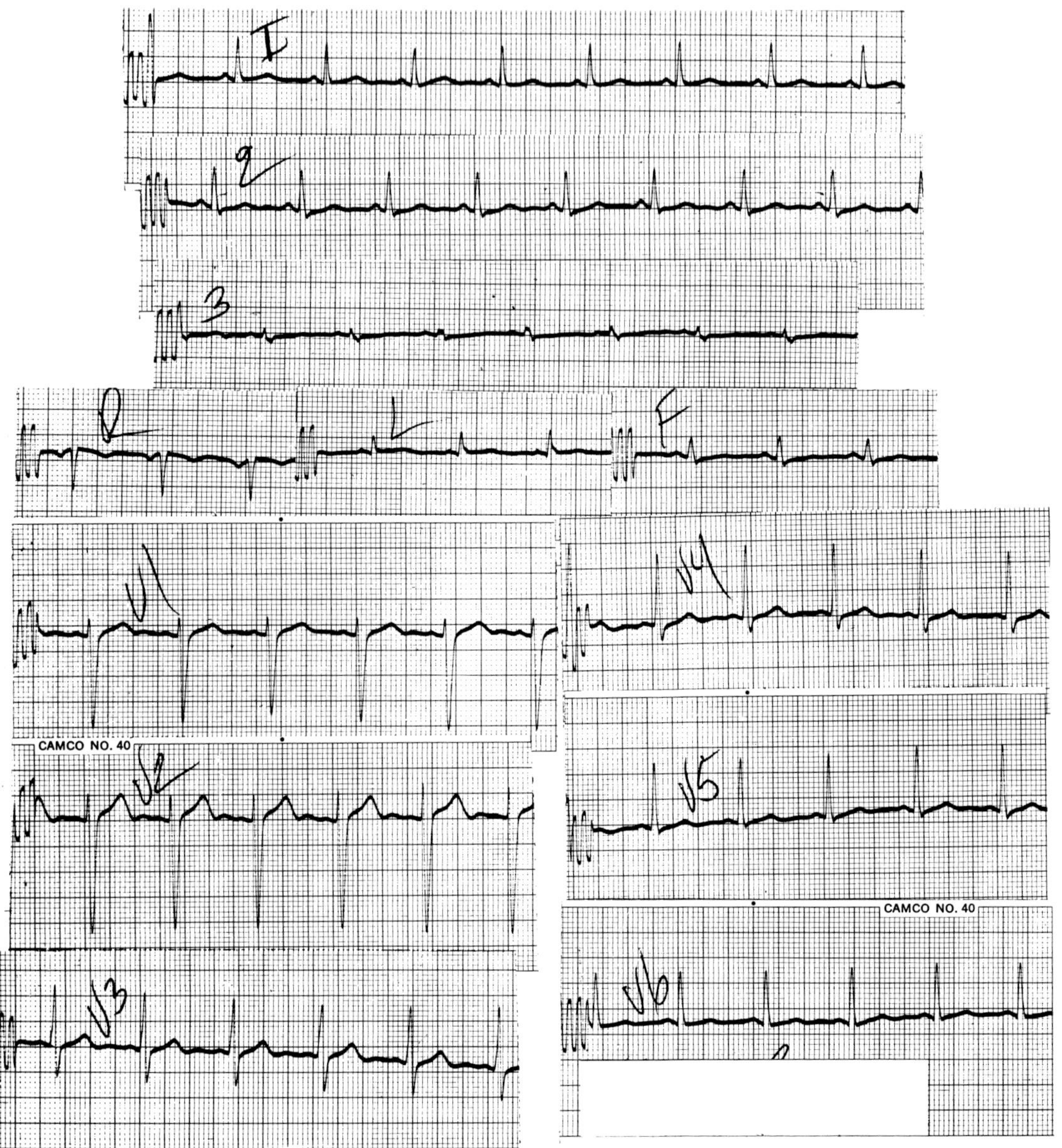

FIGURE 5

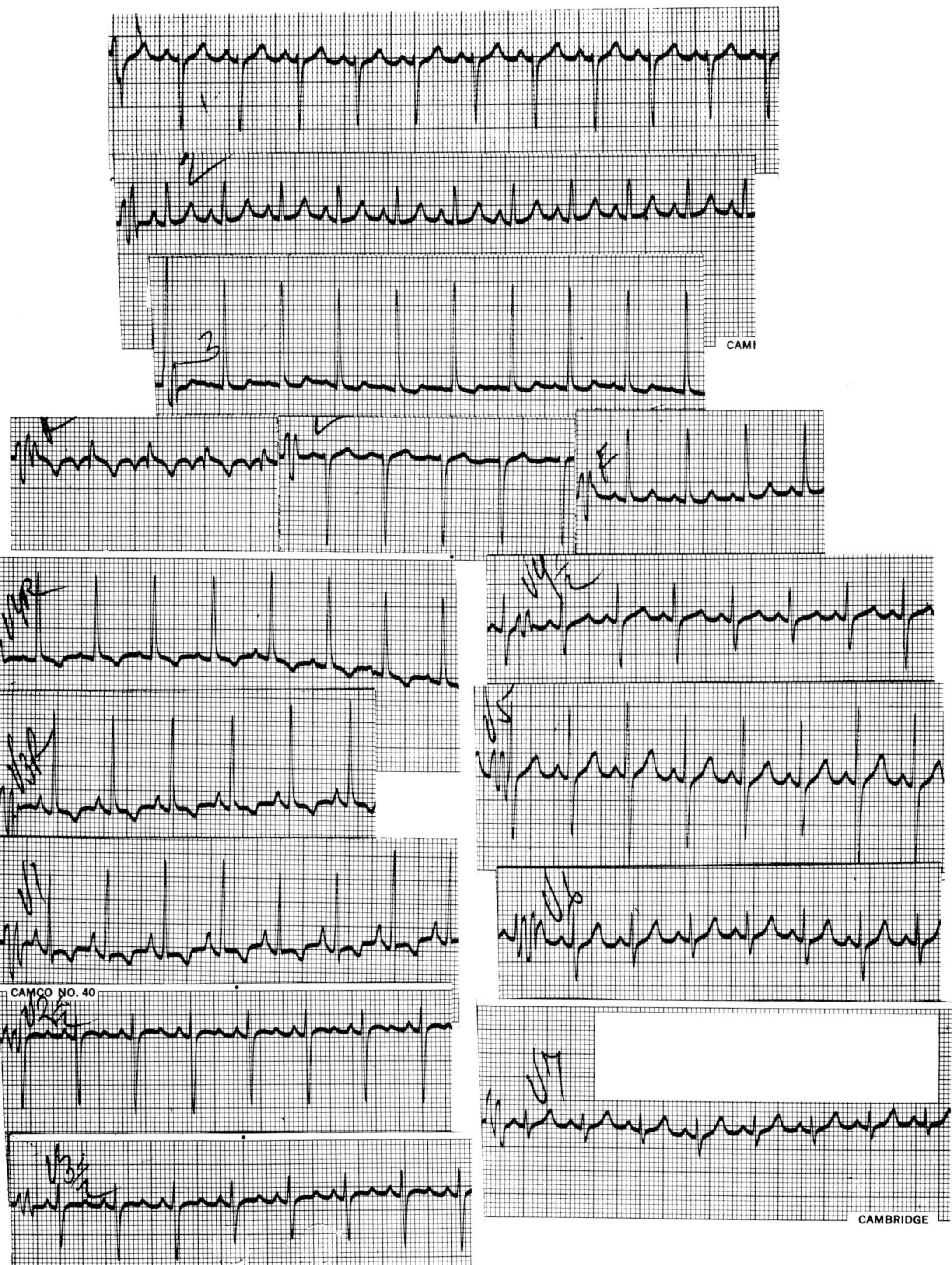

FIGURE 6 Note: Patient became extremely agitated during procedure.

AUDIOMETRIC RESULTS

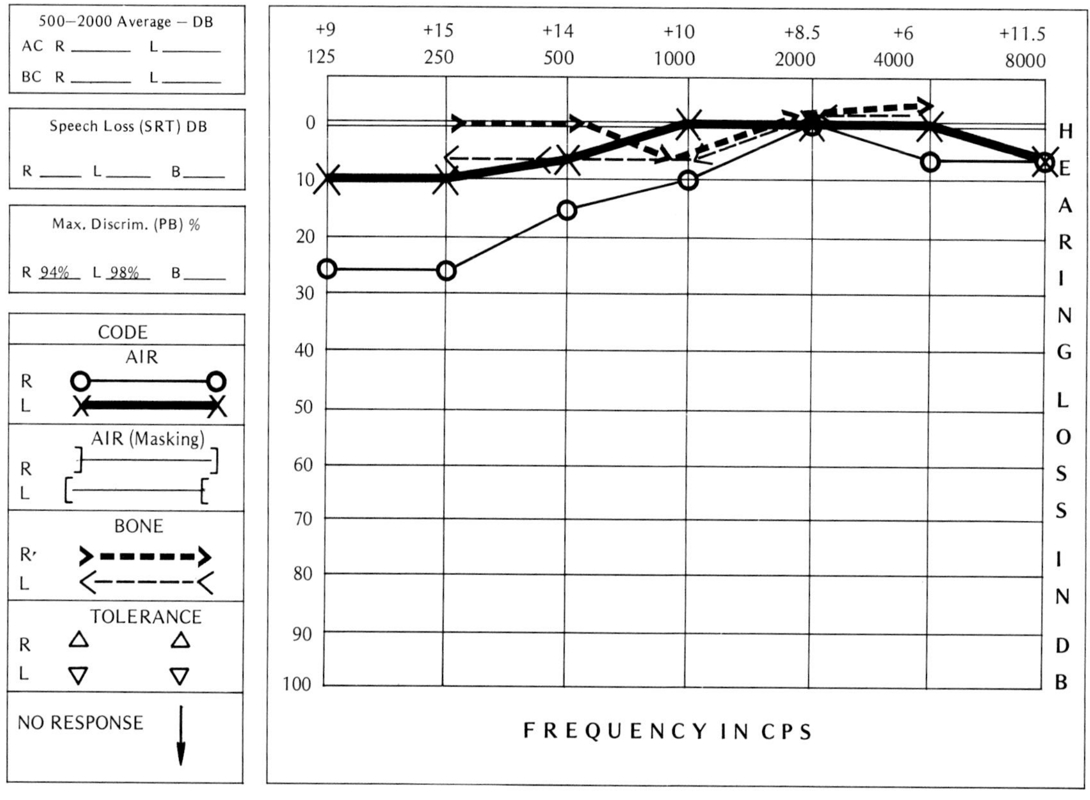

REMARKS ______

FIGURE 7

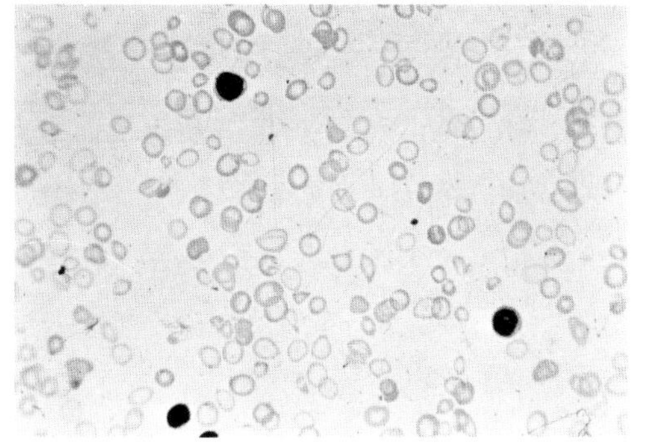

FIGURE 8

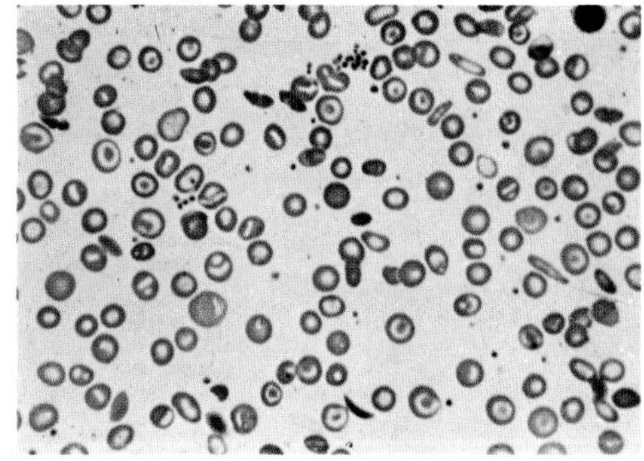

FIGURE 9

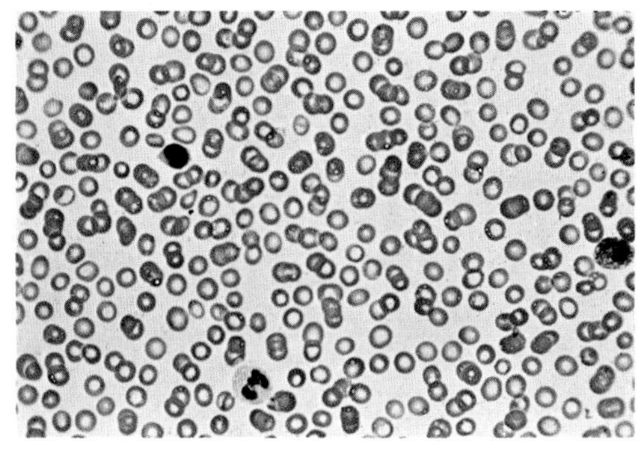

FIGURE 10

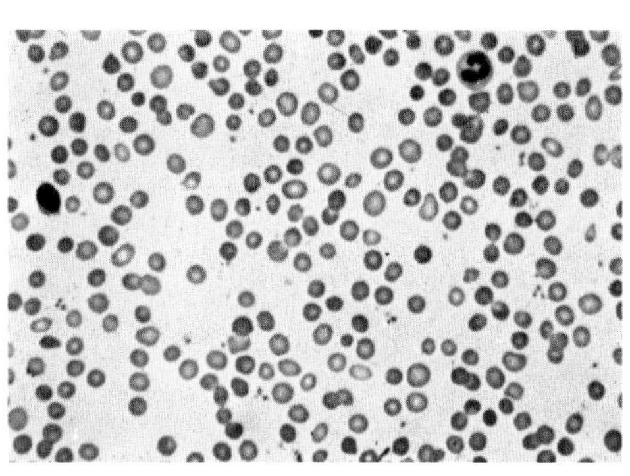

FIGURE 11

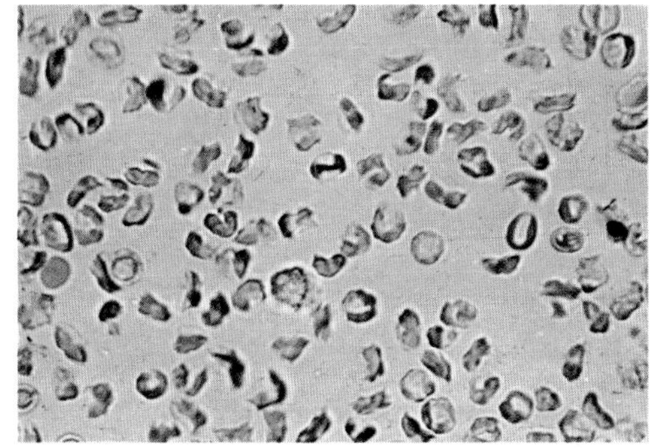

FIGURE 12

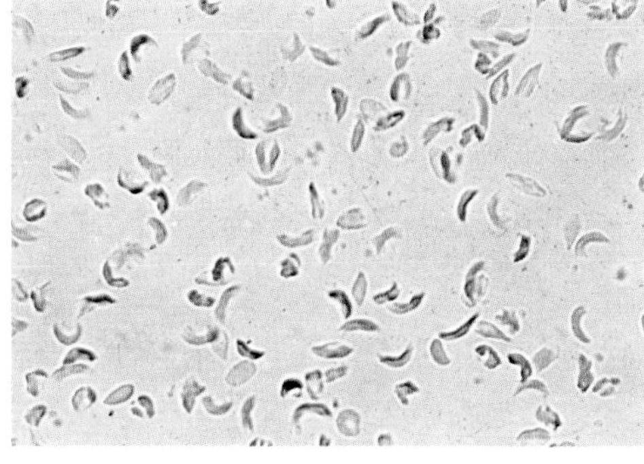

FIGURE 13

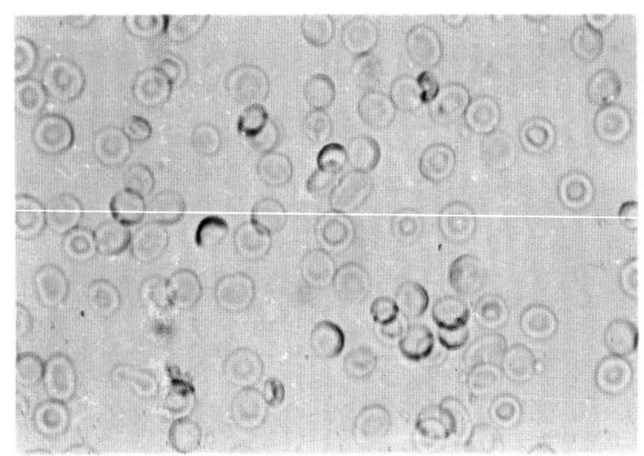

FIGURE 14

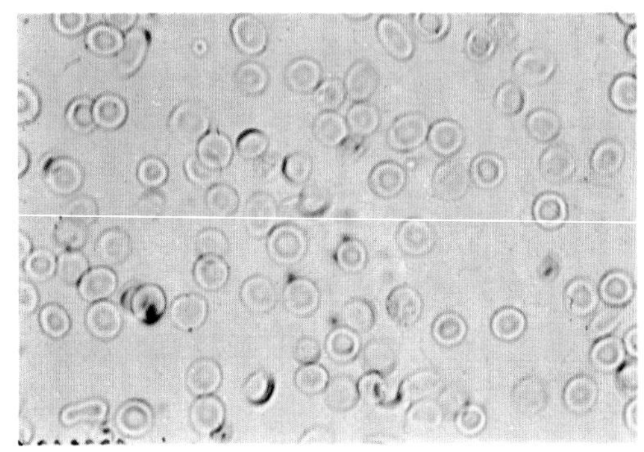

FIGURE 15

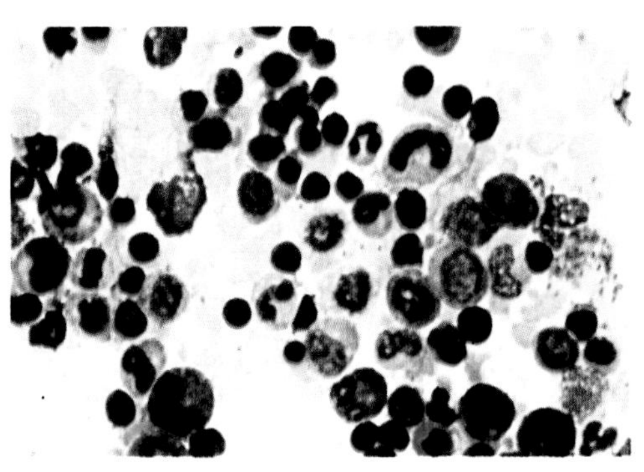

FIGURE 16

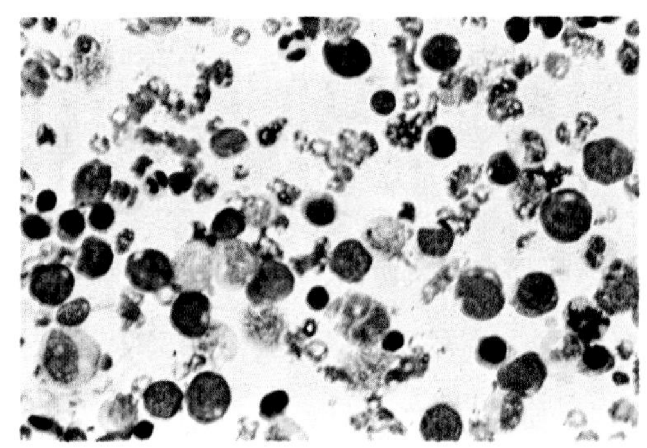

FIGURE 17

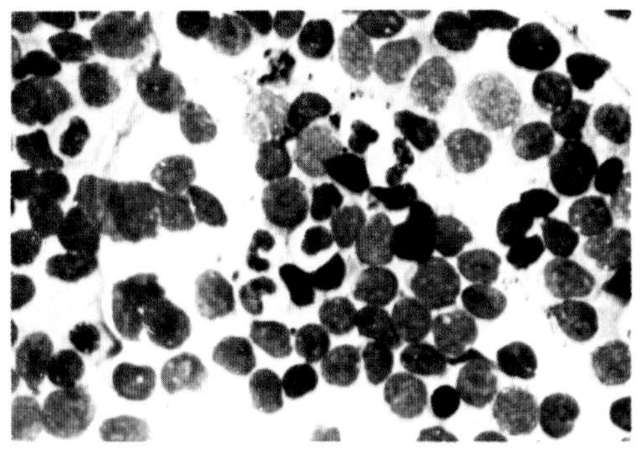

FIGURE 18

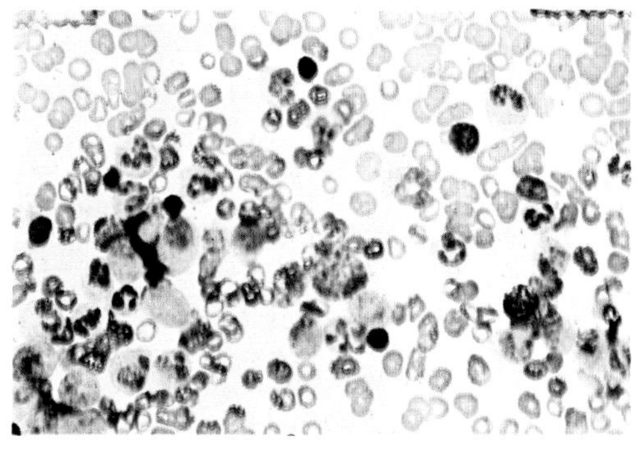

FIGURE 19

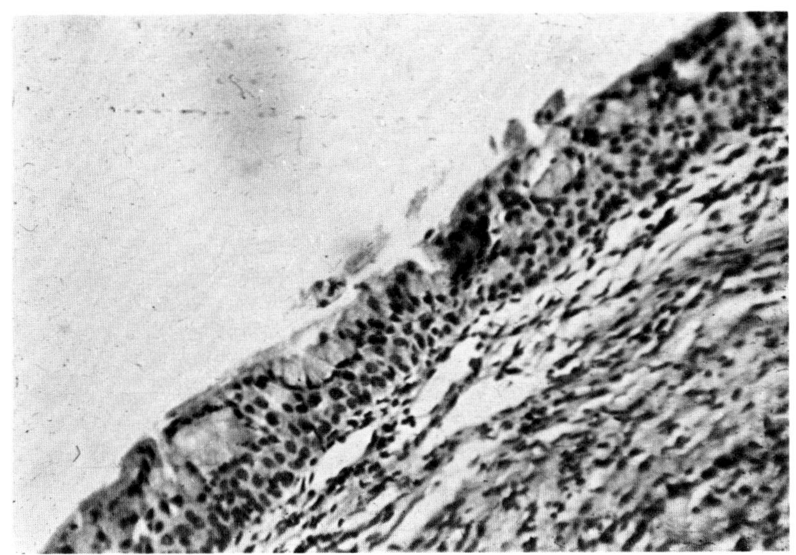

FIGURE 20

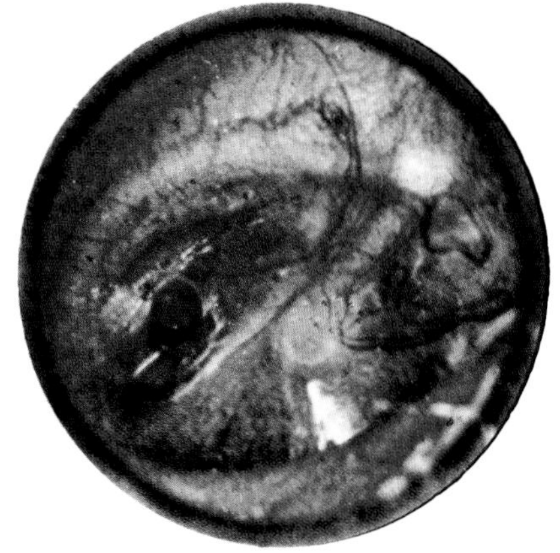

FIGURE 21

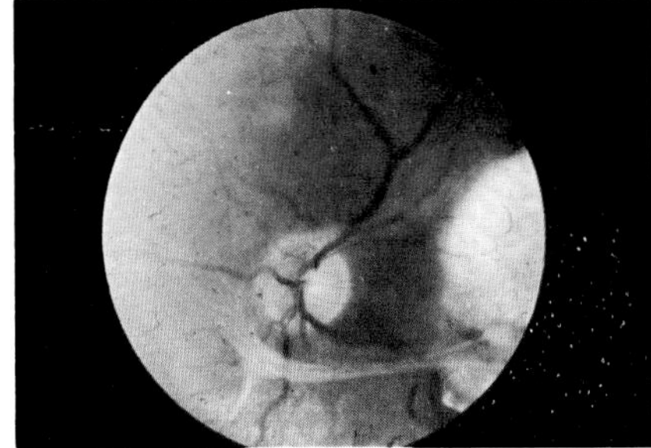

FIGURE 22

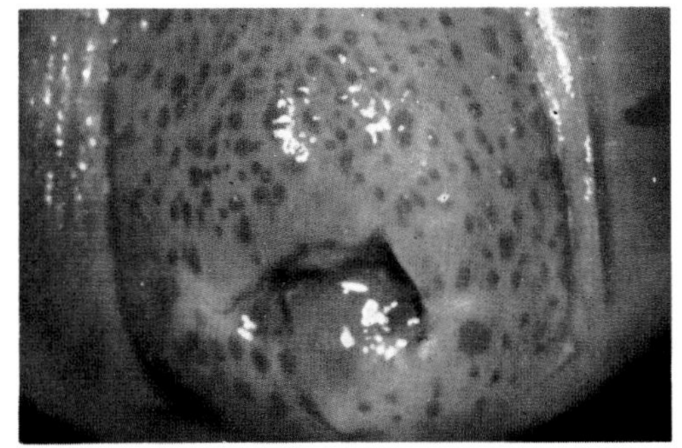

FIGURE 23

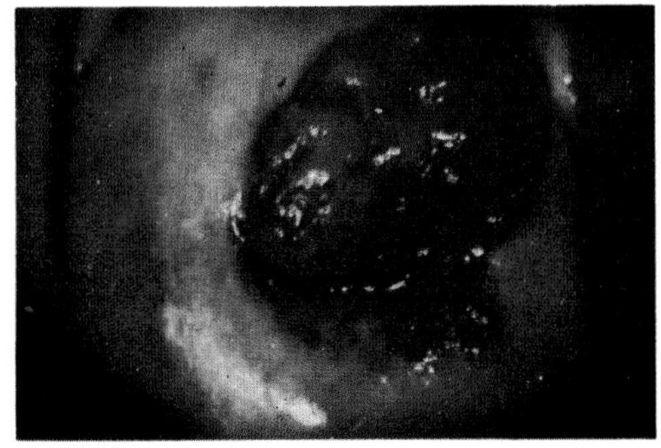

FIGURE 24

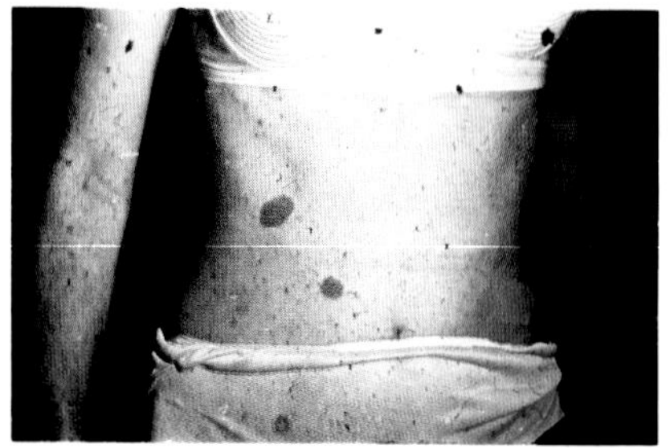
FIGURE 25

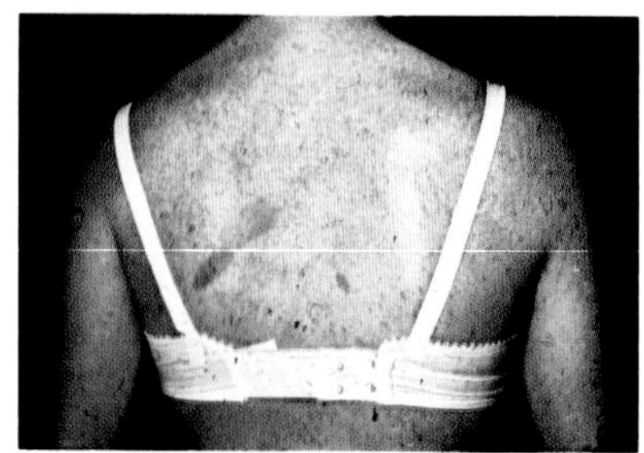
FIGURE 26

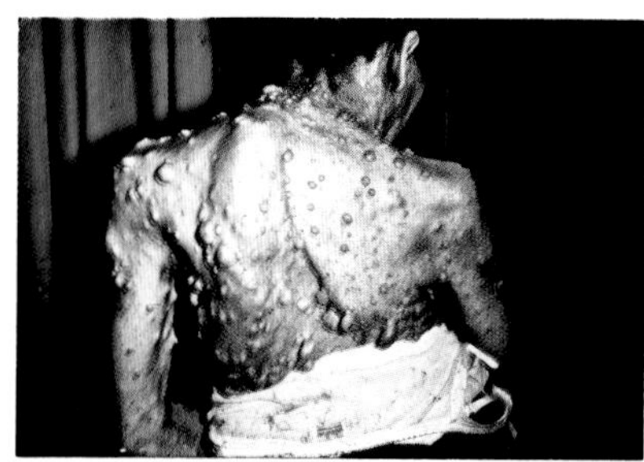
FIGURE 27

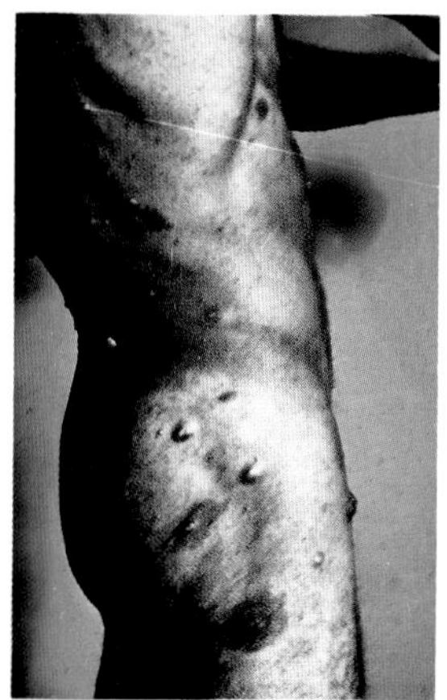
FIGURE 28

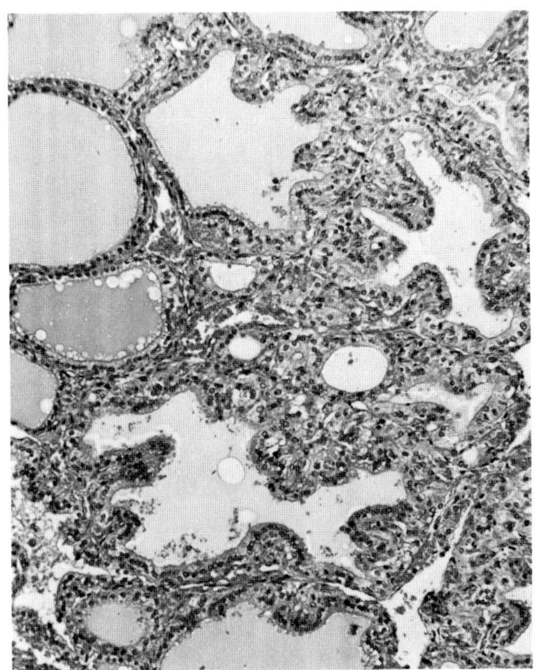

FIGURE 29

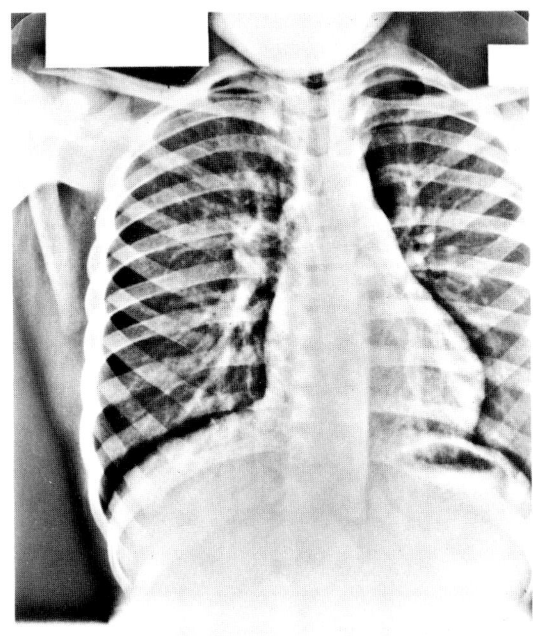

FIGURE 30

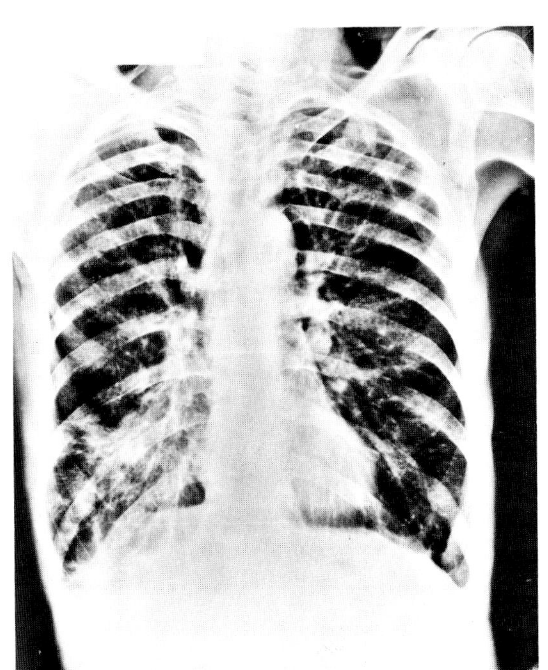

FIGURE 31

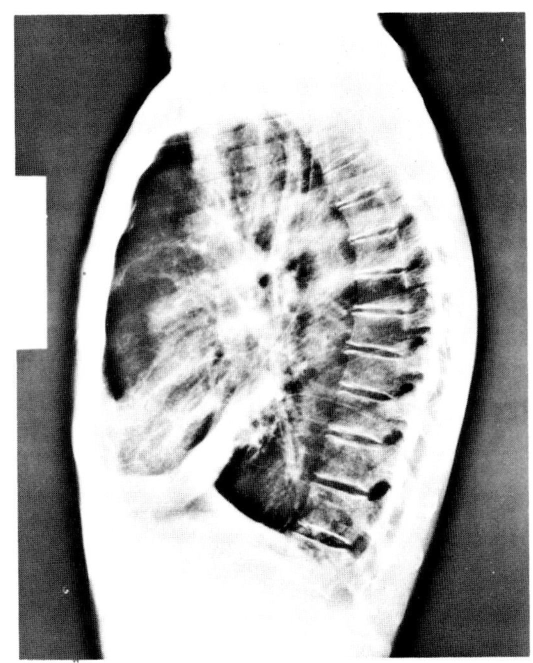

FIGURE 32

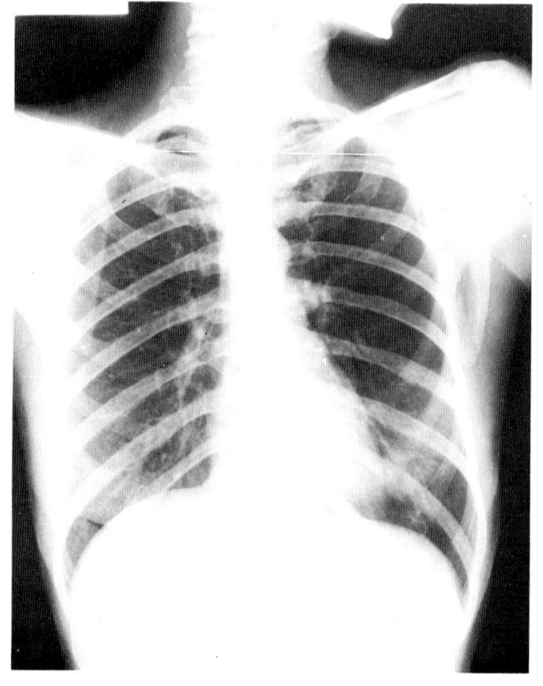

FIGURE 33

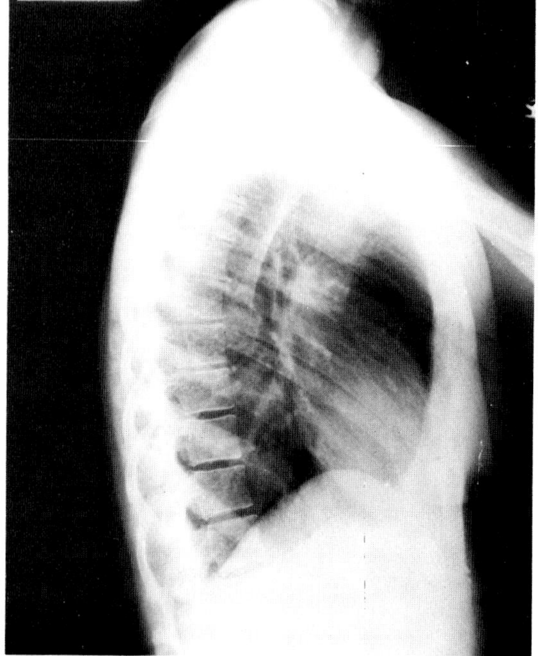

FIGURE 34

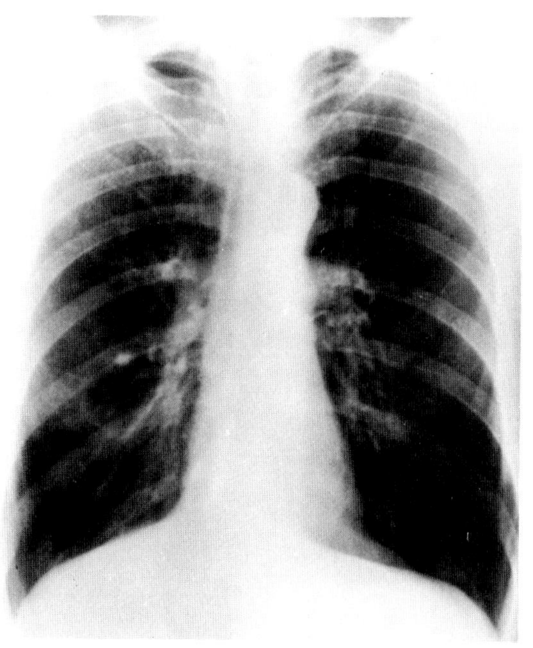

FIGURE 35

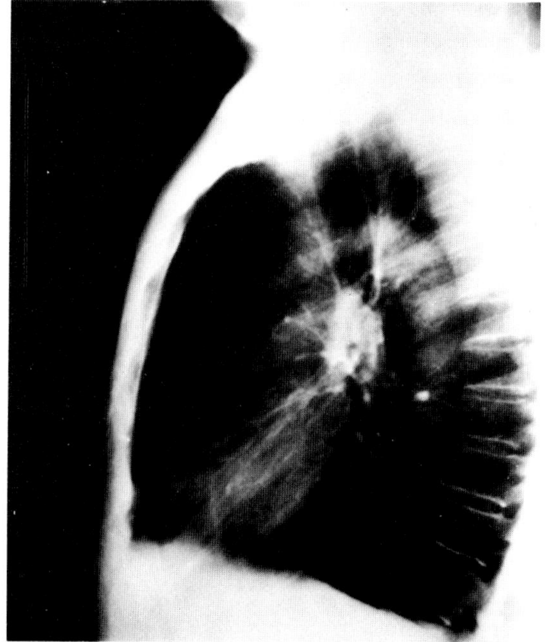

FIGURE 36

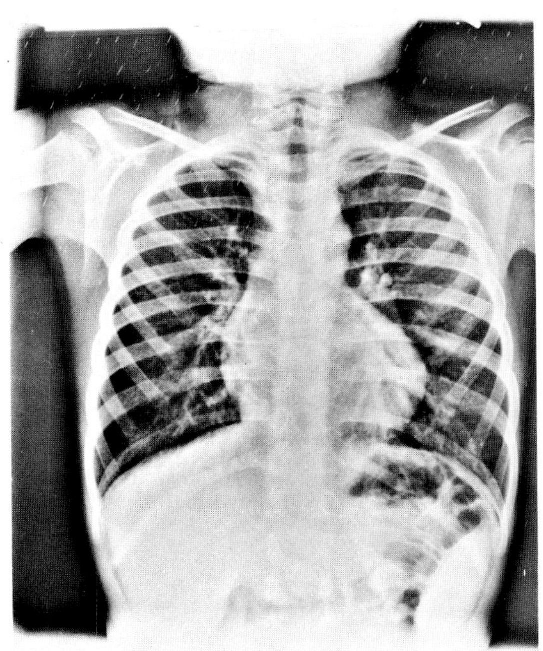

FIGURE 37

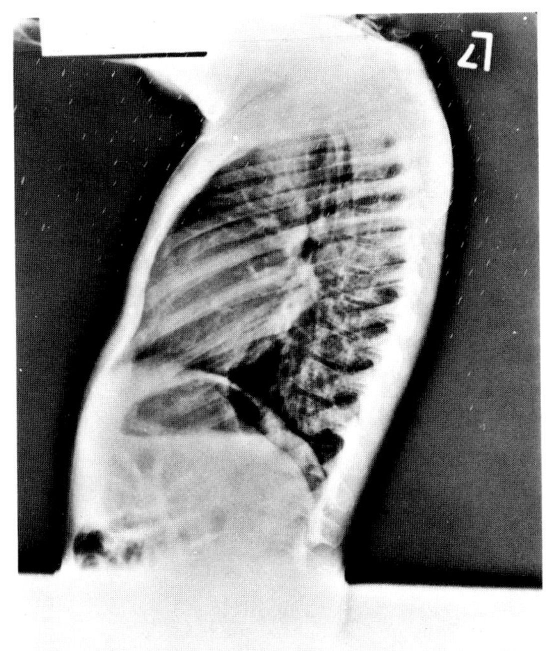

FIGURE 38

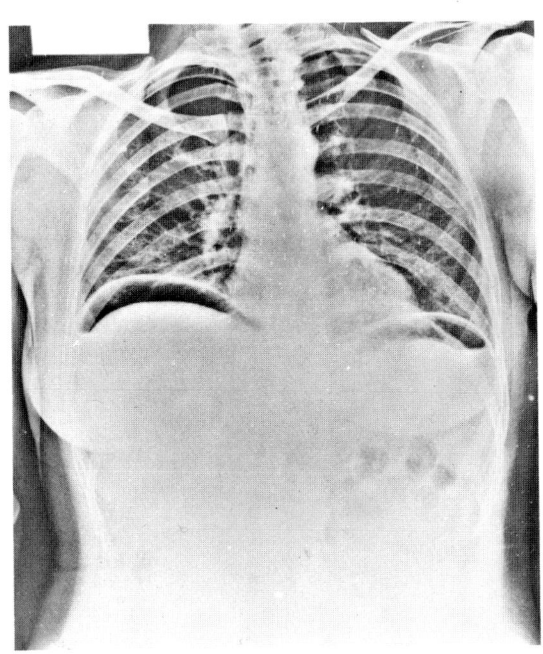

FIGURE 39

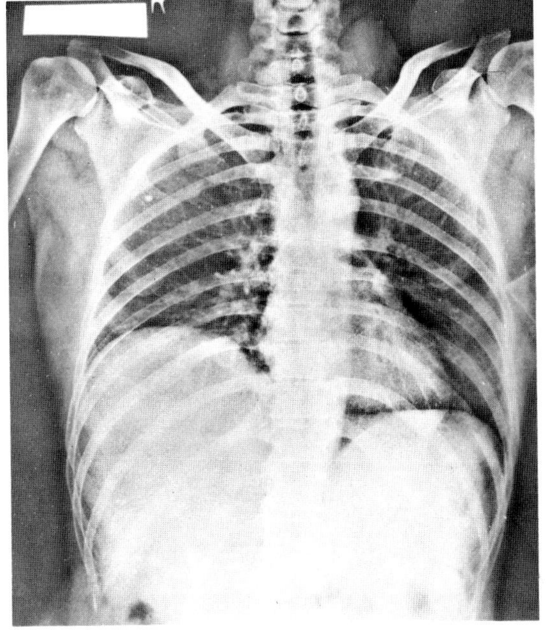

FIGURE 40

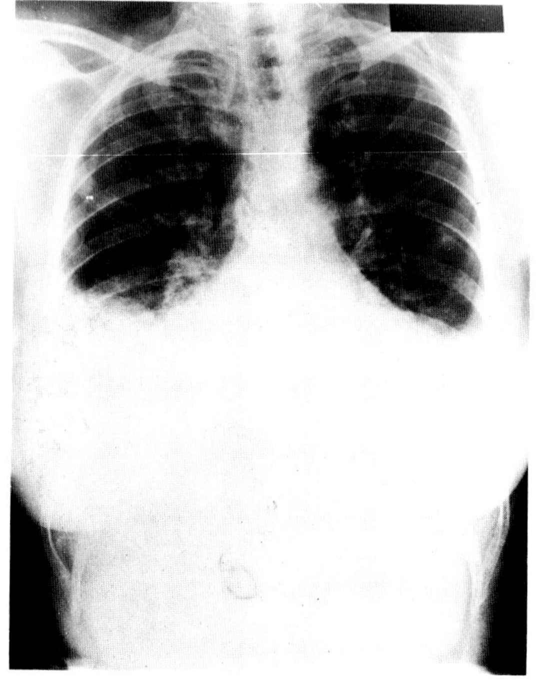

FIGURE 41

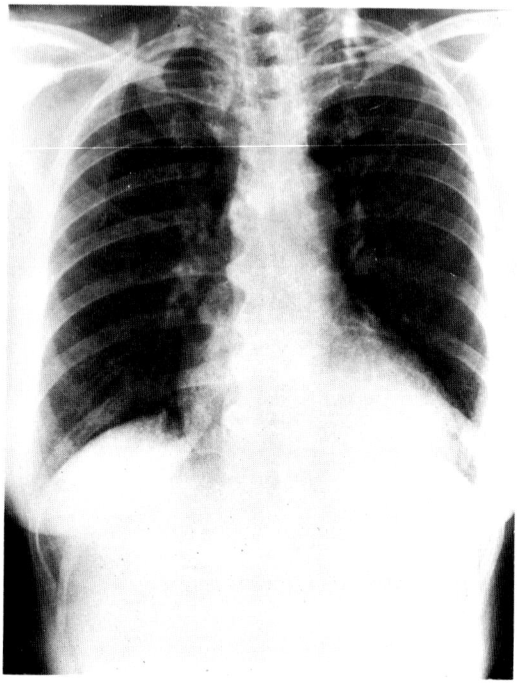

FIGURE 42

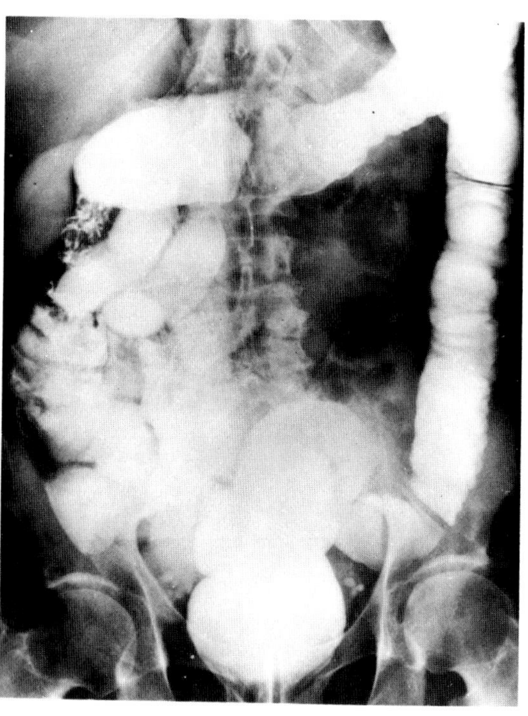

FIGURE 43

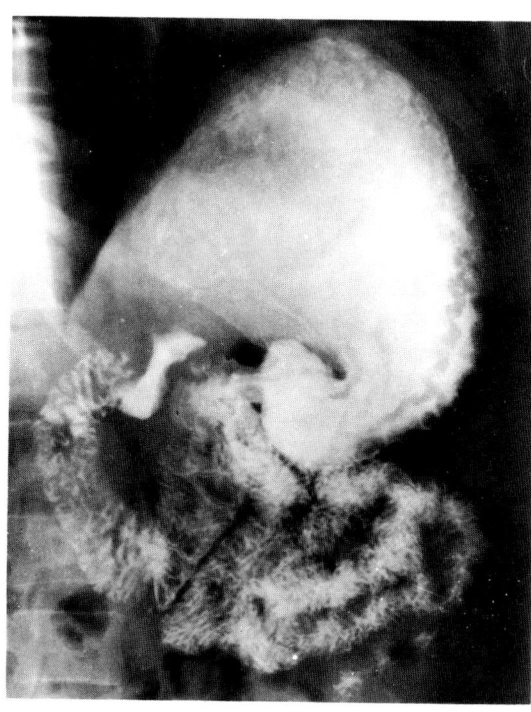

FIGURE 44

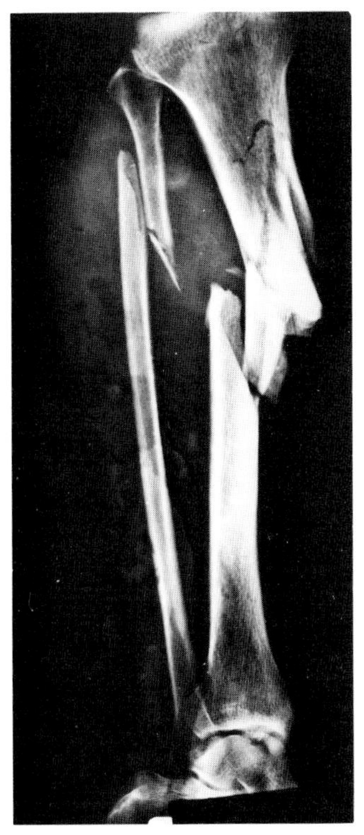

FIGURE 45

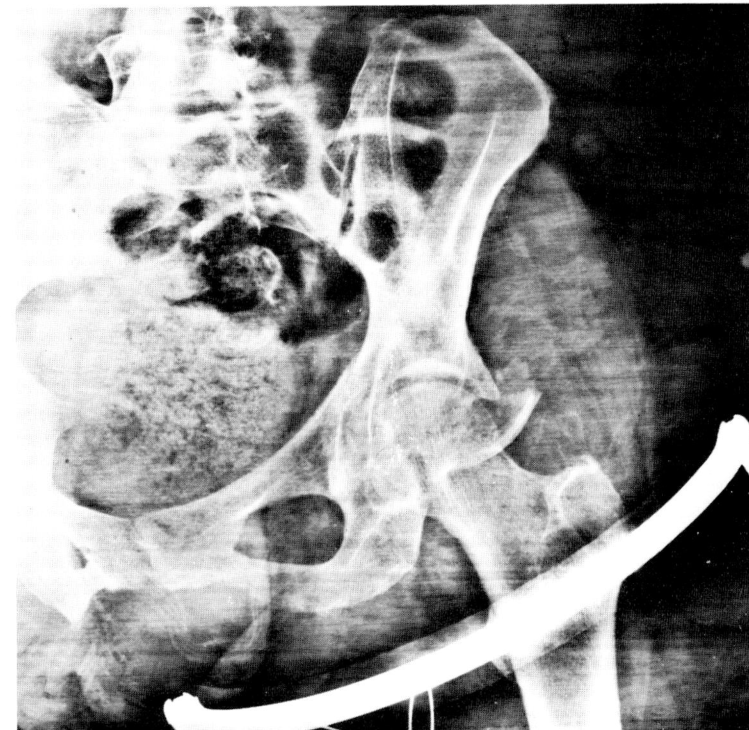

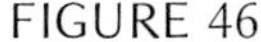

FIGURE 46

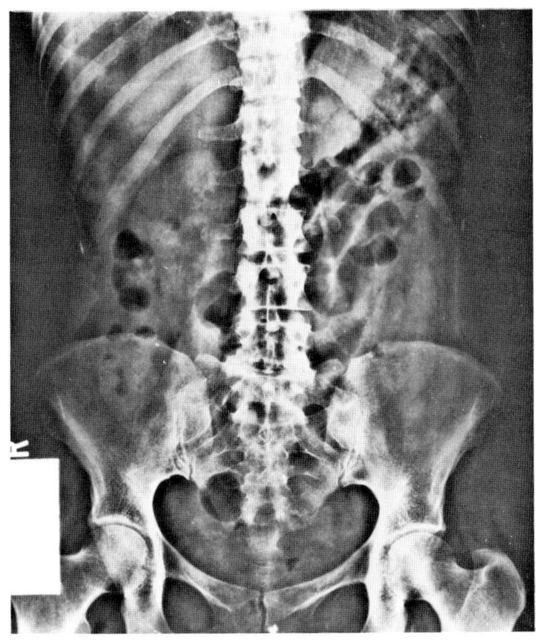

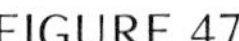

FIGURE 47

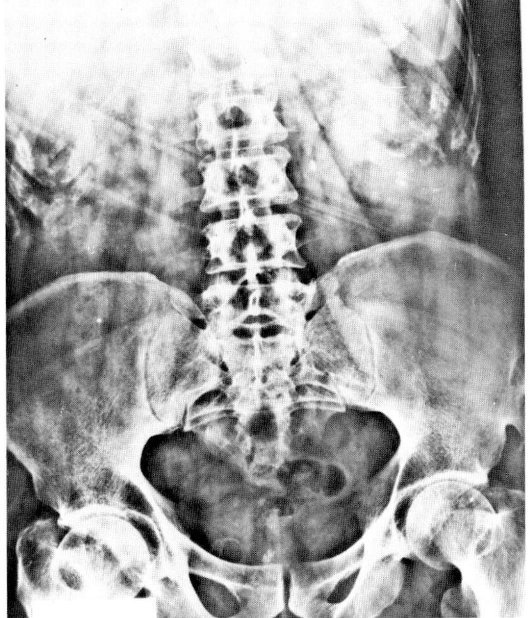

FIGURE 48

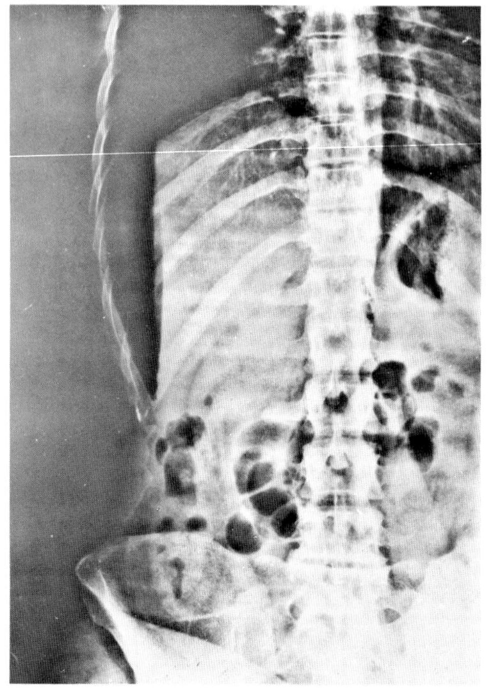

FIGURE 49

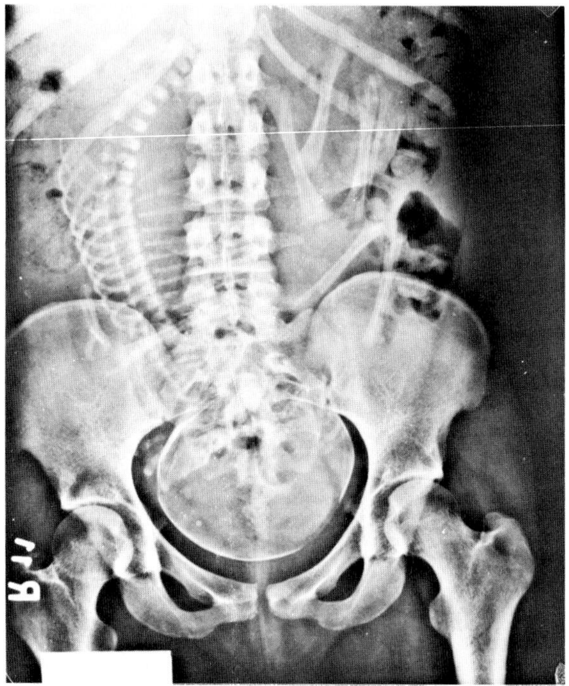

FIGURE 50

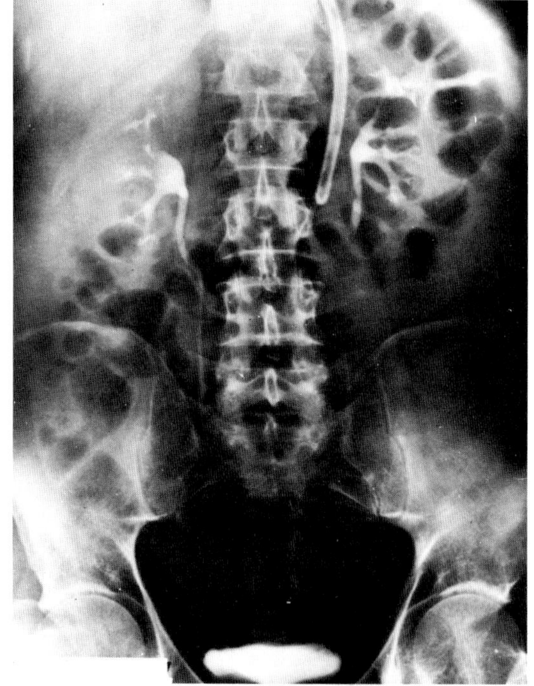

FIGURE 51

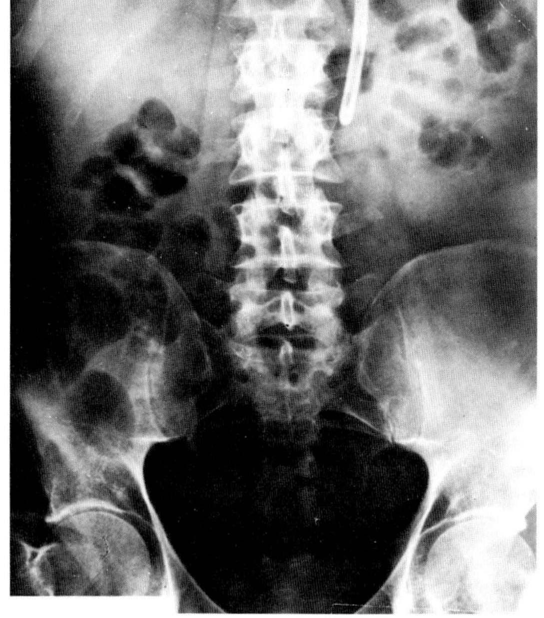

FIGURE 52

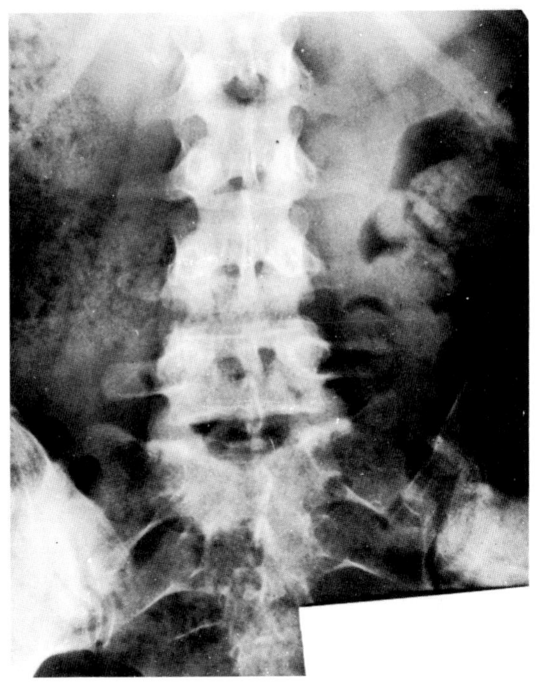

FIGURE 53

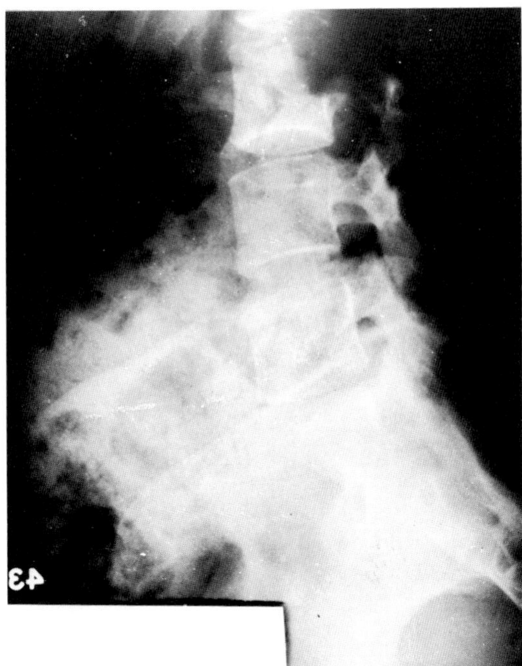

FIGURE 54

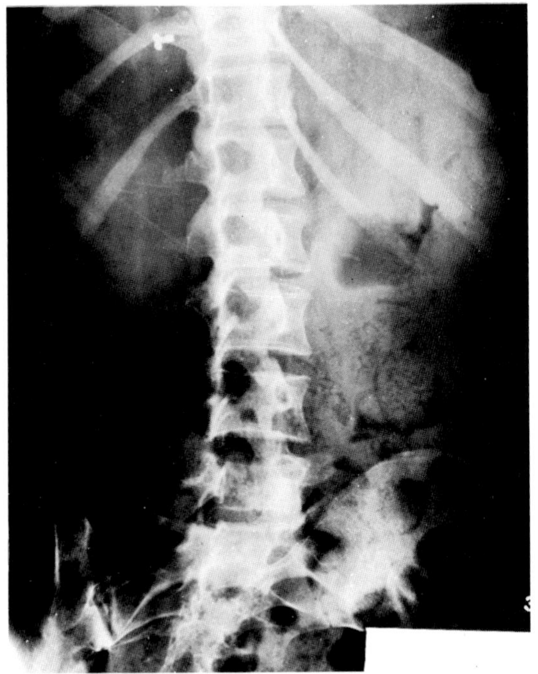

FIGURE 55

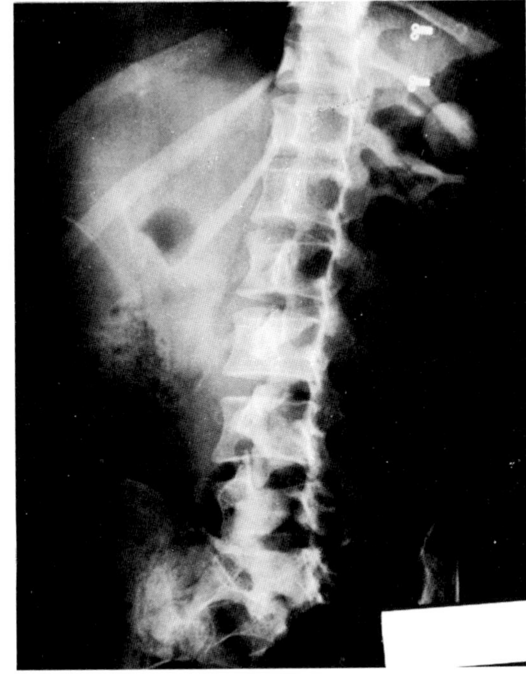

FIGURE 56

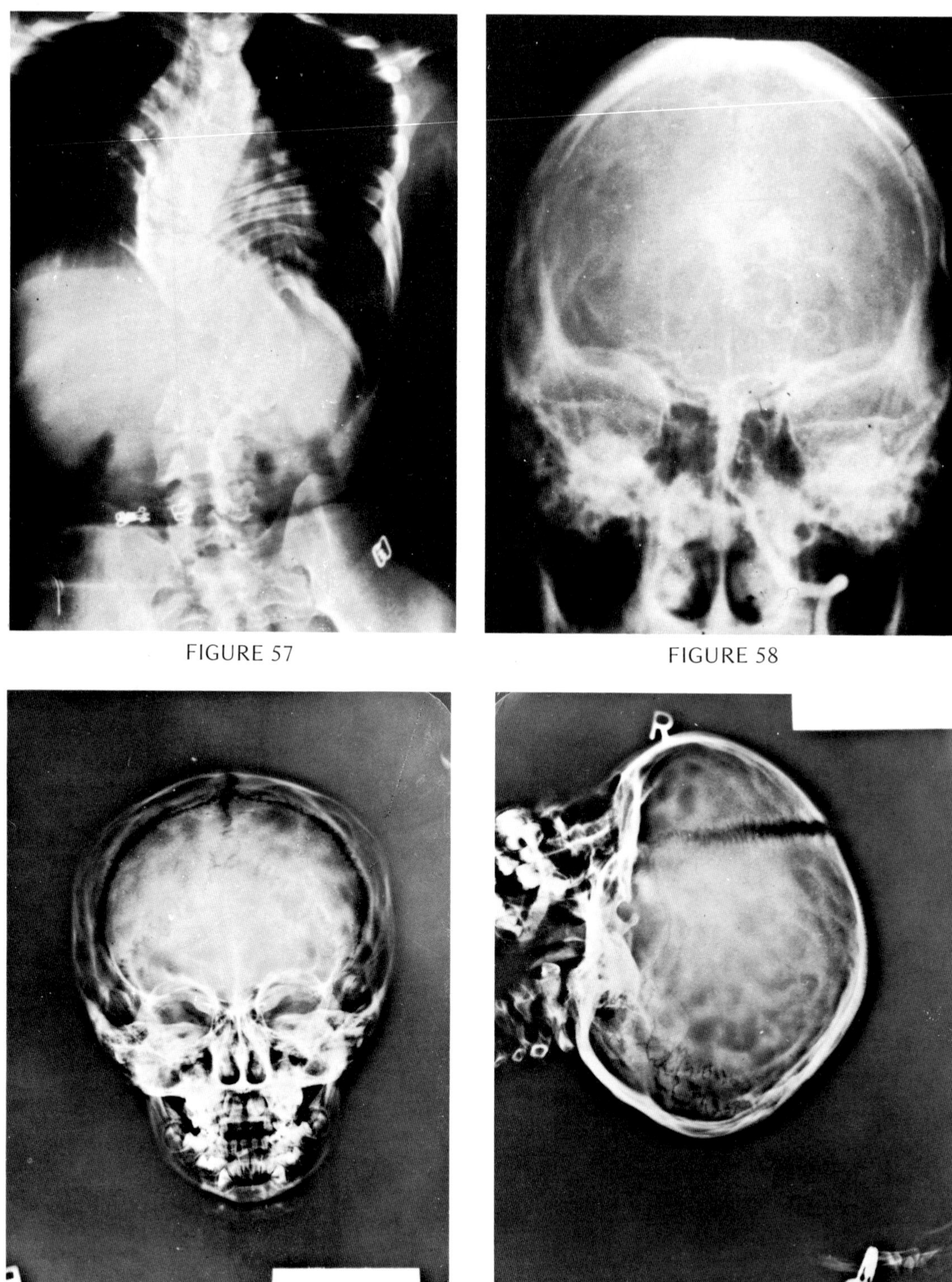

FIGURE 57

FIGURE 58

FIGURE 59

FIGURE 60

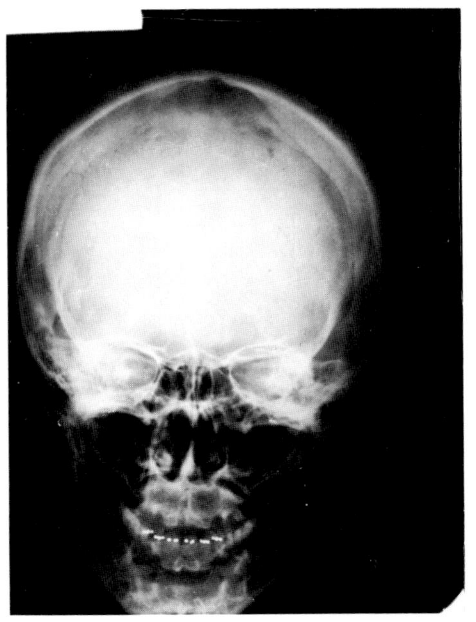

FIGURE 61

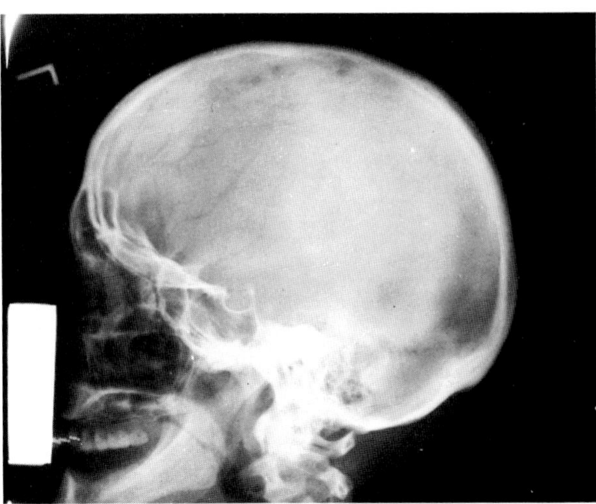

FIGURE 62

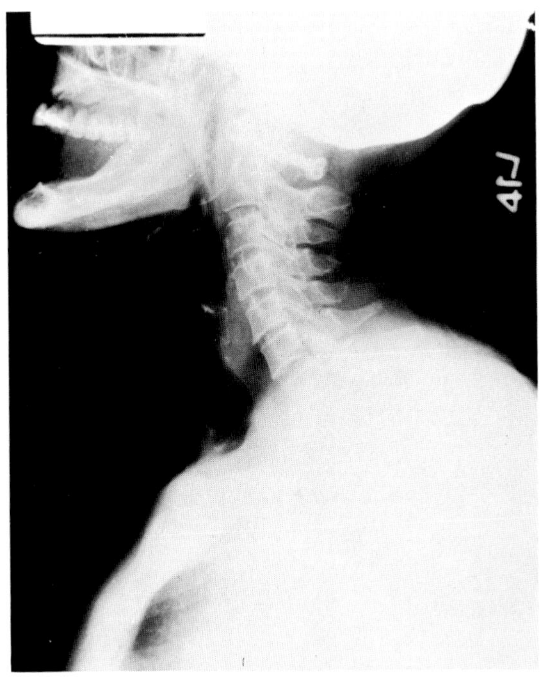

FIGURE 63

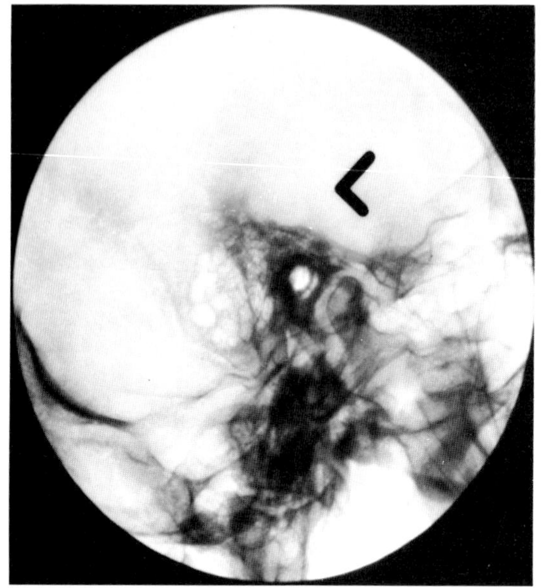

FIGURE 64

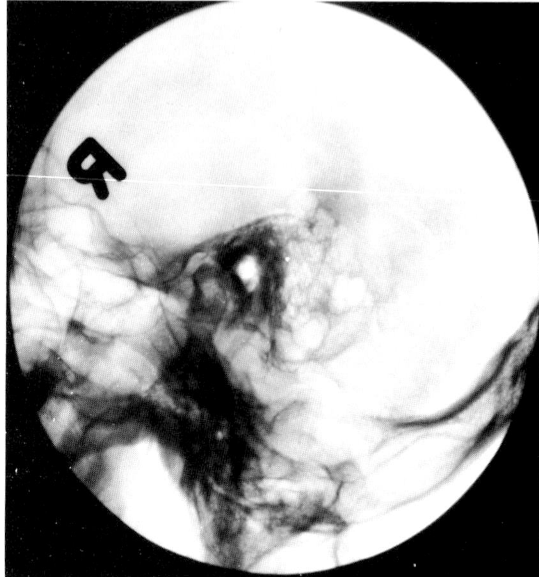

FIGURE 65

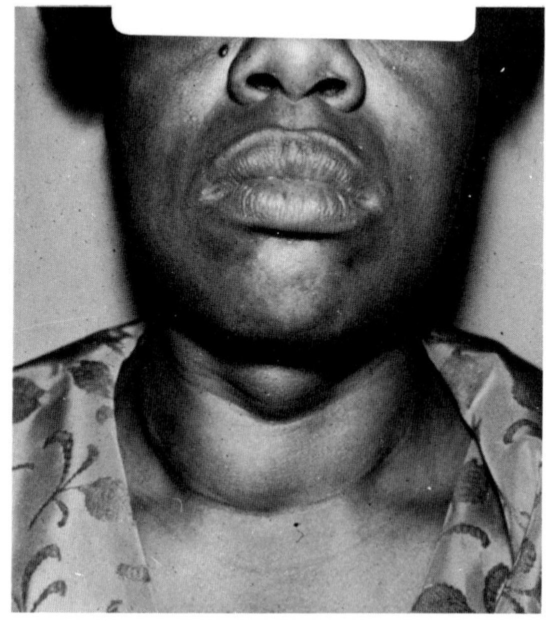

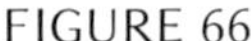
FIGURE 66

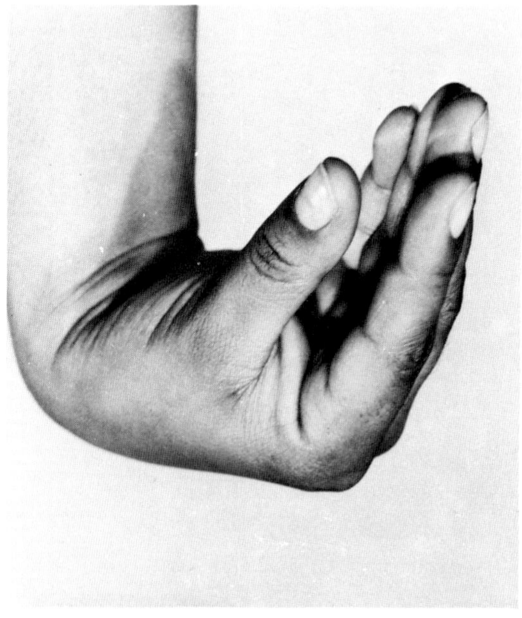

FIGURE 67